Color Atlas of

Gynecological Surgery

Volume 3: Operations for Malignant Disease

David H. Lees

FRCS(ED), FRCOG
Consultant Obstetrician and Gynecologist,
Jessop Hospital for Women, Sheffield

Honorary Clinical Lecturer,
University of Sheffield

Albert Singer

Ph.D, D.Phil (OXON), MRCOG
Senior Lecturer in Obstetrics and Gynecology,
University of Sheffield

Honorary Consultant Obstetrician and Gynecologist,
Jessop Hospital for Women, Sheffield

Year Book Medical Publishers, Inc.
35 East Wacker Drive, Chicago

To our wives
Anne & Talya

Acknowledgements

This six-volume colour Atlas of Gynaecological Surgery was produced at the Jessop Hospital for Women, Sheffield as part of a postgraduate project to teach operative surgery by edited colour slides. We are indebted to all who took part in this exercise, but there are some whom we would like to mention particularly.

Mr Alan Tunstill, Head of Department of Medical Illustration, Hallamshire Hospital, Sheffield Area Health Authority (Teaching), organised the whole of the photography. Mr Stephen Hirst, of the same Department, took nearly all of the photographs; the colour diagrams are all the work of Mr Patrick Elliott, Medical Artist of the Department.

Professor I. D. Cooke generously gave full access to clinical material in his unit. Mr K. J. Anderton and Mr B. Rosenberg of Rotherham, England referred cases of vulvar malignancy from which photographic material is used in Chapter 2. Mr Joseph Jordan of Birmingham, England contributed the photographs to the section on the use of laser in Chapter 3 while Dr Tom Powell of the Weston Park Hospital, Sheffield, England allowed us to reproduce the lymphograms as shown in Chapter 7.

Dr Frank Neil, Consultant Radiotherapist at the Weston Park Hospital, Sheffield, England accepted our invitation to write Chapter 7 on radiation therapy for gynaecological cancer. Although management of malignant disease is a matter for close liaison between surgeons and radiotherapists, the radiation techniques in some fields have become so sophisticated and complex that the radiotherapist, necessarily, must take charge of treatment.

The anaesthetists at all levels were very co-operative. Dr A. G. D. Nicholas, Dr D. R. Powell and Professor J. A. Thornton were the consultants involved. Of the numerous senior registrars we remember particularly Drs Bailey, Birks, Burt, Clark, Dye, Mullins, Saunders and Stacey.

Miss J. Hughes-Nurse, Mr I. V. Scott, Miss P. Buck and Dr H. David were the senior registrars and lecturers in obstetrics and gynaecology during the time and greatly assisted by keeping us informed of suitable cases and in the organising of operations. Drs Katherine Jones, E. Lachman, Janet Patrick, K. Edmonds, A. Bar-Am and C. Rankin were involved in the management of the cases and assisted at operations.

Miss M. Crowley, nursing officer in charge of the Jessop Hospital operating theatres ensured that we had every facility, and Sisters J. Taylor, M. Henderson, E. Duffield, M. Waller and A. Broadly each acted as theatre sister or 'scrub' nurse at the individual operations. Mr Leslie Gilbert and Mr Gordon Dalton, the operating room assistants, were valuable members of the team. We particularly wish to thank the whole theatre staff for their courtesy and efficiency.

A large amount of secretarial work was involved. We are grateful to

Mrs Gillian Hopley of the University Department who dealt with most of it. Mrs Valerie Prior and Mrs Talya Singer were responsible for typing the manuscript and both gave much genial/general help and constructive advice throughout.

The photographs in this book were taken on Kodachrome 25 colour reversal film. The camera was a 35 mm Nikkormat FTN fitted with a 105 mm f2.5 Nikkor auto lens. A PK-3 extension ring was used for close-ups and a 55 mm f3.5 Micro-Nikkor auto lens for general views. Illumination was provided by a Sunpak auto zoom 4000 electronic flash unit, set on full power. An exposure setting of 1/60th of a second at f16 was used.

Contents

Introduction

There is probably no substitute for the type of personal tuition provided by teacher and pupil working together in the operating theatre as surgeon and assistant, with knowledge and experience being passed on directly. There is, however, the disadvantage that such a relationship is not available to everyone and is, at best, transient. In addition the learner is frequently not at a stage in his career when he can take full advantage of what is available. The majority, therefore, have to look elsewhere for such instruction.

Textbooks of operative surgery provide the principal source of information, but these are only as good as their illustrations. The occasional colour plate does not instruct and there is something unreal about the well-executed drawings prepared by a medical artist to the specification of the author. The one worthwhile teaching aid is the simple line diagram or sketch, which demands considerable skill and ingenuity and allows the student to see and follow what is required. But to carry that information in one's mind and apply it in practice is another matter. In surgery, with all its accompanying distractions, the real life structures are frighteningly different from those which the simple diagrams have led one to expect, and these same structures obstinately refuse to adopt the position and behaviour expected of them.

Cine films are excellent but the cost of their production in time and money is high, besides which they are clumsy to use. This series of atlases offers what we consider to be the next best thing: a series of step-by-step colour photographs accompanied by an appropriate written commentary. This form of presentation follows almost exactly the colour slide plus commentary method most often used to teach surgery. Using slides, of course, it is necessary to have projection apparatus and access to a library or bank of suitable material. The method adopted in this series – of using high quality colour reproduction processes – retains the advantages of the slide and commentary method while avoiding its drawbacks.

The present series of atlases sets out to provide detailed instruction in the techniques of standard gynaecological operations. Its methodology is straightforward. The technique of each operation is clearly shown, step-by-step, using life-size photographs in natural colour, and with liberal use of indicators and accompanying diagrams. Where a step is repetitive or there is a natural sequence of steps, grouping has sometimes been used, but the natural size of the structures is maintained.

The accompanying commentary is concise and is printed on the same page as the photograph or photographs to which it refers. Every effort has been made to include only necessary material, but in situations where experience and special training have provided additional information and knowledge, that has been included.

The illustrations are selected and the accompanying commentaries so arranged as to carry the reader forward in a logical progression of thought and action in which he becomes involved. Occupied with one step he is at the same time anticipating the next, and in due course confirms his foresight as logical and correct. The photographs are those of a real patient having a real operation and the picture seen is exactly what the reader will see in the operation theatre when he does it himself. Interest is concentrated on the one step of the operation being taken at that time.

In any form of medical teaching there is the inevitable problem of pitching instruction at the level required by the audience and the presumption that the reader has insight into the specialist knowledge of the author is just as irritating as being patronised. We do not think there is a problem in this context because an atlas is by definition a guide and therefore for general use. It is just as likely to be consulted by a junior house surgeon about to assist at his first hysterectomy as by a senior colleague seeking an alternative method of dealing with a particular problem. That, at least, is the spirit in which it has been written.

Certain assumptions have had to be made to avoid verbosity, tediousness and sheer bulk of paper. It is hoped that the reader will be kind enough to attribute any omissions and shortcomings to the acceptance of such a policy. No one should be embarking on any of the procedures described without training in surgical principles, nor should he attempt them without knowledge of abdominal and pelvic anatomy and physiology.

Several areas have purposely been avoided in preparing the Atlas. There is no attempt to advise on the indications for operative treatment and only in the most general terms are the uses of a particular operation discussed. Individual surgeons develop their own ideas on pre- and post-operative care and have their personal predilections regarding forms of anaesthesia, fluid replacement and the use of antibiotics.

Even on the purely technical aspects the temptation to advise on the choice of instruments and surgical materials is largely resisted and it is assumed that the reader is capable of placing secure knots and ligatures. Each volume of the Atlas contains a photograph of the instruments used by the authors and some of these are shown individually. Most readers will have their own favourites but the information may be useful to younger colleagues. We do not consider the choice of suture material to be of over-riding importance. The senior author has used PGA suture material since its inception and although generally preferring it to catgut does not consider it perfect. It has disadvantages and can be very sore on the surgeon's hands but it does have advantages in that it is particularly suitable for vaginal work and for closing the abdomen.

There are, of course, several methods of performing the various operations but those described here have consistently given the authors the best results. It need hardly be reiterated that the observance of basic surgical principles is probably more important than anything else.

The Atlas is produced in six volumes, each of which relates approximately to a regional subspecialty. This is done primarily to keep the size of the volumes convenient for use but also to allow publication to proceed progressively.

From what has been written it might appear that the authors think of gynaecologists as necessarily male. The suggestion is rejected: the old-fashioned usage of the inclusive masculine gender is merely retained for simplicity and neatness. Anyone questioning the sincerity of this explanation would have to be reminded that every gynaecologist must, in the very nature of things, be a feminist.

Introduction to Volume 3

The surgery of gynaecological malignant disease has somehow gained the reputation of being difficult and dangerous and, at the same time, quite different from normal operative work. A mystique has grown up around it and the radical operations with their rather awesome reputations have tended to become the prerogative and responsibility of chiefs of service or senior consultants. As a result, apprenticeship and experience can be hard to come by and young specialists sometimes embark on their careers woefully inexperienced in cancer surgery and fearful of their inadequacies. The authors are determined, if possible, to demolish this misleading concept by setting out the realities of the situation.

It can be stated quite firmly that there are very few special techniques in the surgery of gynaecological malignancy that should tax a competent practising gynaecologist. There are certain recognised pitfalls in radical operations such as the danger posed by surgical dissection of certain blood vessels or urinary structures. These are well recognised and in the hands of a careful operator can all be anticipated. Such matters will be emphasised as they are dealt with in the text and a safe method of dealing with each will be illustrated. The authors believe that they can safely conduct their readers through these operations by employing well-tried and completely orthodox methods.

It can be said with equal force that matters can go badly wrong in the surgical selection of malignant cases and these are points which have to be very carefully considered. Preoperative preparation is equally important and readers need not be reminded of the dire penalties for omissions in this regard.

With the case carefully selected and prepared for operation, the techniques described in the Atlas need only be carefully and unhurriedly followed. As a final reassurance at this stage, the reader is reminded that these radical operations gained their disconcerting reputations before the benefits of modern anaesthesia, blood transfusion and antibiotics were available. The scene is now completely transformed and the anxieties previously associated with cancer surgery have largely been removed.

In previous volumes of the series some comment on the contents and their presentation has been made and that policy is continued here.

There are areas in the management of non-malignant disease where one operation is suitable for several different conditions. Abdominal and vaginal hysterectomy are obvious examples and the only problem facing the writers is to select the most suitable procedure of its type. It is then a comparatively straightforward matter to instruct the reader in the operative technique. For brevity and other reasons the authors have not become involved in the indications for any particular operation. However that may be, it is not possible to maintain an attitude of complete non-involvement in dealing with malignant disease because it is widely agreed that individualization of treatment is an essential element in successful management. The various modalities of treatment have all been fully developed and evaluated; the problem is to choose the correct one or the correct combination for the individual case, and some guidance should be available.

The authors have therefore continued their policy of selecting the operations considered of most value in the management of malignant disease but have also indicated in the text the type of case which might be suitable for a particular procedure. Surgical treatments of graded complexity are offered for vulvar, cervical, endometrial and ovarian cancer and this also allows a choice of treatment to suit the general condition of the patient. Recurrences sometimes demand further surgery of more specialised or perhaps palliative type procedures and some such operations are described. As examples, a procedure for an extensive recurrence of vulvar epithelioma is shown and a hysterectomy for cases of failed radiotherapy in uterine carcinoma is described.

The Atlas is largely based on personal records of work done by the authors. Sometimes proven methods, though not universally known and which may be of interest to the reader, are described. For example, the results of an extended hysterectomy with partial vaginectomy which has given the senior author consistently good results in over 100 cases of endometrial carcinoma is discussed. Another such example is the techniques used in the treatment of epithelioma of the vulva, where much benefit can be conferred on the patient while saving a large amount of hospital time by immediately covering the raw vulvar area with a split skin graft.

The authors pondered over the question of pelvic exenteration and decided against its inclusion. These formidable operations are fortunately only rarely required. They are specialist procedures in the sense that, apart from the difficulties of technique, unique hazards and obstacles may be encountered during the operation. Post-operative management demands special nursing skills, careful blood and electrolyte control and a considerable measure of psychological support for the patient. The latter is probably the most demanding requirement and is generally the least likely to be available. Sometimes a gynaecologist will share with a urologist the surgical management of an anterior exenteration or combine with a rectal surgeon in doing a posterior exenteration. By such co-operation the patient may be very effectively treated and we are aware of the satisfaction engendered by such procedures. Unless one has the support of the very best facilities, however, and particularly if there is any question of total pelvic exenteration, it is better to direct the case to a centre specially equipped to deal with it.

Readers will obviously wish to know what kind of results should be obtainable with surgical treatment and in each chapter we have tried to provide some information on the particular cancer under consideration, although it can only be in very general terms. We have sought the latest opinion of recognised authorities and freely used the 'Annual Report on the Results of Treatment of Gynaecological Malignancy' (1976) as a source of reference. Ovarian cancers in particular and some of the vulvar growths so often demand individualized treatment that statistics are of limited value and should be accepted as a very general guide to what can be achieved.

1: Surgical anatomy and instruments

SURGICAL ANATOMY

Lymph glands and vessels

In treating any form of malignancy the aim of surgery is to excise the affected organ or group of organs completely, with the excision line well outside the estimated tumour edge. If the tumour is known to spread by the lymph stream the glands on the line of drainage from the structures are also removed. Gynaecologists are fortunate in that the anatomy of pelvic and vulvar lymph drainage is well understood and it is possible to plan and carry out logical procedures with good prospects of success provided the lesion is in an early stage of development.

Pelvic lymph drainage

The lymph drainage from the pelvis is ultimately towards the upper abdomen by the para-aortic glands and follows the direction of the main blood vessels. The glands and lymph vessels in the pelvis itself lie on and surround the common iliac, the external iliac and the internal iliac arteries and veins. These lymph vessels receive tributaries from the vulva which enter through the femoral and sometimes through the obturator canals. Most of these join the external iliac lymph flow. The lymphogram (Figure 1) is shown to indicate the general tide of lymph drainage from the pelvis, vulva and groins, while the diagram (Figure 2) shows the major lymph drainage pathways from the pelvis with the important groups of glands numbered and named.

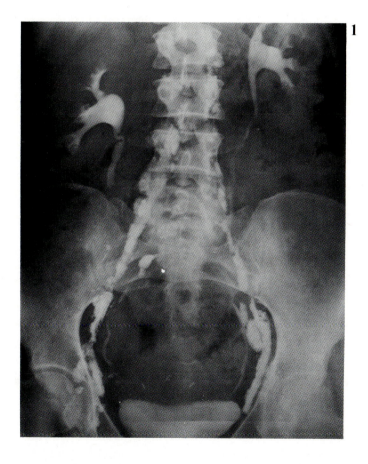

1

1 Normal lymphogram

An A.P. radiograph, lymphogram and I.V.U. of a 48 year-old patient with a stage 1 carcinoma of the cervix. On both sides, the lymph node groups are clearly shown and are normal in size with no filling defects or other evidence of tumour deposits. The I.V. urogram is also normal.

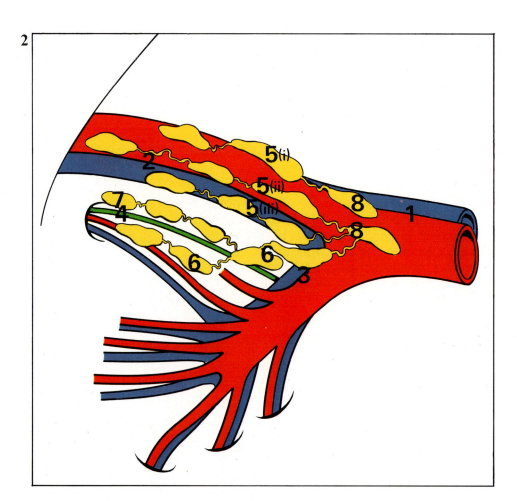

2 Pelvic drainage
1 Common iliac vessels
2 External iliac vessels
3 Internal iliac (hypogastric) vessels
4 Obturator nerve
5 External iliac glands
    (i) lateral chain
    (ii) middle chain
    (iii) medial chain
6 Internal iliac (hypogastric) glands
7 Obturator gland
8 Common iliac glands

In the most general terms, lymph drainage from the uterus and appendages passes through two aggregations of glands which serve as a primary line of defence. These are the middle and medial chains of the external iliac glands and the internal iliac or hypogastric glands which are continuous distally with the obturator glands. The lymph flow from these two primary groups is channelled through the second line of defence which is made up of the common iliac nodes. Thereafter it ascends to the third defence area of the para-aortic glands. There is nearly always a large gland at the bifurcation of the common iliac artery through which the major lymph flow must pass. As shown in the diagram, the external iliac glands lie on and between the external iliac artery and vein while the internal iliac group lies in the space between the external iliac vein on the side wall of the pelvis and the internal iliac artery postero-medially. This latter group of glands surrounds the obturator nerve. The obturator group of glands is usually described separately but is more or less continuous with the internal iliac or hypogastric group, although it may be recognisable separately in the region of the obturator foramen. There is no other recognisable organised lymph defence of the intra-pelvic genital organs, either in or on the parametrium, along the ureters or in the postero-lateral aspect of the pelvis. The authors make this statement categorically and advisedly, because the pursuit of such mythical glands has sometimes led inexperienced surgeons into trouble.

Lymph drainage of vulva

The lymph drainage of the skin of the vulva is of great importance in relation to epitheliomatous growths and their treatment and is shown in the form of a simple diagram (Figure 3). The grouping of these lymph glands is not constant but they generally present in two bands lying at right angles to each other. One is parallel to and just below the inguinal ligament and the other lies along the great saphenous vein and the femoral vein. They meet at and form a right angle which opens laterally and has its apex over the femoral canal. These groups are referred to as the superficial inguinal and the superficial femoral groups respectively and they drain into the deeper femoral glands at the entrance to, and in the femoral canal. The gland of Cloquet is alleged to be the largest of this latter group and it has always been said to transmit the main lymph flow through the femoral canal. The gland is certainly not constantly present and Way (1977, 1978) disputes its importance. Our experience leads us to the same conclusion. On entering the pelvis the lymph flow is via the external iliac chains to the common iliac glands. The skin of the vulva has lymphatic drainage to contralateral as well as to ipsilateral glands. That from the clitoris and the vestibule bypasses the superficial inguinal glands and goes direct to the external iliac group. When the urethra and vagina are involved, lymph drainage is to the obturator and internal iliac glands through the obturator foramen.

These are the essential points in relation to lymph drainage and it is not proposed to go into greater detail except where relevant to treatment in particular operations.

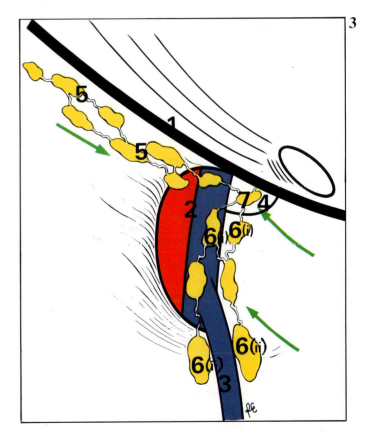

3 Lymph drainage of vulva

1 Inguinal ligament
2 Femoral vessels
3 Great saphenous vein
4 Femoral canal
5 Superficial inguinal glands
6 Superficial femoral glands
    (i) on femoral vessels
    (ii) around great saphenous vein
7 Deep femoral gland (Cloquet)
The green arrows indicate the general direction of the lymph flow

Pelvic vascular circulation and venous drainage

In the surgery of pelvic malignancy, haemorrhage and difficulty in controlling it can be major problems. Apart from the effects on the patient's condition, the surgeon's view is clouded so that it becomes difficult or even impossible accurately to define and excise the growth. Danger then increasingly threatens bladder and ureters. It is essential to know the anatomy of the pelvic blood circulation in order to understand why these dangers arise and how to avoid them.

Bleeding from deep in the pelvis is nearly always venous and the diagram (Figure 4) shows a very rich venous plexus draining into the internal and the common iliac veins. The veins are much larger and more numerous than the arteries they accompany and they are thin-walled with minimal support from areolar tissue, so that they are easily torn. Many of them enter the pelvis from the gluteal region and if divided the distal ends retract into the pelvic foramina, where they cannot be secured by forceps or stitches. In most cases it is not even possible to obtain haemostasis by pressure.

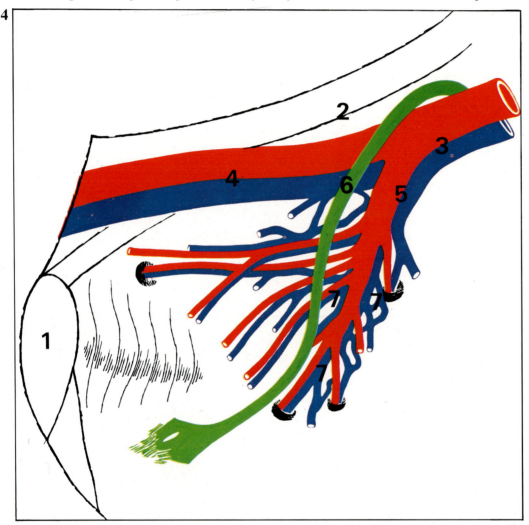

4 Venous drainage from pelvis

1 Symphysis pubis
2 Inguinal ligament
3 Common iliac vessels
4 External iliac vessels
5 Internal iliac (hypogastric) vessels
6 Ureter
7 Venous plexus posterior to ureter, drainage into internal iliac vein

Since there are no recognisable lymph glands posterior or medial to the line of the ureter in the pelvis it is unnecessary to disturb the vascular system in that area. Pelvic lymph-adenectomy is fully adequate if the chains of the external iliac group have been cleared and the aggregation of internal iliac and obturator glands have been removed from the pelvic side wall and obturator fossa.

Despite all possible care and precautions, profuse bleeding may be encountered and the surgeon should always remember the value of pressure in haemostasis. If a swab is held directly and firmly over the bleeding point for a full two minutes nearly all such bleeding will cease. This procedure should always be tried in the first instance and repeated where necessary. If bleeding stubbornly persists, the internal iliac artery may be ligated on the affected side or on both sides. The bleeding, however, comes from vessels which have a collateral circulation through the sacro-sciatic notch so that ligation is not always effective. In ligating the internal iliac artery the whole trunk should be tied and not just the anterior branch as is sometimes advised. If bleeding still persists, it may be necessary as a last resort to pack the area with gauze and bring the end of the gauze roll out through the abdominal wound. Forty-eight hours' later and under a short general anaesthetic the pack can be removed with safety.

Another and more spectacular type of bleeding occurs if a large vein, usually the femoral or external iliac, is torn during the removal of an adherent lymph gland or group of glands. This is infrequent because even in advanced malignancy, gland metastases almost always remain within the capsule of the gland and do not invade the actual vessel wall. Nonetheless the accident can happen and is rather frightening. The first step is to control bleeding by digital pressure above and below the lesion and immediately remove the blood from the wound. The injury to the vessel must then be defined and arrangements made to repair it.

In circumstances where the operator must deal with the problem himself the following principles apply. The circumference of the vein is gently defined at a distance of 2.5 cm above and below the injury, disturbing it as little as possible from its bed. Tapes are passed under it at both points to expose the lesion and to control bleeding as required. The defect is closed by interrupted fine silk or prolene mattress sutures on a No. 0000 round-bodied needle. They are placed in such a way as to evert the edges and leave the lumen smooth. The general principles are shown diagramatically in Figure 5.

5 Repair of damaged large vein

1 Injury to vessel wall
2 Tapes to define defect and control bleeding
3 Fine mattress prolene sutures
4 Inset showing method of everting vessel wall

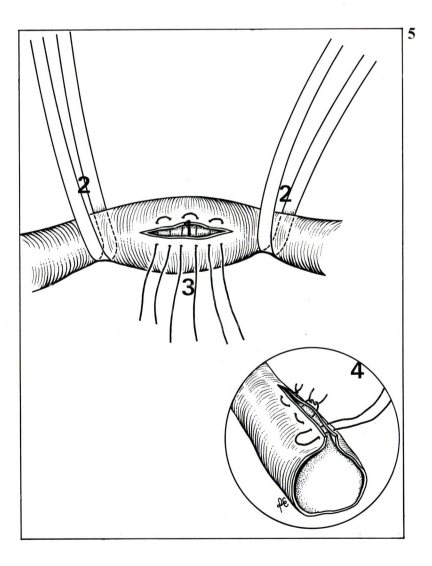

Bladder and ureters

The ease with which the ureters and the bladder can be damaged during pelvic surgery was noted in Volume II of this series (pages 10–13). The possibility of such mishaps is considerably greater in the surgery of malignant conditions. The average incidence of vesico-vaginal and uretero-vaginal fistulae in Wertheim's hysterectomy is between one and three per cent. (Buchsbaum and Schmidt (1978), Mattingly and Borkowf (1978), Lawson (1978).)

The best safeguard against damage to the bladder and ureter is a concise knowledge of the anatomy of the lower urinary tract and especially of the ureter; it is essential to know the exact course of the ureter in normal circumstances, its relationship to other structures and its blood supply.

The bladder is closely applied and adherent to the anterior aspect of the lower uterus and the cervix and the two organs frequently have to be separated by sharp dissection. Cervical growths are always infected to some degree and the surrounding area of inflammatory reaction frequently extends to the adjacent bladder, making separation of that structure hazardous. The necessary precautions will be referred to in the text.

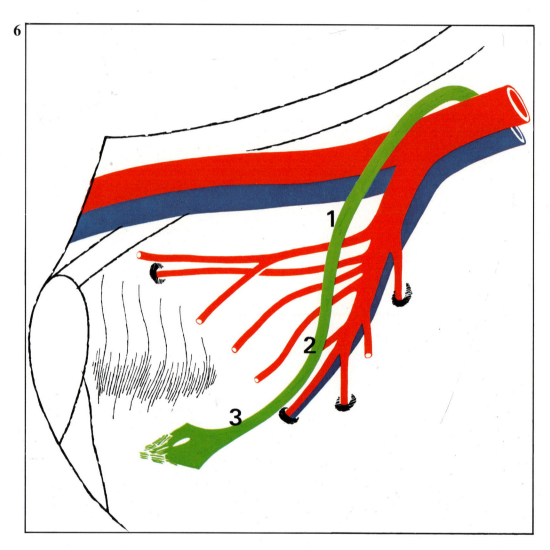

6 Relationship of ureter to blood vessel of pelvic side wall showing areas liable to surgical damage

Danger to ureter at different levels:
1 When clamping ovarian pedicle
2 When mobilising an adherent pelvic tumour
3 During hysterectomy when parametrium invaded or cervix enlarged by growth

The ureters present a greater problem. They are vulnerable over a considerable distance and at certain specific points, which are indicated on the diagram (Figure 6), but it must be remembered that the greatest danger to the ureter is the vulnerability of its own blood supply. The ureter enters the true pelvis at the level of the bifurcation of the common iliac artery. It is external and adherent to the parietal pelvic peritoneum and runs downwards slightly medially on a converging course with a number of parallel blood vessels. It picks up part of its blood supply from each vessel as it crosses it. The ureter is surrounded by its own areolar tissue mesentery and by a closely enmeshed network of blood vessels which are fed from the vessels it encounters throughout its length. In the iliac fossa it receives branches from the iliolumbar and the ovarian arteries and it picks up further branches from the internal pudendal and middle rectal arteries as it descends into the pelvis. In the rest of its course and where it particularly concerns the gynaecologist, it receives contributions from the uterine, the vaginal and the middle and inferior vesical arteries. As it nears the bladder, the superior and other vesical arteries send back branches along the ureter to anastomose with those from above. The concept of distinct and visible arteries running towards the ureter to furnish a blood supply is erroneous. Advice to preserve this or that vessel is confusing and dangerous because such branches will not be immediately visible and searching for them may cause tissue disturbance and bleeding.

The safest approach to the ureter is to disturb it as little as possible from its bed and certainly refrain from stripping it from its mesentery. Otherwise the damaged blood supply may well lead to necrosis and subsequent fistula formation. This afferent blood supply is maintained intact by avoiding separation of the ureter and so preserving the mesentery. The distributive network of nutrient vessels is preserved by gentle handling, care with diathermy coagulation and avoidance of any kinking or constriction when reconstituting the pelvic peritoneum. Where it is necessary to displace the ureters laterally, this can always be done without disturbing the surrounding leash of vessels. Figure 7 shows the surrounding network of vessels which, incidentally, also have attachments to the peritoneum. The mesentery is clearly shown in Figure 8, where the ureter and its accompanying leash of blood vessels are supported on the forceps.

There are three points of potential danger to the pelvic ureter during hysterectomy or pelvic surgery and these are indicated by the numbers 1, 2 and 3 on the diagram (Figure 6). At (1) the ureter lies in the base of the infundibulo-pelvic ligament and unless care is exercised in clamping that structure, the ureter can be caught up and damaged or divided. At (2) the ureter is extra-peritoneal but otherwise uncovered. It is particularly liable to become adherent to or involved in any malignant growth occupying the pelvic floor and this includes many ovarian tumours. At (3) the ureter skirts the uterus on each side at a distance of only 2 cm from the cervix and is fixed in position in its parametrial tunnel. Since the aim of many radical pelvic operations is to remove as much parametrial tissue as possible, the ureters must always first be defined and displaced laterally if they are to be safe. Intra-cervical growths which produce a barrel-shaped enlargement of that structure are very close to the ureters and constitute a major risk to their safety. In addition to these recognised hazards the ureters have a propensity to congenital aberrations and are not always constant in their course.

This list of dangers is formidable but, with precise knowledge of where they lie, it is a straightforward matter to take the appropriate precautions and the risks of damage should be minimal. *The main precautions to be taken are:*

1 When clamping the ovarian pedicle it is important to check that the ureter is below and clear of the chosen point of clamping. See (1) on the diagram.

2 When removing a pelvic tumour which is adherent to the pelvic floor, and especially if there are firm adhesions, one must remember that the ureter may be involved. This corresponds to (2) on the diagram. Ovarian growths usually present so great a problem in their removal that the only really safe procedure is to define the ureter at the pelvic brim and to follow its course downwards to ensure that it is not menaced by the dissection. The problem of large ovarian cysts (whether benign or malignant) which make safe access impossible is referred to under the appropriate headings. In these cases, aspiration of the contents may be advisable.

3 The operator must never try to remove a vaginal cuff of tissue or parametrial tissue without first releasing the ureters from their tunnel and displacing them laterally, because they are tethered in position and will inevitably be damaged. The dangers are greatly increased where there is an intra-cervical growth causing the barrel-shaped type of cervix referred to. See (3) on the diagram. Unless the ureters are very clearly defined and displaced they are particularly liable to damage in these latter cases.

4 It is absolutely essential to have preoperative intravenous pyelography done on all cases having major pelvic surgery. A congenital defect such as renal agenesis, horse-shoe kidney, double ureter or abnormal course is always possible. There may also be unsuspected hydro-nephrosis, hydro-ureter, non-functioning kidney, renal calculus, or even renal neoplasm. Quite apart from the clinical importance of having an intravenous pyelogram, the surgeon could otherwise find himself in a totally indefensible medico-legal situation.

There is a further danger to the ureter which is less related to its surgical anatomy than to overzealous attempts at reperitonisation. Following radical hysterectomy there is a bilateral upward extension from the usual transverse peritoneal opening and, at the same time, an actual reduction in the area of available peritoneum.

The usual method of closing the pelvic peritoneum is by a continuous transverse suture which gathers the peritoneum in purse string fashion over the lateral pedicles on one side, continues across the vault and ends by doing the same on the other side. In the circumstances of a radical hysterectomy, this method can so distort the adherent ureter as to obstruct urine flow and interfere with ureteric blood supply.

There are two safe procedures available. One is to use a small number of interrupted sutures to approximate obvious peritoneal leaves loosely, accepting that there will be uncovered raw areas. The neater and safer alternative is to approximate the bladder and rectal leaves of peritoneum transversely across the vault of the vagina, and then quite separately make a sagittal closure on each side along the general line of the large vessels and ureter. Completion of the transverse stitch has already brought the edges into relaxed opposition and the sagittal suture causes no distortion. Details of the method are described and illustrated in relation to Wertheim's and extended hysterectomy (pages 190, 219).

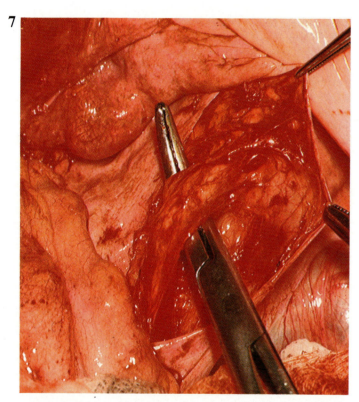

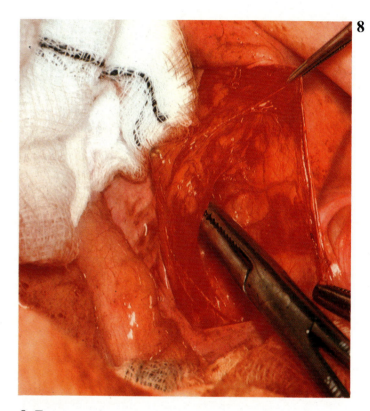

7 Exposure of ureter to show vascular network on its surface
This figure shows the enveloping network of blood vessels on the lower ureter which, contrary to accepted opinion, has a very rich blood supply. The branches from the various pelvic arteries anastomose to form this continuous and tortuous chain which also has attachments to the peritoneum. At a slightly lower level than shown here the ureter is surrounded by a dense plexus of veins which communicates with the internal iliac plexus and vein. There is no lack of blood supply to the actual ureter; the problem is that it is particularly vulnerable during surgery.

8 Exposure of ureter to show its surrounding and attached mesentery
The word 'mesentery' has been used in relation to the blood supply of the lower ureter, although it is not one that will be found in anatomical textbooks. The figure shows a leash of vessels loosely surrounding the ureter and with a firm attachment deep to it to form a sub-ureteric bed. Forceps are used to elevate the ureter and the blood vessels are thrown into relief. Nearer the bladder the wall of the ureter becomes even more bound up with surrounding structures and blood supply as there is an aggregation of longitudinal muscle fibres on the surface of the muscular coat and referred to as the 'sheath of the ureter'. In view of all these anatomical considerations, it is clearly of great importance that the ureter be disturbed from its bed as little as possible and certainly never stripped of its mesentery.

Classification of gynaecological malignant tumours by staging

Classification of pelvic malignant tumours by stages is of great importance since correct treatment, choice of appropriate operation and evaluation of results of therapy all depend on its accuracy. Staging is based entirely on clinical findings except in the case of ovarian cancer where laparotomy is done prior to classification. The system of staging is international and is laid down by F.I.G.O.

Most surgeons are familiar with the major subdivisions but, unless engaged exclusively in oncological work, have to make reference to the definition tables from time to time. The Annual Report on the Results of Treatment in Carcinoma of the Uterus, Vagina and Ovary (1976) sets out the requisite information and gives guidance on clinical and pathological aspects of the subject. The actual tables of the classification and staging of pelvic malignant tumours as they appear in the report are reproduced as an appendix on pages 337 to 339. It is convenient and helpful to have them easily available in outpatient and operation departments.

In the practical sphere there are some constantly recurring dilemmas in regard to staging, and advice based on experience is offered on the more common examples.

In the staging of cervical cancer, the most important parameter is vaginal examination and it may be very difficult to decide whether or not the growth has reached the side wall of the pelvis especially if there is accompanying inflammation. The problem can be resolved frequently by the subsequent rectal examination which gives much better access posterior to the cardinal ligaments, enabling them to be felt at a higher level. Extension of growth along the utero-sacral ligaments has a considerable bearing on operability and must be assessed rectally. From every point of view, therefore, this examination is very important.

When a growth involves both the cervical canal and the lower endometrial cavity it may be difficult to know whether it is primarily uterine or cervical. A compromise diagnosis of *carcinoma corporis et cervicis* was used for a time but was never satisfactory and it is now considered essential to allocate the growth to the cervix or the body of the uterus. The histology of the tumour is taken into consideration in doing so and, if there is no clear indication of origin after all investigations are complete, it is accepted that the case should be classified as *carcinoma corporis* if adenomatous and *carcinoma cervicis* if epidermal.

When lymphography is available unexpected involvement of common iliac or para-aortic glands may be reported. Although interpretation of such radiographs is not an exact science, such a discovery could make surgical treatment inadvisable in some cases and these difficult decisions have to be made on all the available evidence. The staging of the growth is not influenced by such lymphographic evidence which is not considered a routine investigation by the Cancer Commmittee of F.I.G.O.

Ovarian growths are notoriously difficult to assess as regards primary site and the decision often depends on the histological findings. Ovarian cancer is defined as an apparent primary malignant tumour sited in the ovary and this is the only clear guidance available. The main groups of the F.I.G.O. classification are shown for the results of treatment in ovarian cancer (page 244); the reader, having made the major classification, can then allocate the case to one of these groups.

SURGICAL INSTRUMENTS

The authors' views on surgical equipment were discussed in the Introduction to the Atlas. The general abdominal set in use at the Jessop Hospital for Women, Sheffield, is shown in Figure 9, but most readers will be accustomed to their own choice of instruments and there is no desire to dissuade them from that choice. Those illustrated are of the simplest possible design and have been developed for standard hospital use over a number of years by a succession of exceedingly good and careful surgeons.

For identification purposes we have attached to some instruments the names we have learnt to associate with them, but we fully expect that some readers will recognise these items as those they have always linked with the name of someone else.

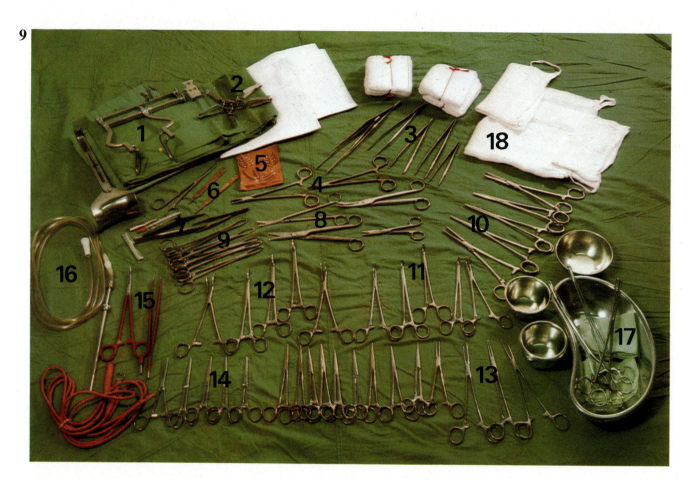

9 Standard abdominal instruments
 1 Self-retaining retractor
 2 Ureteric dissecting forceps
 3 Dissecting forceps
 4 Needle holders
 5 Assorted needles
 6 Scalpels
 7 Michel clip forceps
 8 Scissors
 9 Littlewood's forceps
10 Straight Oschner forceps
11 Curved Oschner forceps
12 Miles-Phillips' forceps
13 Allis' tissue forceps
14 Spencer-Wells forceps
15 Diathermy forceps
16 Sucker
17 Sponge forceps and catheterisation equipment
18 Intra-abdominal packs and swabs

A few instruments of particular value in radical surgery are shown in Figure 10; some of these might be included in the routine abdominal set.

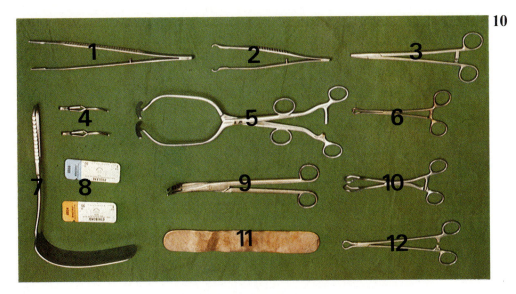

10 Additional instruments for radical surgery
1 Extra-long dissecting forceps
2 Ureteric dissecting forceps
3 Extra-long Mayo-type needle holder
4 Arterial clamps
5 Berkeley-Bonney clamp
6 Babcock's forceps
7 Kelly retractor
8 Fine silk and prolene sutures
9 Extra-long curved scissors
10 Gland-holding forceps
11 Malleable retractor
12 Ureter-holding forceps

The ureter-holding forceps are useful in defining that structure and Babcock's or Duval's forceps are suitable for the gentle handling of urinary and vascular structures. It is helpful to have purpose-made forceps to hold gland tissue securely without compressing it. The other instruments shown are used to obtain better access in a deep pelvis. Most surgeons like to have a malleable retractor to hand, and a large Kelly retractor, although clumsy, is sometimes the only possible method of exposing the anterior vaginal wall in a Wertheim hysterectomy. A long needle holder and dissecting forceps to match sometimes makes the placing of a deep stitch possible where it could not otherwise be done. It is prudent to have some arterial clamps and fine silk sutures available for repair of possible damage to large blood vessels.

Suggested reading
Annual report on the results of treatment in carcinoma of the uterus, vagina and ovary (Vol. 16, 1976), edited by H. L. Kottmeier. Radiumhemmet, Stockholm.
Buchsbaum, H. J. & Schmidt, J. D. (1978). The urinary tract in radical hysterectomy. *Gynecologic and Obstetric Urology*, 113–127. W. B. Saunders, Philadelphia.
Lawson, J. (1978). The management of genito-urinary fistulae. *Clinics in Obstetrics and Gynaecology*, 5, 1, 209–236.
Mattingley, R. F. & Borkowf, H. I. (1978). Acute operative injury to the lower urinary tract. *Clinics in Obstetrics and Gynaecology*, 5, 1, 123–150.
Way, S. (1977). The lymphatics of the pelvis. *Scientific Foundations in Obstetrics and Gynaecology*. Second edition, 118–126, edited by E. E. Philip, J. Barnes & M. Newton. Heinemann (William) Medical Books, London.
Way, S. (1978). The surgery of vulval carcinoma: an appraisal. *Clinics in Obstetrics and Gynaecology*, 5, 1, 623–628.

2: Carcinoma of the vulva

The treatment of a vulvar carcinoma is essentially surgical. The disease is a multi-centric one usually preceded and often accompanied by dystrophic skin lesions. The collateral circulation of the vulva is poor while the skin has a rich lymphatic network and a multitude of sweat glands. For these various reasons radiation is an unsuitable form of therapy.

Stanley Way (1977, 1978) has done much to develop the modern surgical treatment of the condition and, on a basis of 347 cases of vulvar cancer treated and studied over 40 years, is convinced that the ideal treatment is radical vulvectomy with superficial inguinal and deep pelvic node dissection.

While in agreement with this general assessment, the authors must point out that some patients neither require nor are medically fit for such radical treatment. Cases can be divided into separate clinical groups as judged by the severity of the disease and general fitness; such groups are indicated. The various available surgical treatments are then listed and it is reasonably simple to assign to the patients in each group the most appropriate surgical operation from those available.

The clinical groups of patients are:

1 Those with vulvar dystrophic lesions where a periodic biopsy has revealed an *in situ* or even early micro-invasive carcinoma.
2 Relatively young women (around 50) who present with an early single centre lesion. Their general condition is good and symptoms are few.
3 Elderly but not unfit patients with a large cancer of the vulva which has been concealed until it caused severe symptoms or was accidentally discovered.
4 Elderly and frail patients with advanced growths who are often in the terminal stages of illness.
5 Young women with a particularly locally aggressive lesion involving not only vulva but also the anorectal and vaginal regions. This growth is a variant of squamous carcinoma and is referred to as a verrucous carcinoma and has a peculiar geographic and racial distribution.

The available surgical treatments are:

1 *Local vulvectomy* i.e. removal of the skin of the vulva and including the clitoris.
2 *Radical vulvectomy* i.e. wide removal of the whole vulva including the superficial inguinal and superficial femoral gland groups. Lymph glands and vessels are removed only as far as the entrance to the femoral canal. Some of the deeper femoral glands in the lower femoral canal will be removed.
3 *Radical vulvectomy with pelvic lymphadenectomy* This is the operation recommended by Way and, in addition to the surgery carried out in operation 2, the inguinal canal is opened, the transversalis fascia divided, the peritoneum swept medially and the pelvic glands dissected downwards off the vessels from the bifurcation of the common iliac artery to the inguinal ligament.

Matching the clinical groups with the operations

Clinical group 1 is adequately dealt with by operation 1.
Patients in clinical group 2 are best treated by operation 3 (radical vulvectomy and pelvic lymphadenectomy) but, if the growth is of low histological grading (which means that the incidence of involved iliac glands is very small) it may be reasonable to treat such cases by operation 2 (radical vulvectomy without pelvic lymphadenectomy).

Clinical group 3 unfortunately includes the majority of patients seen and many are grossly obese. Inguinal glands are palpable in some cases although this may be from inflammatory rather than neoplastic cause. The operation of choice for such cases is operation 3 (radical vulvectomy with pelvic lymphadenectomy). Although major, the operation is associated with remarkably little shock and patients do extraordinarily well.

Clinical group 4 presents major problems but the situation is desperate and palliative treatment must be attempted. Operation 2 is generally possible after a period in hospital to clean up the growth, correct anaemia and to build up the patient's general health on a high protein diet.

Clinical group 5 frequently requires colostomy prior to vulvectomy because of anal involvement. Operation 2 (radical vulvectomy) seems to be adequate because of infrequent lymph node metastases.

To cover the field of possible requirements the following six operations are described:

1 Local vulvectomy
2 Radical vulvectomy without pelvic lymphadenectomy
3 Radical vulvectomy with pelvic lymphadenectomy
   i Advanced fungating growth in an obese patient with distal urethral involvement and semi-fluctuant inguinal nodes (inguinal ligaments detached during operation)
   ii Localised primary lesion without added complications in a fit patient where radical operation was indicated (inguinal ligaments not divided)
   iii Straightforward case where the raw area of the vulva is immediately grafted with split skin
4 Excision of recurrent vulvar growth

Biopsy of the vulva

Biopsy of the vulva in relation to clinical malignancy is straightforward and the naked eye appearances leave little doubt as to the diagnosis. The nature of the malignant change must be confirmed histologically as this is very important both in prognosis and in choice of treatment. Premalignant changes require a different approach. For example, some *in situ* vulvar lesions may look clinically as dangerous as invasive disease but require considerably less radical treatment. The degree of cell differentiation may even decide whether or not to embark on any form of surgery in a very advanced case. Way (1977) showed that in anaplastic growths, the overall node involvement was 62 per cent compared with 35 per cent with differentiated lesions. There was bilateral node involvement in 35 per cent of the former as compared with 12 per cent in the latter growths. The superficial and deep nodes were involved in 22 per cent of anaplastic and 8 per cent of the differentiated group. Individualization of treatment is, therefore, particularly applicable in vulvar malignancy and, as can be seen from Way's figures, the degree of cell differentiation is by far the most important factor in choosing treatment.

The difficult question of the chronic vulvar dystrophies as precursors of vulvar malignancy is dealt with in Volume 4 of this series but, for general guidance, it can be said that clinical lesions which are under observation because of their recognised danger should have regular biopsy.

Vulvar biopsies are taken from the most active area of the growth; they need not be large or unduly deep and it is generally possible to avoid stitches. In the case of a localised growth not considered necessarily malignant, it is reasonable to remove the growth with a surrounding 1 cm of healthy skin and thereby possibly complete treatment at the same time. The case chosen for illustration here was not clinically malignant although it was judged and subsequently proved to be so.

The actual taking of the biopsy is only part of a careful examination of the vulva and adjacent structures to assess the extent of the disease and its involvement of surrounding organs or tissues. The degree of involvement of the urethra, vagina and anus is noted and vaginal examination should be made by speculum as well as digitally. These growths usually stop short of invading the actual vaginal canal but the authors remember one case where the epithelioma progressed right up the posterior vaginal wall as far as the posterior fornix so that not only the vulvar but the vaginal skin also had to be removed before the operation could be called complete.

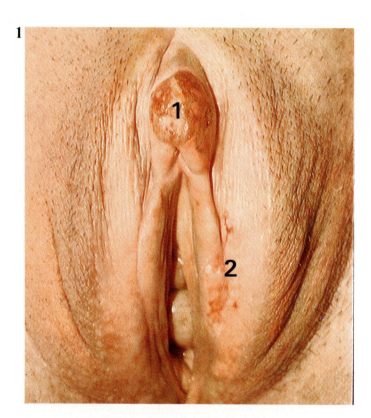

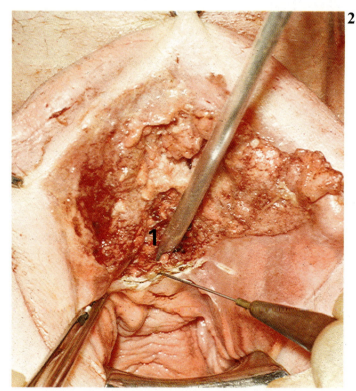

1 and 2 Epithelioma of vulva – typical lesions

Figure 1 shows a clinically recognised growth involving the clitoris (1) and with accompanying dystrophic change in the skin of the labia (2). The patient was 45 years old and the tumour cell differentiation was poor, thus the prognosis was also poor. Figure 2 shows an advanced growth with involvement of the distal urethra (1) (metal catheter *in situ*). The diathermy needle shows the point at which the distal urethra will have to be excised.

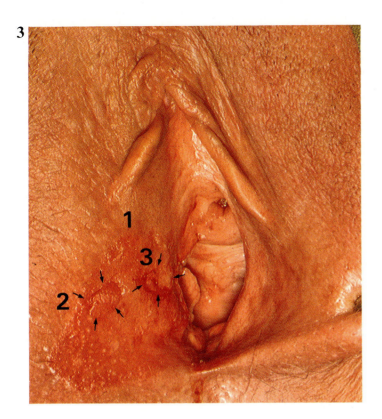

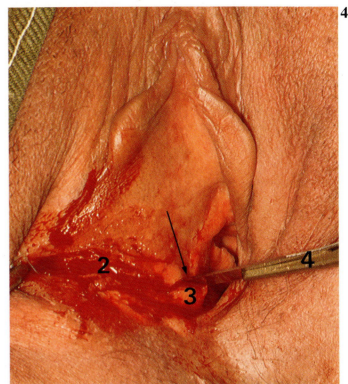

3 to 5 Vulvar biopsy for suspected malignancy

This observed case of chronic vulvar dystrophy with clinical leukoplakia progressed to an atrophic stage which obliterated both labia on the right side of the vulva (1). At the same time hard nodules ((2) and (3) and arrowed in Figure 3) developed on the inner aspect of the right labium majus and were considered almost certainly malignant. Biopsy is best done under general anaesthesia in these cases and specimens are taken from all suspicious areas. In Figure 4 the area 2 has been removed completely by the biopsy and a curved incision is made with the scalpel (4) just clear of the growth in area 3 (arrowed) and is matched by a similar curved incision below it in Figure 5 (arrowed), to remove a wedge of full thickness skin and some superficial fat for histological examination. The nodule is steadied with the dissecting forceps (5) while the second curved incision is completed. It is preferable not to insert stitches which are rarely necessary as bleeding is minimal.

Even if the malignancy is obvious as in the growths shown in Figures 1 and 2, vulvar biopsy should always be done because it is important to know the histological grading of the tumour; also, the opportunity should be taken to define the extent of the growth and make plans for subsequent operation. Vulvar cancers do not usually invade the vagina but they sometimes do so and it is essential to make a full speculum examination.

Local vulvectomy

There are two groups of cases where local vulvectomy may be used. The first is where the symptoms resulting from chronic vulvar dystrophy or clinical leukoplakia are so severe and medical treatment in the form of local steroids and/or hormones so unsuccessful that surgery becomes necessary. The management of such cases will be considered in Volume 4 of the Atlas. In the other group, biopsy has shown a carcinoma *in situ* lesion, usually in a previous dystrophic lesion under observation.

The case illustrated here belongs to the latter group.

Since any vulvar malignancy is likely to be multicentric the aim must be to remove the whole of the vulvar skin.

There is no necessity to remove more than the thickness of the skin and the defect can be closed by a single layer of carefully placed sutures. Removal of the underlying fat confers no advantage and may cause haematomata.

The area of skin to be removed lies between two parallel oval incisions. It extends laterally to the labio-crural fold, includes the clitoris anteriorly and generally takes the anterior half of the perineal skin. There may be some tension on suturing the skin posteriorly and it is advisable to under-cut the lower edge of the skin of the posterior vaginal wall so that it can be drawn down to cover the perineum without tension.

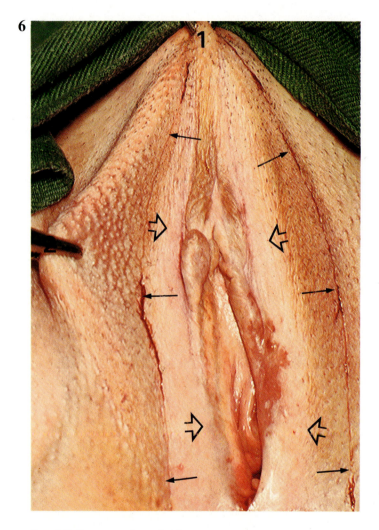

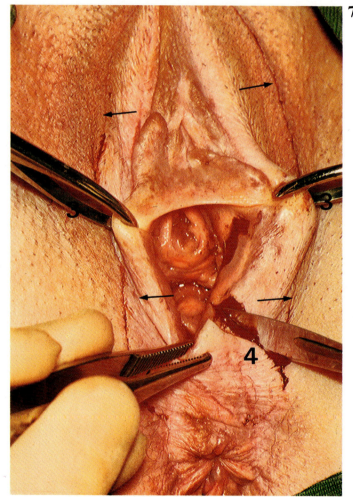

6 and 7 Demarcation of skin area for removal

With the patient in lithotomy position, the skin over the pubis is held upwards by forceps (1) in Figure 6, while the tip of the diathermy needle is used to outline superficially the area for subsequent removal. Dissecting forceps (2) keep the skin taut while this is done. The broad arrows indicate the extent of the lesion. In Figure 7 the labia are steadied by forceps (3 and 3) while a radial skin incision is made postero-laterally (4) to give access to the introitus, so that an inner parallel incision can be made. The outer line of skin removal is arrowed on both photographs.

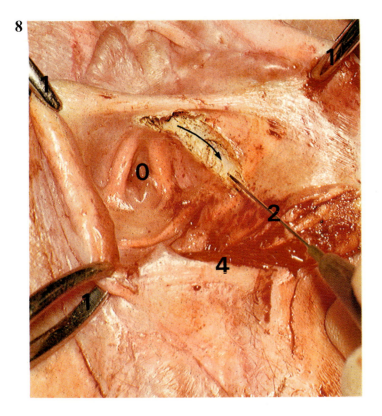

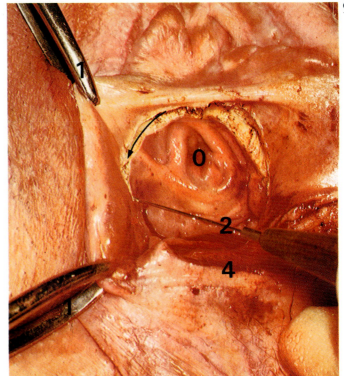

9

8 to 10 Release of vulvar skin at inner (introital) edge

Having obtained adequate access to the vulvo-vaginal junction the labia are retracted with tissue forceps (1, 1, 1) in Figure 8, while the diathermy needle (2) commences the incision anterior to and 1 cm clear of the external urethral orifice (0) and carries it posteriorly along the left introital edge (arrowed). The procedure is repeated on the right side in Figure 9 as arrowed, and in Figure 10 the circle is completed posteriorly (arrowed). The number 4 denotes the relief skin incision on each photograph.

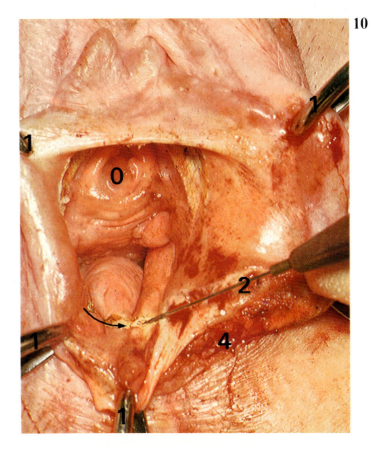

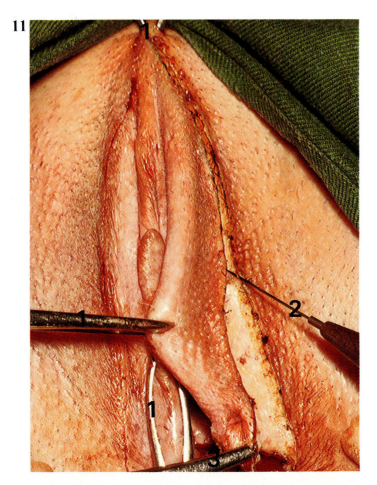

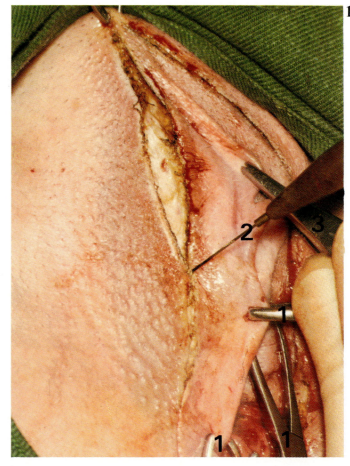

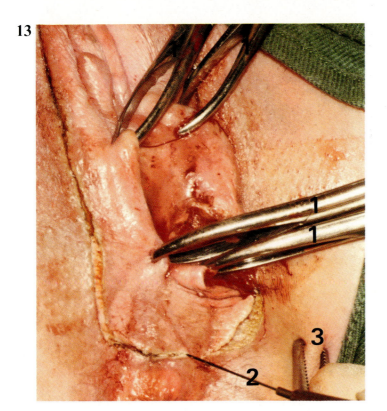

11 to 13 Completing lateral skin incision

The skin is held taught where required by tissue forceps (1) and dissecting forceps (3) while the diathermy needle (2) divides the skin in its full thickness on the left side in Figure 11, on the right in Figure 12, and across the perineum in Figure 13.

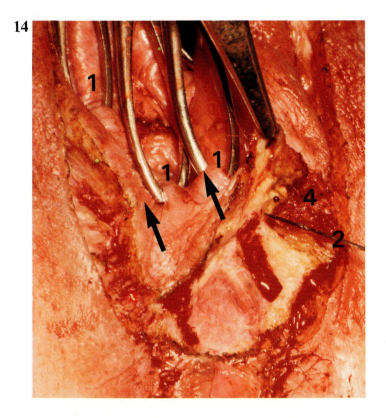

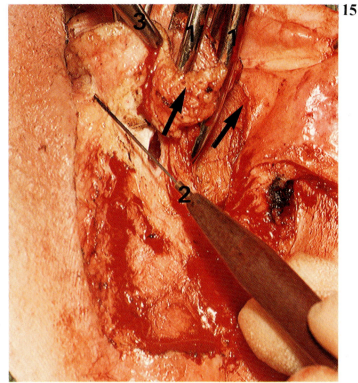

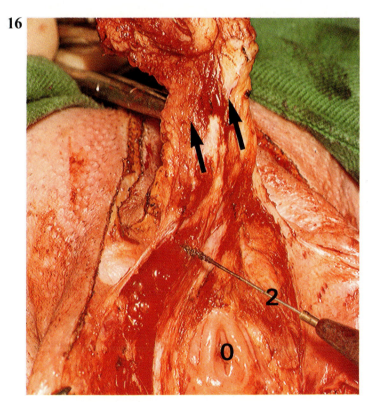

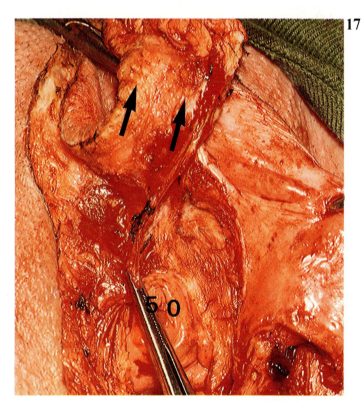

14 to 17 Raising skin area in anterior direction

The skin for removal is held in tissue forceps (1) and the whole area is lifted up and detached in a forward direction from the underlying superficial fat by gentle strokes of the diathermy needle (2) and in the general direction of the arrows. The posterior edge is freed at the area of the radial incision (4) in Figure 14. The right side is elevated in Figure 15, the left side in Figure 16. In Figure 17 the forceps (5) secure a bleeding point to the right of the external urethral orifice (0) while the flap is lifted anteriorly. The direction in which the excised skin is held is indicated by arrows.

18

19

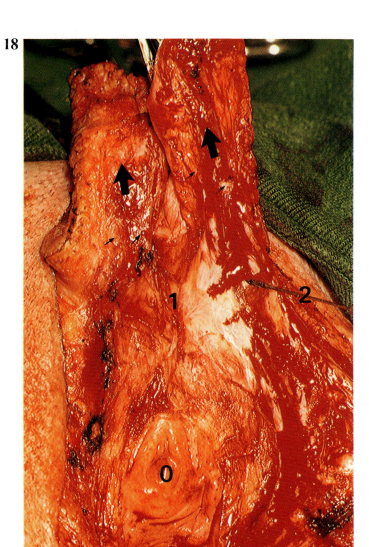

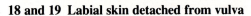

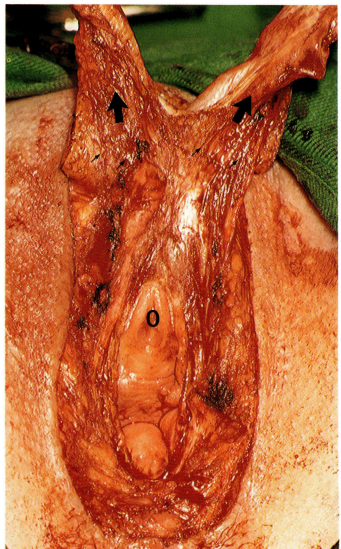

18 and 19 Labial skin detached from vulva

Both illustrations show the full thickness skin and an attached thin layer of superficial fat (fine arrows) being lifted in the general direction of the broad arrows. Figure 18 gives a close-up view and the external urethral orifice is at (0). The vascular area of the clitoris lies in the area of (1). These clitoral vessels require definitive attention and are

more suitably dealt with from above as shown on the opposite page. Figure 19 shows the vulva denuded by the removal of labial and perineal skin. It will be seen that the lower posterior vaginal wall (2) is sufficiently lax to provide cover for the perineum if required. This appearance is constant. The blackened areas are the result of diathermy coagulation of small blood vessels.

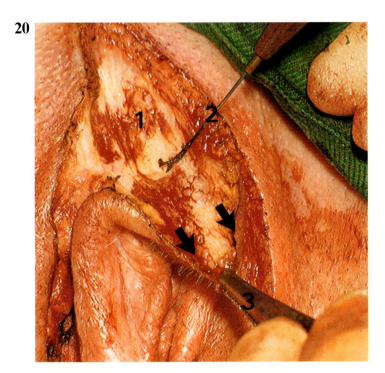

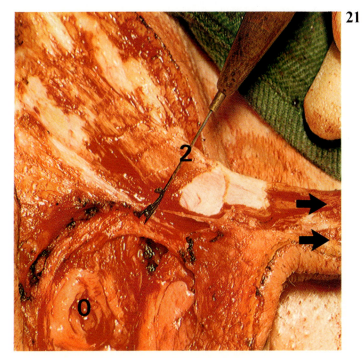

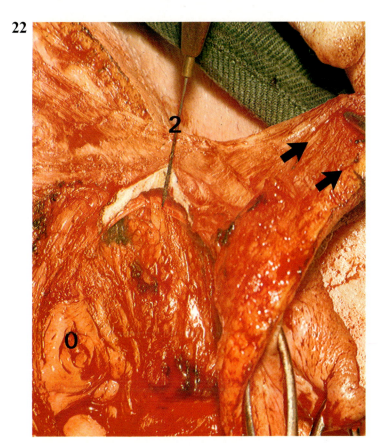

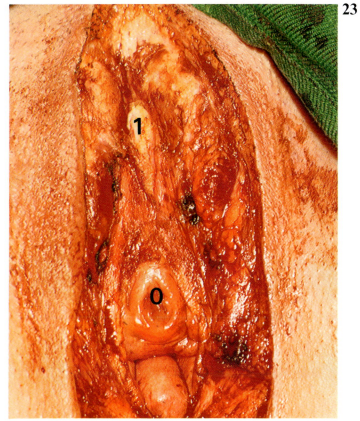

20 to 23 Removal of vulvar skin including clitoris

While the vulvar skin is held posteriorly by dissecting forceps (3) in the general line of the arrows in Figure 20, the diathermy needle (2) cuts across the suspensory ligaments and blood supply of the clitoris (1). In this instance, the coagulation efficiently sealed the clitoral vessels but if bleeding is persistent it is sometimes better to use a fine ligature or underrun the bleeding point with a fine figure-of-eight haemostatic stitch. Rather more superficial fat is removed from this area than elsewhere but the periosteum is not breached. Figures 21 and 22 show further stages in separation of the vulvar skin and Figure 23 shows the denuded anterior vulva with the suspensory ligaments of the clitoris (1). The external urethral orifice is designated (0) where visible.

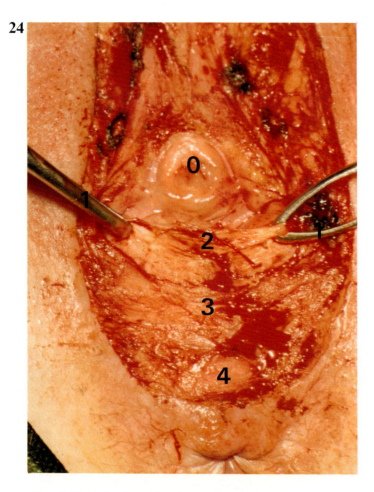

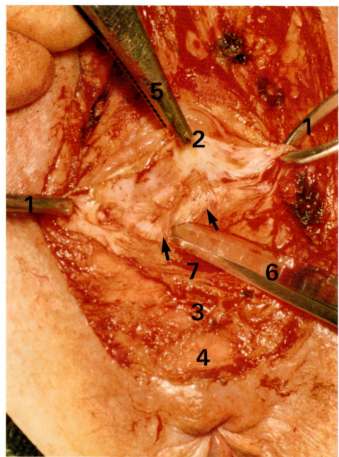

24 and 25 Releasing skin of posterior vaginal wall

The possibility of covering the denuded perineum by posterior vaginal wall skin has already been mentioned; in Figure 24 it is clear that the amount of perineal skin removed will cause tension on the suture line unless this is done. The lower edge of vaginal skin (2) is held in tissue forceps

(1) and (1) in both photographs displaying the superficial perineal muscles (3) and the external anal sphincter (4). In Figure 25 the edge of the vaginal skin is held in dissecting forceps (5) while the scissors (6) find a plane of cleavage (arrowed) to separate it from the perineal muscles (3) and the anterior aspect of the rectum (7).

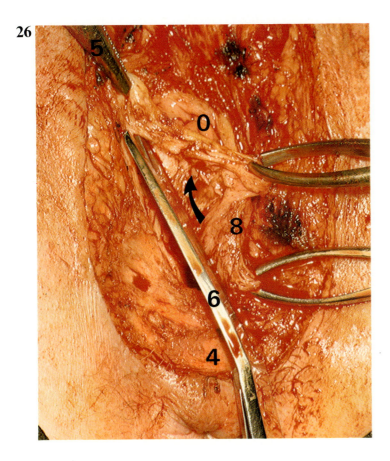

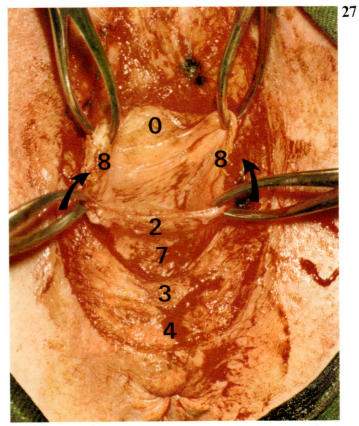

26 to 28 Undercutting vaginal skin laterally and posteriorly

It is usually sufficient to release the skin of the posterior vaginal wall but sometimes (as in this case) there is the prospect of some tension on the lateral suture lines and it is a simple matter to release the lateral vaginal skin. In Figure 26 this is being done with the scissors in the direction of the arrow. The process has been completed on both sides in Figure 27; in Figure 28 it is seen that there is adequate mobile skin to give a relaxed closure all round. The numbers used on the previous page are repeated here with the addition of the lateral vaginal edges designated (8).

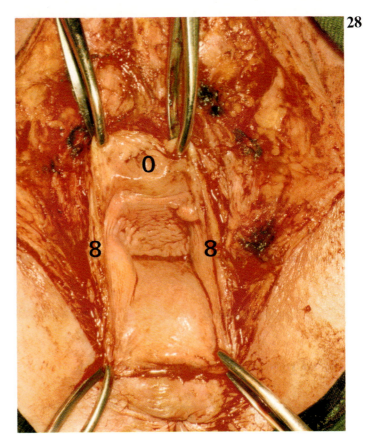

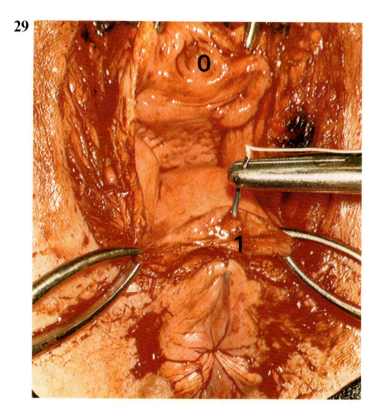

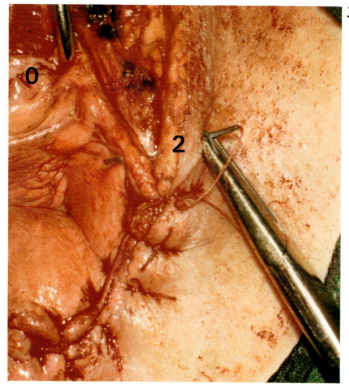

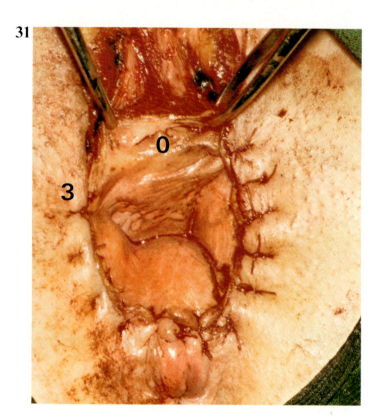

29 to 31 Skin suture to cover raw area of vulvectomy (i)

The suture should always commence in the midline posteriorly and proceed forwards symmetrically on each side in turn. This brings any redundant lateral skin anteriorly to the area of the urethral orifice where it can always be used to advantage in making a neat skin closure without tension. The first interrupted vertical mattress suture of PGA No. 0 material is being placed at (1) which is the midpoint posteriorly in Figure 29. The left side has been sutured as far forward as (2) in Figure 30. In Figure 31 this is being matched by a similar line of sutures on the right side which has reached (3). The external urethral orifice is still designated (0) for orientation.

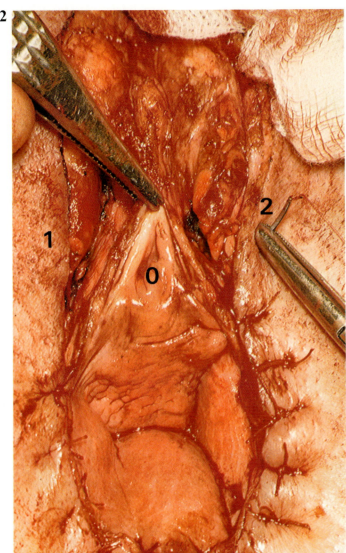

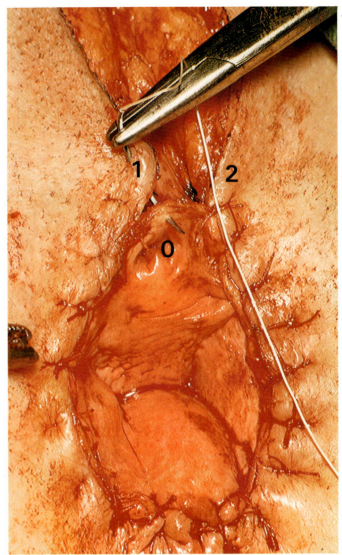

32 and 33 Skin suture to cover raw area of vulvectomy (ii)

Sutures alternately placed on each side attach the lateral skin flaps to the skin around the external urethral orifice to make a complete closure. In Figure 32 this step commences and there is seen to be surface skin at (1) and (2). The step is nearing completion in Figure 33 and the needle is seen to bring the right lateral skin flap (1) to the midline without tension. The left side is also relaxed (2). Although the patient is in the lithotomy position it is obvious at this stage that vulvectomy leaves the introitus and vagina abnormally open and this prompts the question of possible complications. Contrary to expectations, these patients do not appear to be more liable to vaginitis or discharges but it is generally accepted that there is an increased propensity to vaginal wall prolapse. Local vulvectomy is a comparatively uncommon operation so that statistics are not available but following radical vulvectomy, a sizeable proportion of women develop prolapse, apparently as a result of the removal of introital support. The usual surgical treatment of vaginal prolapse is applicable and results are entirely satisfactory.

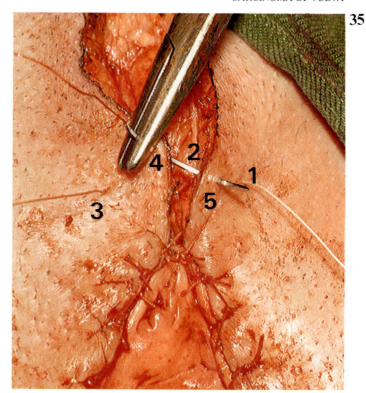

34 and 35 Skin suture to cover raw area of vulvectomy (iii)
The lateral skin flaps are approximated in the midline up to the mons pubis. In Figure 34 the needle has traversed the left skin thickness just behind the needle holder at (1) and is taking a bite of fascia to eliminate dead space at (2). In Figure 35 it has already traversed the right skin thickness at (3) and is returning through the skin edges at (4) and (5) to complete the vertical mattress stitch.

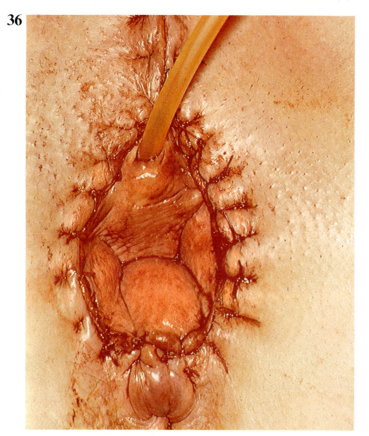

36 Skin closure completed
The Foley catheter is retained for five days. No dressing is necessary, the patient is ambulant and has a daily bath.

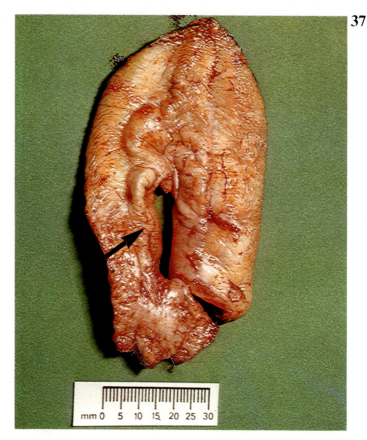

37 Local vulvectomy specimen
The site of the area of carcinoma *in situ* is arrowed.

Radical vulvectomy

The operation now described is that usually referred to as radical vulvectomy although it is radical in a local sense only and does not include intra-pelvic lymphadenectomy. That procedure is described subsequently and the indications for the various operations have been discussed in the introduction to the chapter.

The aim of the operation now described is to remove:

1 The entire vulva with all the area of skin liable to contain present or future malignant change.
2 The superficial inguinal group of glands including the overlying skin.
3 The superficial femoral glands *en bloc* with the segment of the great saphenous vein which they surround.
4 The deeper gland group at the entrance to the femoral canal. The canal is regarded as the upper limit of the operation but removal of accessible glands in the lower canal is always attempted.
5 The superficial fascia and fatty tissue of the vulva and lymph drainage area. It is removed entire and is swept medially from each side in turn.

The operation is carried out in two stages.

1 The patient is in the dorsal position with the legs abducted. The various lymph gland groups, fatty tissue and great saphenous vein segments are dissected clear and reflected medially from the femoral triangle on each side. The lateral part of the groin wounds are then closed by sutures.
2 The patient is in the lithotomy position and the whole vulva is removed between two parallel oval incisions: the inner surrounds the vaginal introitus and the outer is formed by extending the inner ends of the groin incisions round the vulva in the labio-crural fold on each side so that they meet on the perineum posteriorly. The question of wound closure is dealt with in the text but apart from a few stitches posteriorly to prevent contamination from the anus, the wound is left open to heal by granulation. Other methods of wound management will be described subsequently.

Results of Radical Surgical Treatment

Plentl and Friedman (1971) provide striking and convincing evidence that surgery seems to be the correct treatment and that the more radical procedures give the best results (Table 1).

Table 1
Vulvar Cancer Survival by Treatment Plan

Modality	Patient Treated	5-Year Survival	
		Number	Per cent
Radiotherapy	836	109	13.0
Simple vulvectomy	334	103	30.8
Vulvectomy plus radiotherapy	659	214	32.5
Radical vulvectomy and femoral lymphadenectomy	449	250	55.7
Radical vulvectomy and femoral and pelvic lymphadenectomy	440	278	63.2

Cases collected from 36 series from 1934–1965.

Way (1978) performed radical vulvectomy on 367 cases, thirteen of which did not include deep node dissection. The crude 5-year survival rate was 48.1 per cent but when corrected to exclude known intercurrent deaths, the figure was 57.9 per cent. If the nodes were found to be negative, the corrected 5-year survival rate was 90.6 per cent; if the superficial nodes were positive, it was 62.1 per cent; if both superficial and deep were involved, it fell to 24.1 per cent. Twenty-two per cent of all patients subjected to operation had involvement of deep nodes and slightly less than one quarter survived. These figures emphasise how little can be achieved if deep nodes are involved.

Both authorities raise the question of whether it is justifiable to dissect the deep nodes since gland involvement is comparatively rare and the results are bound to be poor. The case for not doing so is stronger if the operator is inexperienced, but the surgeon concerned is in the best position to make these decisions.

From his own experience, Way discourages hopes that postoperative radiotherapy has anything to offer and he also finds that the results of two-stage operations are inferior to those of single stage procedures.

The question of results will be taken up again when considering extended radical vulvectomy, i.e. when operation includes deep node dissection.

Stage 1: Skin incision

The extent of vulvar excision and skin removal is of great importance and while it must be complete, unnecessary mutilation should be avoided. Apart from an area on the perineum, the whole lymph flow from the vulva is in an anterior and cephalad direction along the length of the labia majora towards the superficial inguinal glands and the femoral canal (Figure 3). The catchment area does not extend lateral to the labio-crural fold where drainage is towards the anterior aspect of the thigh. Above the line of the pubic crest, drainage is towards the abdominal wall. There is therefore no need to remove vulvar skin lateral to the labio-crural fold or to place the upper inguinal skin incision more than 1 cm above the level of the pubic crest and the inguinal ligament.

Vulvar lymph return towards the femoral canal may traverse medial glands of the superficial inguinal group so that the overlying skin may be involved by growth. This skin area should be removed with the glands and Way emphasises this in his writings. The superficial femoral glands surrounding the great saphenous vein are not on the direct lymph drainage route from the vulva and only contain metastases in the most advanced cases. The overlying skin does not become adherent and infiltrated as it does over the inguinal glands; the authors have not seen it in over 100 cases. It is not necessary to remove the skin overlying the superficial femoral glands surrounding the great saphenous tributary of the femoral vein. This is important because retention of this area of skin means that the lower flap of the inguinal skin incision is of adequate size to cover any inguinal defect and the only remaining raw area is over the pubic bones anteriorly. Diagram 1 shows the gland groups concerned. The heavy broken line indicates the outline of a groin incision which will remove any skin likely to be infiltrated by growth.

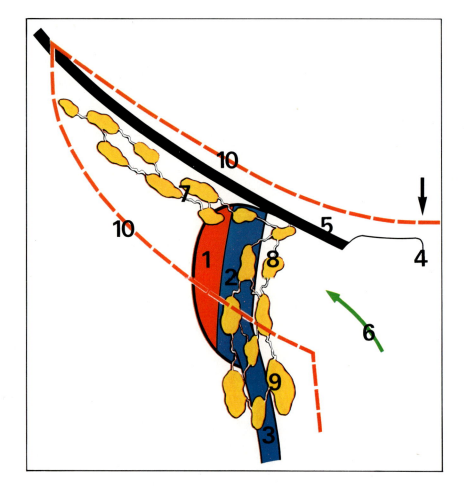

Diagram 1
1 Femoral artery
2 Femoral vein
3 Great saphenous vein
4 Symphysis pubis
5 Inguinal ligament
6 Lymph drainage from vulva
7 Superficial inguinal glands
8 Superficial femoral glands
9 Superficial femoral glands (great saphenous group)
10 Outline of skin incision

1 Outline of skin area for excision

For reasons already stated the incisions are made as shown in the photograph. To preserve symmetry, especially in an obese patient, the complete skin incision outlines are best made before commencing gland dissection on each side and any superficial bleeding vessels are controlled by diathermy. Incision (1) runs transversely 1 cm above the inguinal ligament and the pubic crest to within 3 cm of the anterior superior iliac spine on each side. Incisions (2) and (2) are so placed as to include the vulva widely and continue posteriorly in line with the labio-crural fold. Incisions (3) and (3) commence at the outer ends of incision (1) and deviate from it medially to a distance of 2 cm when they meet incisions (2) and (2). The superficial inguinal glands underlie the general skin area (4) and superficial and deep femoral glands underlie the area (5). The flap or angulated areas (6) cover those glands at the junction of the great saphenous vein and the femoral vein. They will be retracted in the direction of the arrows to give adequate access during the operation.

Diagram 2 is inserted to recall the deeper structures exposed within the outlines of the skin incision just described; the main ones are numbered. Superimposed on the diagram of the area is a grid which divides the area into twelve regions (I–XII). Where there could be any doubt about the actual location when describing any stage of the operation, the grid number is stated or indicated on a black-and-white miniature of the diagram.

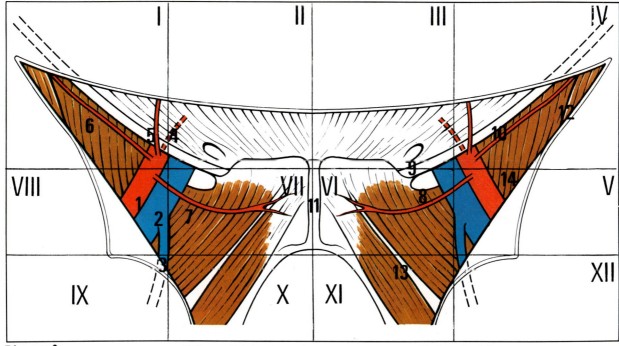

Diagram 2

1 Femoral artery	5 Superficial epigastric artery	10 Inguinal ligament
2 Femoral vein	6 Superficial circumflex iliac artery	11 Symphysis pubis
3 Great saphenous vein	7 Superficial external pudendal artery	12 Sartorious muscle
4 Deep epigastric artery	8 Femoral canal	13 Adductor muscles
	9 External inguinal ring	14 Lateral aspect of femoral triangle

Stage 2: Gland dissection

A complete and relatively avascular clearance of the vulvar glands and lymphatics is possible if the operator knows where to expect bleeding and, at the same time, has a precise knowledge of the lymph drainage of the area.

Blood vessels of the vulva

The vulva is necessarily a vascular organ. The large vessels emerging from and returning to the pelvis are at the centre of the operative area but they are at a relatively superficial level and, unless accidentally injured at gland separation, they should not be a source of bleeding. The deep epigastric vessels are important but are definitively controlled when working above the inguinal ligament. None of the other vessels is large and the operator does not waste time in identifying each of them separately. There are, however, three groups which are constant and which radiate from the femoral triangle to serve as signposts to the anatomy of the region. The *superficial epigastric artery* runs up over the inguinal ligament at the lateral end of its inner third; the *superficial circumflex iliac artery* runs laterally 1 cm below the inguinal ligament towards the anterior superior iliac spine; the *superficial external pudendal artery* runs medially towards the vulva on the front of the pubes. These arteries come from the anterior aspect of the femoral artery and pierce its sheath; the accompanying veins drain into the terminal portion of the great saphenous vein. It is reassuring to recognise each group in turn during the operation and thereby know that one's surgical orientation is correct. The various vessels are shown in Diagram 3.

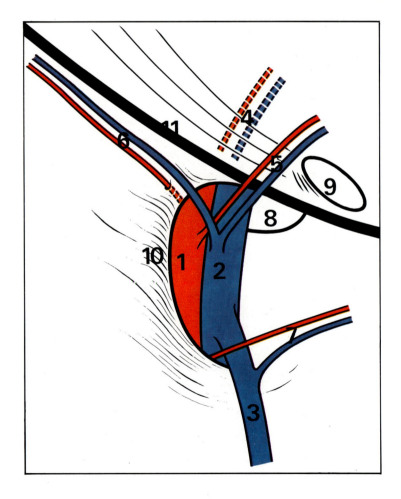

Diagram 3

1 Femoral artery
2 Femoral vein
3 Great saphenous vein
4 Deep epigastric artery and vein
5 Superficial epigastric vessels
6 Superficial circumflex iliac vessels
7 Superficial external pudendal vessels
8 Femoral canal
9 External inguinal ring
10 Femoral triangle
11 Inguinal ligament

Lymph drainage of vulva

Parry Jones (1976) and others studied the lymphatic system of the vulva and established that it is on a regional anatomical basis, the main features of which are shown in Diagram 4. The total area of vulvar skin drainage has already been defined (page 13) but the reader is reminded of some alternative routes taken by part of the lymph return and this must be taken into account at operation. Drainage from the clitoris and vestibule flows laterally towards the femoral canal and may enter it directly without passing through any superficial inguinal gland. Lymph return from the medial aspect of the labia minora is towards the vestibule and continues with the lymph flow from there. The terminal urethra is not infrequently involved in the vulvar growth and the lymph drainage is to the obturator and internal iliac glands through the obturator foramen.

Diagram 4
1 Superficial inguinal glands
2 Superficial femoral glands
3 Deep femoral glands (in femoral canal)
4 External iliac glands
5 Lymph drainage from labia majora
6 Lymph drainage from labia minora, vestibule and clitoris
7 Lymph drainage from perineum

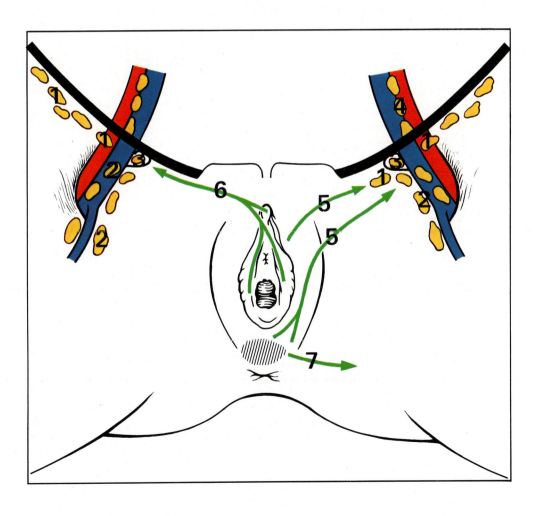

2

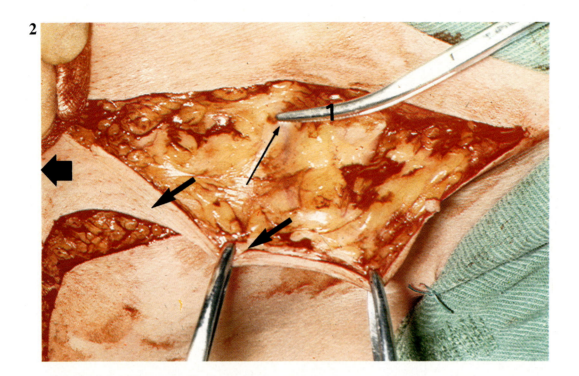

3

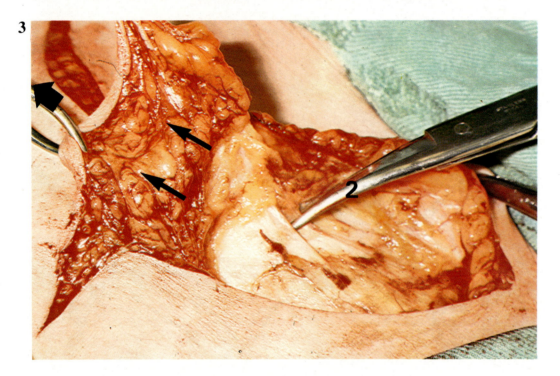

2 and 3 Block dissection of left superficial inguinal glands (i)

The skin incisions are deepened to the muscle aponeurosis and commencing laterally the whole wedge of skin, fat and glands is dissected off the muscles in a medial direction, as arrowed. In Figure 2 the incision has cut branches of the superficial epigastric vessels which are being secured by forceps (1). In Figure 3 the full thickness of the wedge is being dissected medially and upwards off the muscles by scissors (2), as arrowed. The short broad arrows point towards the symphysis pubis in each photograph and the operation field corresponds to areas IV and V on the grid.

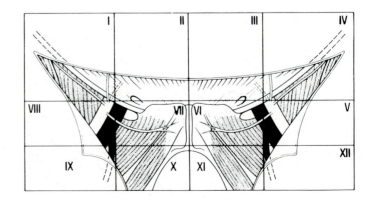

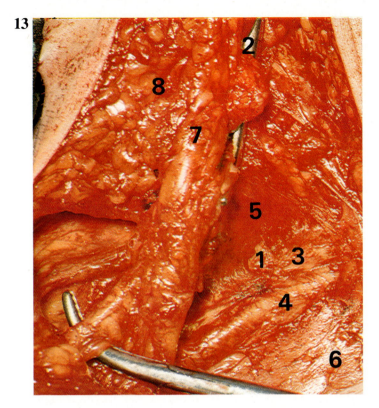

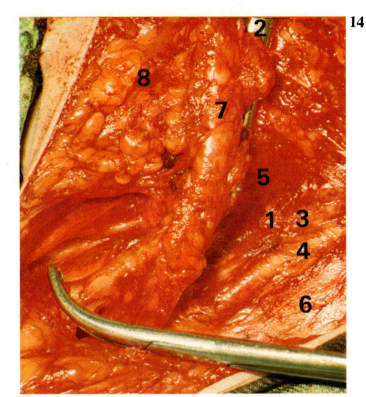

13 to 15 Block dissection of left great saphenous vein and associated lymph glands (ii)

A segment of approximately 5 cm of the great saphenous vein and attached tissue is removed and is shown being defined in Figure 13. The distal end of the vein is secured in Figure 14 and is about to be cut between forceps in Figure 15. It is not unusual for the great saphenous vein to present as two large tributaries rather than as a single trunk in this region and that should be kept in mind, as otherwise bleeding may occur with the dissection being incomplete. The various structures are numbered as on the diagram on the opposite page. The numbers on the grid are V and XII.

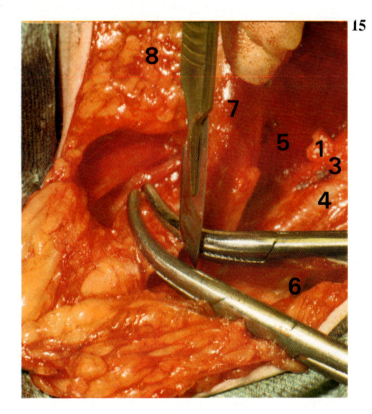

16

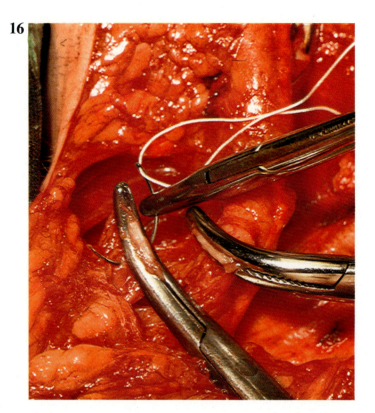

17

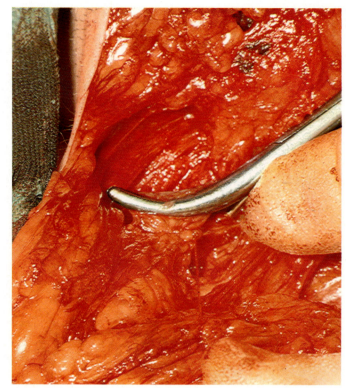

18

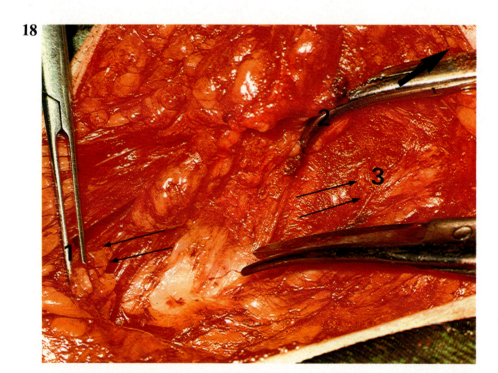

16 to 18 Block dissection of left great saphenous vein and associated lymph glands (iii)

The distal end of the great saphenous vein will retreat under the skin edge when ligated and it is important that it should be properly secured. This is done in the same fashion as proximally and transfixion and tying are shown in Figures 16 and 17 respectively. In Figure 18 the ligated distal end is held in tissue forceps (1) while the forceps on the distal end of the detached segment (2) are retracted in the direction of the arrow, so that the scissors can complete separation of the vein and glands. The ligated upper end of the great saphenous vein is at (3) so that the whole area between (1) and (3) has been cleared of the saphenous vein and its surrounding glands (shown by fine arrows). The relative numbers on the grid are still V and XII.

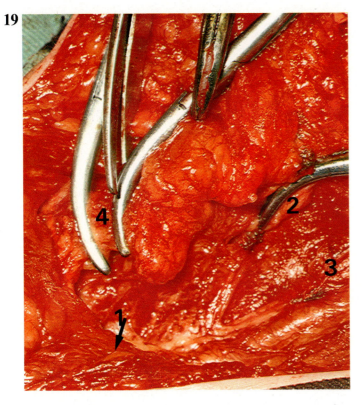

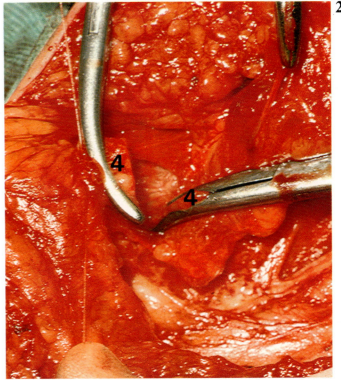

19 and 20 Block dissection of left great saphenous vein and associated lymph glands (iv)

The possibility of meeting a double great saphenous vein was mentioned in relation to Figure 15. In Figure 19, where the distal end of the great saphenous segment is held in forceps at (2), a further large tributary of the great saphenous vein was encountered at (4) and is shown doubly clamped and about to be divided. In Figure 20 it has been cut and the distal end is being ligated. This large vein is rather too medial to be a typical double saphenous and probably represents a large vein of the deep external pudendal group, but it is dealt with in exactly the same way as the double saphenous vein and emphasises that venous drainage here, as elsewhere, is not necessarily constant. The relative grid number is XI.

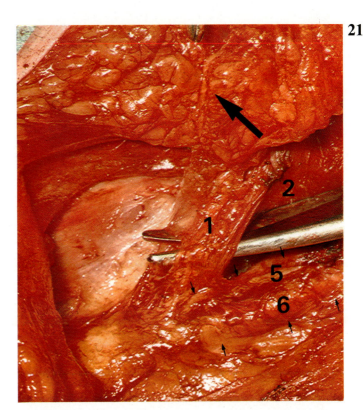

21 Completing separation of gland mass in left groin

The scissors are dissecting off the deep fascia (1) just below the entrance to the femoral canal (2) to sweep the whole gland mass medially in the direction of the arrow and leave the femoral vessels (outlined) exposed in the femoral triangle. The vein is at (5), the artery (6) and the grid number is VI.

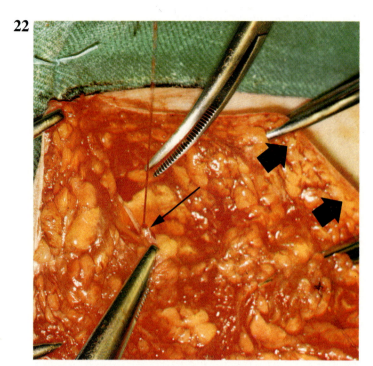

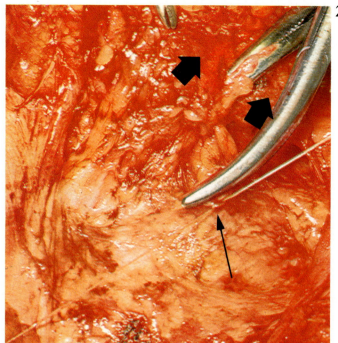

22 to 24 Defining and securing superficial blood vessels during vulvectomy on right side

The three radial groups of vessels were mentioned in the Introduction and are shown in these illustrations. In Figure 22 the superficial circumflex iliac artery (arrowed) declares itself in typical fashion on the fascia lata as the fat and gland mass is swept medially. In Figure 23 and during dissection medially, the superficial epigastric artery (arrowed) has been clamped and is being ligated where it pierces the anterior aspect of the femoral sheath. In Figure 24 a group of superficial external pudendal veins are clearly seen in relation to the great saphenous vein where they enter it at (1). The outline of the superficial external pudendal artery is seen at (2) as it emerges from the femoral sheath. The relative grid numbers are I and VIII.

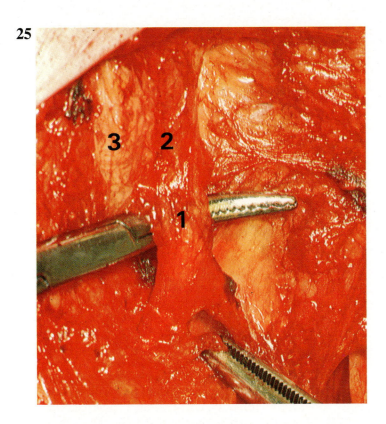
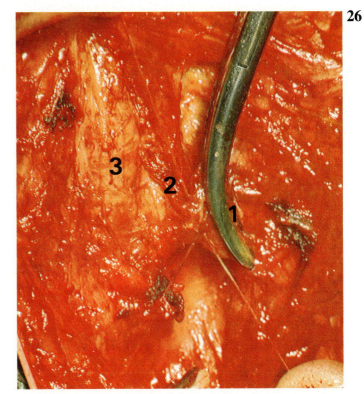

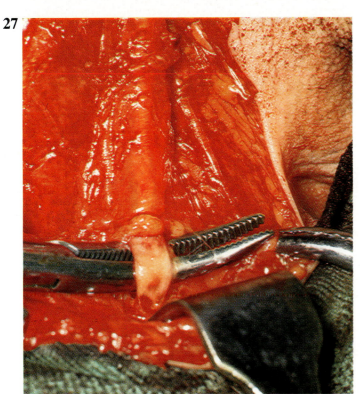
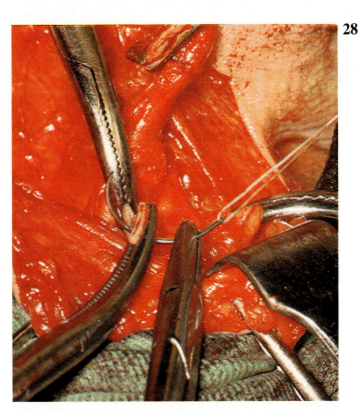

25 to 28 Steps in excising segment of great saphenous vein and its attached lymph glands on right side

The great saphenous vein (1) is raised off the femoral vein (2) with the femoral artery at (3) in Figure 25. It is ligated in Figure 26 and the distal end is defined in Figure 27 and transfixed after having divided in Figure 28. The relative grid numbers are VIII and IX.

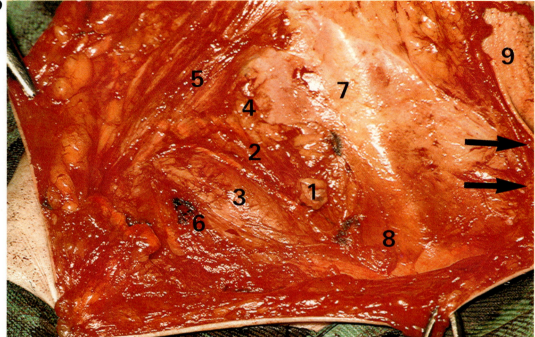

29 Appearance after clearance of glands from right groin

With the wedge-shaped block of skin, fat and inguinal glands swept medially in the direction of the arrows, the great vessels of the thigh and the entrance to the femoral canal are laid bare below the inguinal ligament. The great saphenous vein and its accompanying glands have been removed and the outline of the femoral triangle laterally, and the adductor muscles medially stand out. The various structures are numbered on the diagram and the grid number is VII.

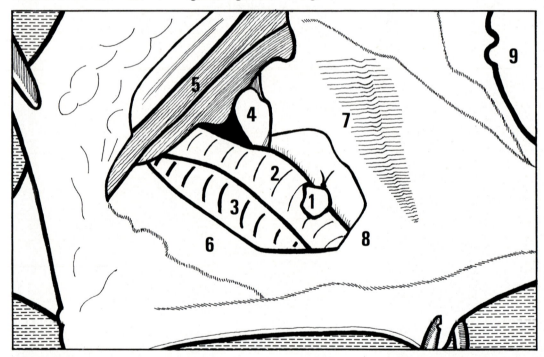

Diagram 6

1 Ligated great saphenous vein
2 Femoral vein
3 Femoral artery
4 Entrance to femoral canal
5 Inguinal ligament
6 Edge of femoral triangle (sartorius muscle underlies)
7 Pubic ramus (right side)
8 Adductor longus muscle covered by fascia
9 Vulva

There is one point worthy of mention at this stage. The tissue covering the muscles of the thigh and the edge of the fossa ovalis is muscle sheath and not deep fascia: the latter has already been removed. Mention of this is made because the authors have seen surgeons attempting to strip the muscles of their covering of fascia lata in the belief that they were removing deep fascia. Apart from being anatomically wrong, this step can be dangerous because it destroys a most efficient natural barrier.

30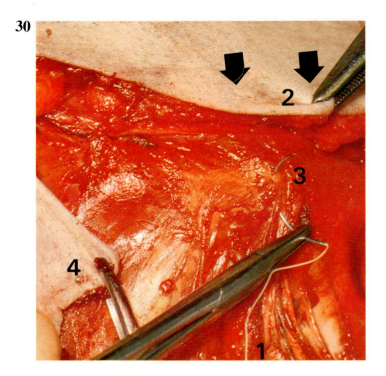

31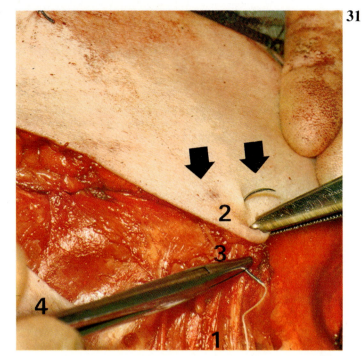

32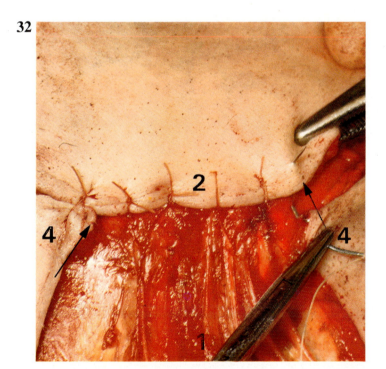

33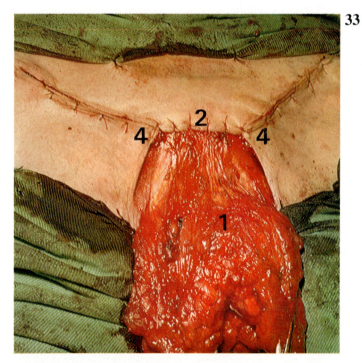

30 to 33 Closure of inguinal incisions

Following bilateral block dissection the separated tissue remains integral with the vulva (1). The upper semilunar skin edge (2) is brought down (broad arrows) and neatly sutured to the fascia across the line of the anterior border of the pubic crest (3). The stitches are detailed in Figures 30 and 31 and the completed suture line is seen in Figure 32. The angle between the lower inguinal incision and the labio-crural incision ((6) on Figure 1) and (4) here is brought medially and upwards (long arrows) and sutured to the semi-lunar edge just lateral to the pubic tubercle. This is shown completed on the right and being completed on the left in Figure 32. The inguinal skin edges are now symmetrical and are closed by a series of vertical mattress sutures of the same PGA No. 0 material. The completed appearance is seen in Figure 33.

Stage 3: Excision of vulva

This stage involves removal of the vulva and the patient is placed in the lithotomy position. This should be done slowly and gently as there is much evidence that patients, especially if elderly, can suffer shock from rapid postural changes in their blood vascular circulation. The vulvar growth which has been excluded from the operative field until now and which almost certainly has a broken and infected surface should be wrapped in a gauze covering secured by forceps as shown in Figure 34. This serves as a 'handle' in the subsequent operation.

The outline of the actual vulvectomy is essentially that described for local vulvectomy and entails removal of all the skin between a circular incision round the introitus and another around the labia majora. The depth of the removal is, of course, greater and skin, superficial fascia, erectile tissue and deep fascia are all removed. It is preferable to make the inner or introital incision first and this can be done with little or no loss of blood. It then remains only to make the outer incision to the requisite depth and work inwards at the correct level to meet the inner incision and remove the vulva. The steps are as follows:

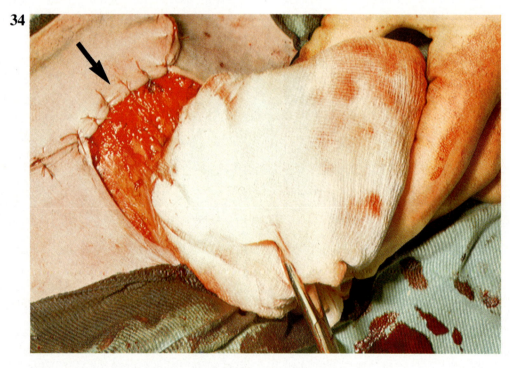

34 Appearance at commencement of vulvectomy
The inguinal incisions have been closed and the detached tissues are covered by a large abdominal pack which is held in position by Littlewood's forceps. The position of the symphysis pubis is shown by the arrow.

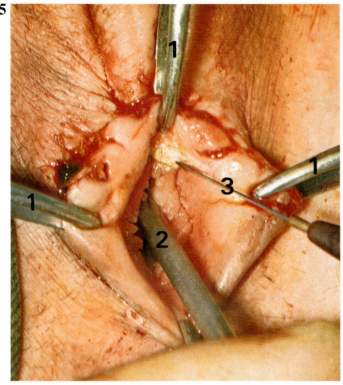

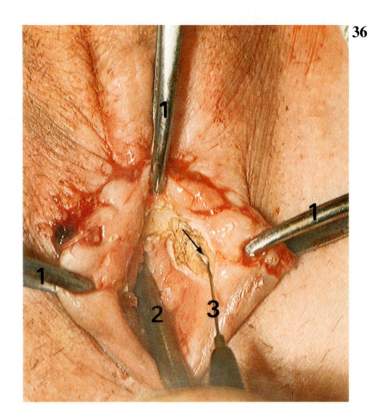

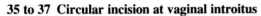

35 to 37 Circular incision at vaginal introitus

Extension of the growth to the vagina is exceedingly unlikely and will have been excluded. A vertical incision of approximately 1.5 cm depth is made around the introitus at the level shown in the illustrations. The labia are retracted with tissue forceps (1), (1) and (1) and the urethra is denoted by the indwelling catheter (2). The diathermy cutting needle (3) commences the incision just anterior to the external urethral orifice in Figure 35 at a distance of 1 cm from it, and it continues round the left side in Figure 36 and on the right side in Figure 37 where the circumcision is almost complete (arrowed). It may appear obvious but the surgeon should consciously note that the incision starts below or 'outside' the external urethral orifice.

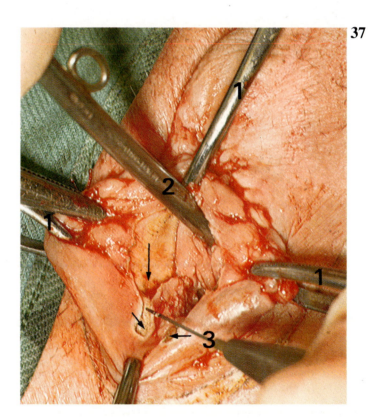

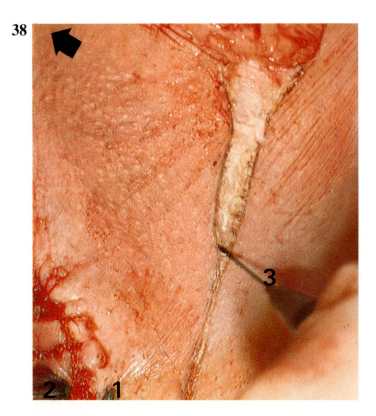

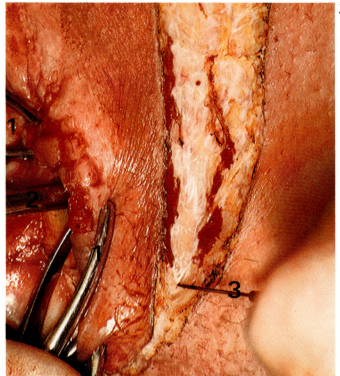

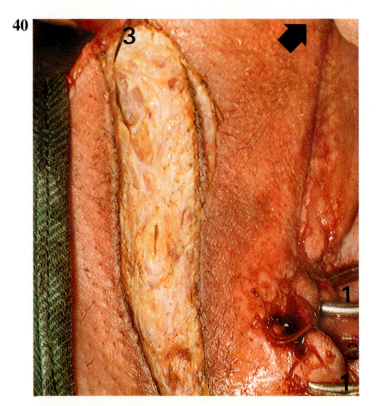

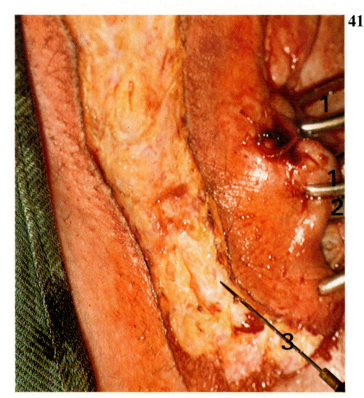

38 to 41 Outlining vulvectomy skin incision

With the inner or introital vulvectomy incision completed and before removing the vulva, it is essential to outline the outer vulvectomy skin incision. The patient is in the lithotomy position and, to aid orientation, a broad arrow points to the symphysis pubis in Figures 38 and 40 while the presence of the urethral catheter (2) acts as a guide in Figures 39 and 41. The procedures are self explanatory. The diathermy needle (3) first defines and then deepens the incision on the left in Figures 38 and 39 and on the right in Figures 40 and 41. The general line follows the labio-crural folds and half of the perineal skin is included.

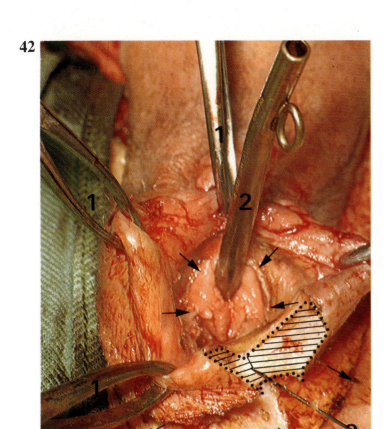

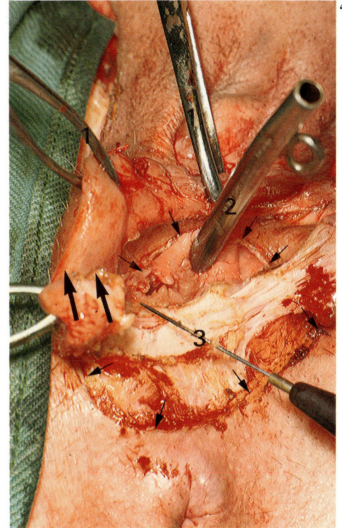

42 and 43 Commencing removal of vulva

The incisions which include the growth between them have been made and are now joined up by cutting across the demarcated area in the five o'clock position as shown in Figure 42. This allows clear access for separating the labial mass from the underlying tissues; a certain amount of bleeding must be anticipated and the surgeon, therefore, must have a clear view. In Figure 43, the right side of the vulva is being elevated and detached in the direction of the arrows. The inner and outer incision lines are indicated by fine arrows in both illustrations; the tissue forceps (1), (1) and (1); the catheter (2); the diathermy (3).

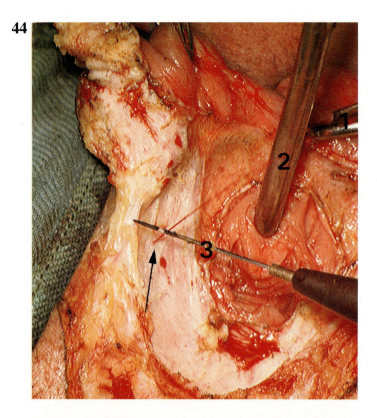

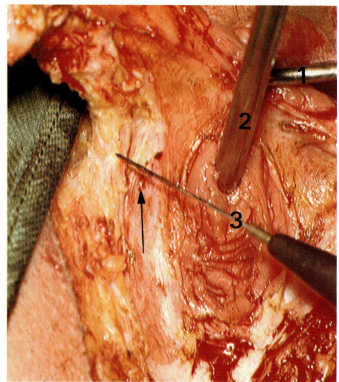

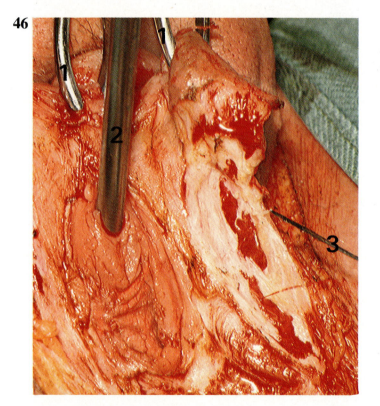

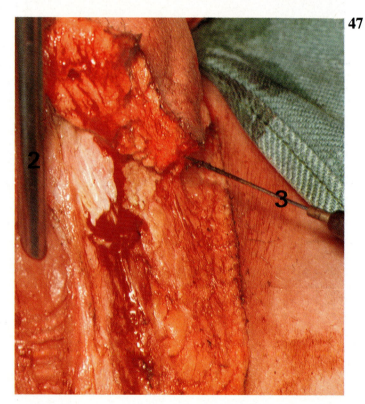

44 to 47 Removing labial portion of vulva

Detachment of the right labial mass proceeds in Figures 44 and 45 and on the left in Figures 46 and 47 and it will be seen that the muscular surface is exposed in the process. The diathermy is generally capable of sealing off any bleeding points encountered as, for example, the spouting artery arrowed in Figure 44 and subsequently sealed in Figure 45. If persistent, a ligature or underrunning figure-of-eight haemostatic stitch is used.

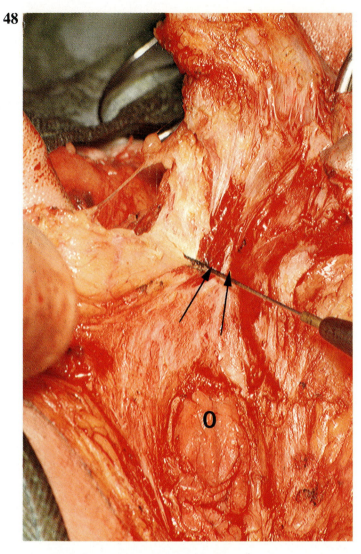

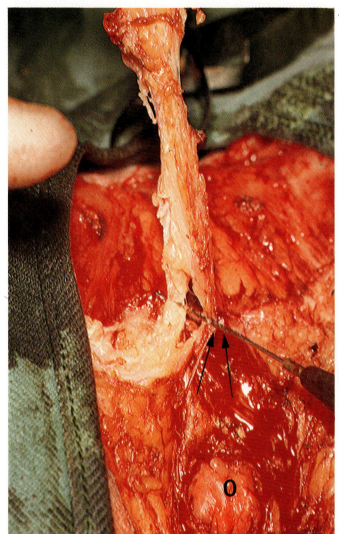

48 and 49 Completing removal of vulva

The final stages in the diathermy detachment of the vulva are shown in Figures 48 and 49. One has to anticipate some bleeding when removing the clitoris and cutting through the clitoral ligaments and vessels. The area concerned is indicated by the arrows in Figures 48 and 49 and it is seen that the diathermy has satisfactorily sealed the vessels. If bleeding is brisk, and to avoid burning the tissues, it is better to use a fine underrunning stitch. The diathermy should not be allowed to burn the fascia lata and periosteum lest it should lead to osteomyelitis. The external urethral orifice is at (0) and helps to orientate the photographs.

Stage 4: Haemostasis – partial closure and drainage of vulvectomy area

There are wide differences of opinion on the management of vulvectomy wounds. The authors cannot agree with those who attempt primary closure and are prepared to employ skin flaps to obtain it. Misfortune and disappointment always seem to follow.

Unless the surgeon employs a split skin graft (the advantages of which are discussed later), the vulvar wound should be left open to heal by granulation. It will do so with surprisingly little resultant mutilation or distortion, but requires ten or twelve weeks for healing to be completed. Leaving the wound open is the orthodox method and is described here. Unless the growth is primarily in the posterior part of the vulva or arises on the perineum, it is possible to make a partial closure posteriorly to prevent soiling and infection of the wound from the anus. Epitheliomata are nearly always sited anteriorly so that a limited closure can usually be made posteriorly.

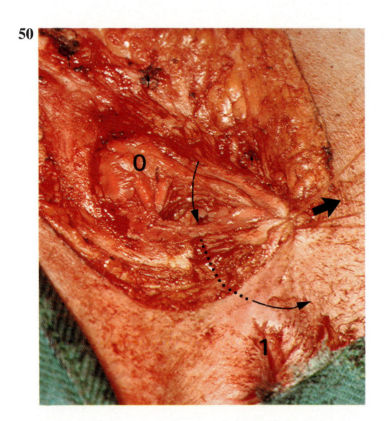

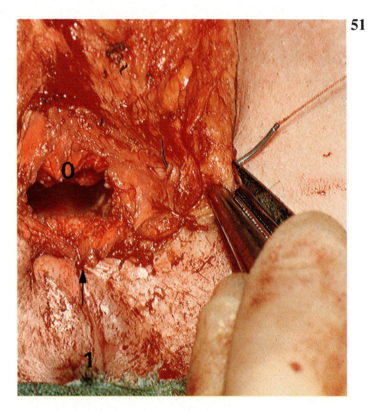

50 and 51 Haemostasis and closing vulvectomy wound posteriorly

Haemostasis has been secured in Figure 50 and the charring from the diathermy shows that there were multiple bleeding points (fine arrows). To obtain symmetry when stitching vaginal skin edge to perineal skin edge, the first stitch is placed exactly in the midline in the line of the arrow; the right and left-sided stitches are added alternately. For demonstration purposes the first left lateral stitch was inserted to keep the skin edges taut while placing the central suture. The external urethral meatus is at (0) and the anus at (1). The process continues anteriorly only for a short distance on the left side in Figure 51 and this is matched with the right side. The initial central stitch is arrowed.

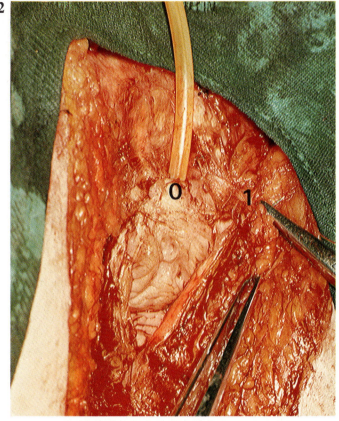

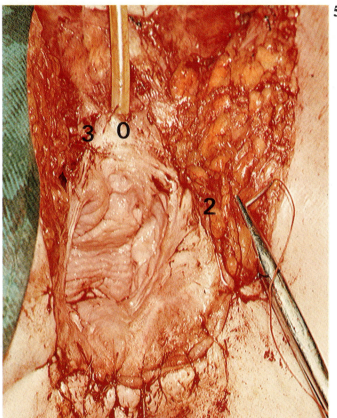

52 and 53 Checking haemostasis and anchoring vaginal skin edge

Any persistent oozing points are underrun with a fine stitch as at (1) in Figure 52 and where the vaginal skin edge is undercut or loose, small tacking stitches are made to anchor it as at (2) in Figure 53. Similar small anchoring sutures are generally used near the urethral orifice as at (3). These various fine stitches are placed to support and prevent distortion of the vulva – not in any sense to try and cover the raw area.

54 Appearance at completion of operation

A Foley catheter (1) is retained for 72 hours. A corrugated plastic drain of 1 cm width (2) lies along the line of and just below the inguinal ligament on each side to drain the whole lateral area. The drains extend along the full length of the wound, immediately under the closed skin edges. Insertion is made at this stage using a sinus forceps to place and direct them accurately in the line of drainage. They are stitched to the skin and have a safety-pin marker.

No dressings are applied and the patient is nursed under a bed cradle to keep the sheets clear of the wound. Mobilisation is immediate and the patient has a daily bath from the second postoperative day.

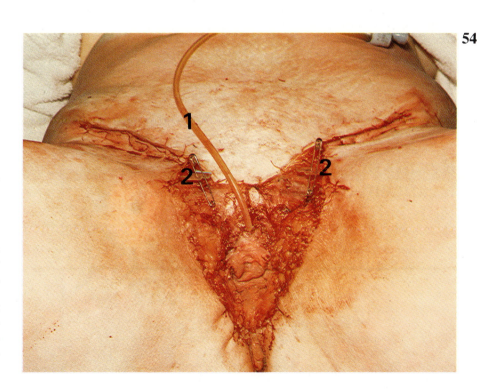

Radical vulvectomy with pelvic lymphadenectomy

Radical vulvectomy and pelvic lymphadenectomy constitute one of the major gynaecological operations. A bilateral meticulous dissection of the whole vulvar lymph drainage system is implicit, with removal of the deep femoral nodes from the femoral canal and the external, internal and common iliac glands from the corresponding blood vessels in the retro-peritoneal space.

The approach is via the inguinal canal and after opening that structure, the transversalis fascia is divided and the deep epigastric vessels are secured. The peritoneum can then be displaced upwards and medially to expose the pelvic vessels and the accompanying lymph glands lying extra-peritoneally. Division of the inguinal ligaments from their pubic attachment gives better general access and ensures clearance of all lymph tissue from the femoral canal. It also enables the whole lymph drainage chain to be removed in one piece and some consider that to be an advantage. Dissection of the glands is carried up as far as the common iliac vessels; the inguinal ligaments are reconstituted and the anatomy of the inguinal canal restored. The actual vulvectomy is done as previously described (page 54) and the wound similarly left open.

There is one matter worthy of comment in relation to the operation. In describing the operation some surgeons take the view that transplantation of the sartorius muscle is an almost essential step in the operation. The muscle is detached from the anterior superior iliac spine and swung medially to be sutured to the external oblique aponeurosis about the middle third of the inguinal ligament and overlying the femoral vessels. This procedure is alleged to give support and a better blood supply to the superficially placed femoral vessels and prevent the development of necrosis and massive haemorrhage in the presence of wound infection. In support of the contrary view, there is the objection that detachment of muscular tissue leads to a diminished blood supply within it, so that it is not ideal tissue for transplantation. Disturbance always necessitates some traumatisation and if this is at the immediate site of a malignant condition, it could provide the ideal conditions for the implantation of spilled cells. The authors consider the latter reasons the stronger and omit the step. In a series of 110 personal cases the senior author has never seen necrosis or inflammation involving the femoral vessel walls.

Results of radical surgical treatment (Radical vulvectomy with pelvic lymphadenectomy)

It is helpful to draw on Way's experience (1977) when contemplating the extended radical operation. In his series, anaplastic tumours showed an overall node involvement of 62 per cent compared with 35 per cent in differentiating growths. Superficial and deep nodes were involved in 22 per cent of anaplastic tumours and in only 8 per cent of the differentiating group, so that node involvement is very important. When the nodes were involved the results of extended radical vulvectomy were much poorer than when

they were not; with less extensive surgery, results were disastrous.

The extent of node involvement at the time of treatment seriously affects the prognosis:

Table 2
Results of Extended Radical Vulvectomy
According to Node Involvement

	Five Year Survivors	Ten Year Survivors	Fifteen Year Survivors
Lymph nodes positive	47%	42%	32%
Lymph nodes negative	70%	38%	27%

From Way (1977)

Plentl and Friedman's figures (1971) are similar:

Table 3
Comparative Survival Rates in Vulvar Cancer
According to Regional Node Involvement

Status of Node	Number of Patients	Five Year Survival Number*	Five Year Survival Per cent
Negative	314	237	75.5
Positive	236	98	41.5

*550 cases collected from 12 series from 1941–1963

It seems inescapable that if the expertise is available and conditions are suitable, radical surgery should be employed.

The case to be described was specifically chosen to illustrate the standard radical operative technique (Way 1977,78). The indications for radical vulvectomy were absolute in that the growth was advanced with clinically involved inguinal glands and the virtual certainty of spread to pelvic glands. Histological examination showed poorly differentiated cells with a grading that offered a poor prognosis unless removal of the growth could be complete. The distal urethra was involved in the growth and this is a not uncommon complication that one should know how to deal with. The patient was stocky and overweight and offered the problems that one frequently encounters in such operations.

This operation requires knowledge of the anatomy of the inguinal canal; the diagram on the page opposite serves as a revision of the structures encountered.

Stage 1: Superficial gland dissection

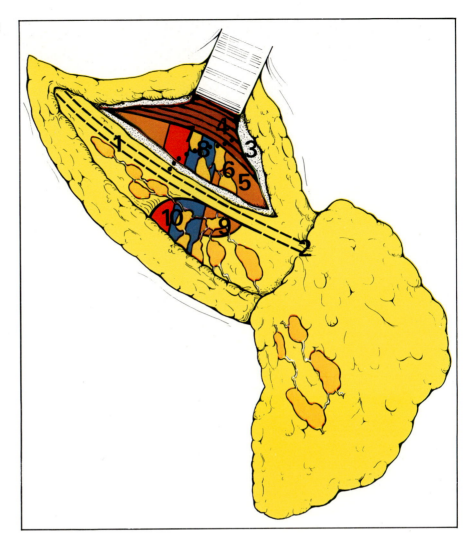

Diagram 7

Anatomy of inguinal canal

1 Inguinal ligament
2 Pubic tubercle
3 External oblique
4 Conjoint tendon
5 Peritoneum
6 Extra-peritoneal fat and glands
7 External iliac vessels
8 Deep epigastric artery
9 Femoral canal
10 Femoral vessels

1 Demarcation of inguinal skin for removal

The amount of skin to remove was discussed on page 38 . It is sufficient that the area between the transverse semilunar incision (1) and the two oblique incisions (3) and (3) be excised. A grossly enlarged gland is seen at (4) and others were palpable. The extension of the incision towards the vulva when the patient is in lithotomy position would commence where arrowed and continue back in the line of the labio-crural fold.

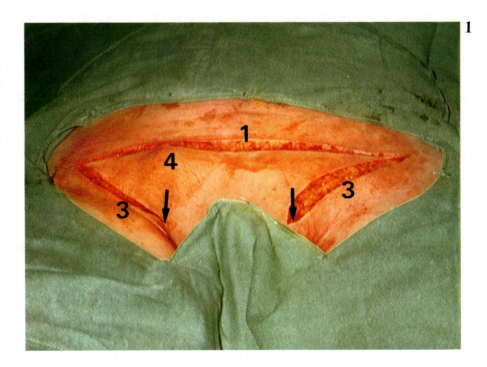

1

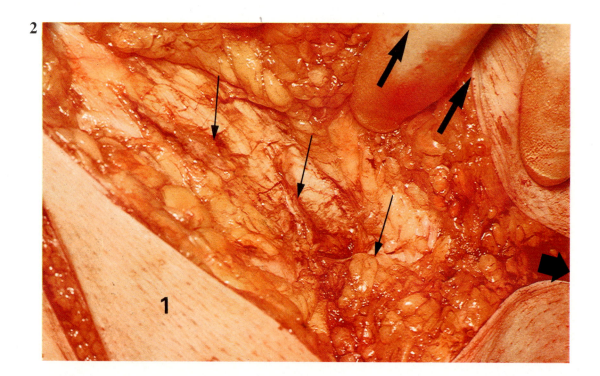

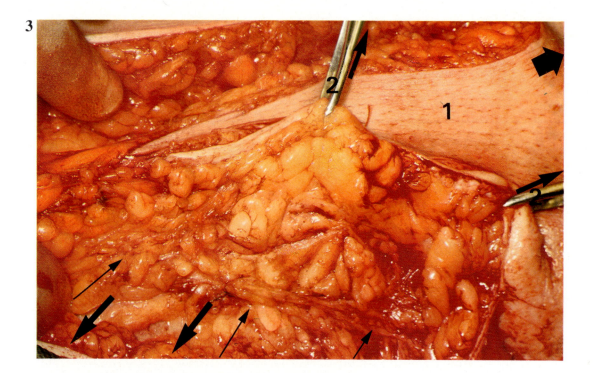

2 and 3 Block dissection of superficial glands (right groin) (i)

The triangular-shaped area of skin with underlying glands and fat (1) is dissected medially off the muscles towards the femoral vessels. In Figure 2 the abdominal edge of the wound is held up (as arrowed) while the surface of the inguinal ligament is cleared in the line of the fine arrows. In Figure 3 the lower lateral edge is retracted as indicated by the arrows and the triangular area held up in tissue forceps (2) and (2). This mass of skin, fat and glands is being cleared in a medial direction along the line of the fine arrows. The very broad arrows point to the symphysis pubis in each photograph and the relative area on the grid is I.

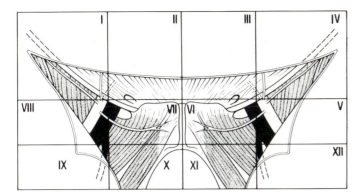

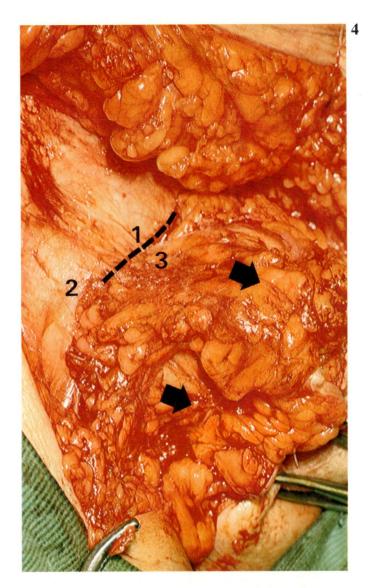

4 Block dissection of superficial glands (right groin) (ii)

The block of tissue has been swept medially (as arrowed) and as far as the lateral border of the femoral triangle ((1) and outlined by broken line); the muscle (sartorius) is shown cleared of fat (2). The femoral artery is medial at (3) and it is necessary to proceed cautiously at this stage because the great saphenous vein joins the femoral vein just medial to that. The relative grid area is VIII.

5 Block dissection of superficial glands (right groin) (iii)

Dissection proceeds with the overlying tissues drawn medially by the dissecting forceps in the direction of the arrows. The junction of the great saphenous vein and the femoral vein is in the general area (4) and the diathermy (5) is sealing off some tributaries of the great saphenous vein (i.e. superficial epigastric, superficial circumflex iliac or superficial external pudendal veins). The grid reference is VIII.

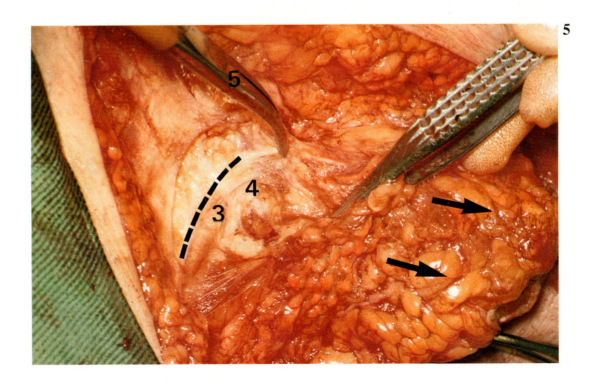

6

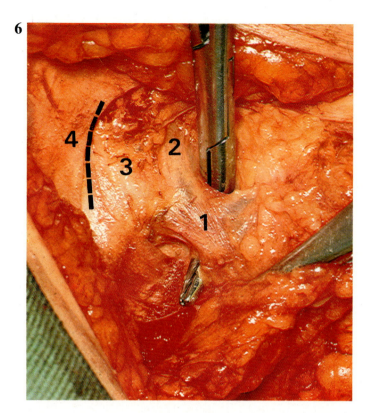

7

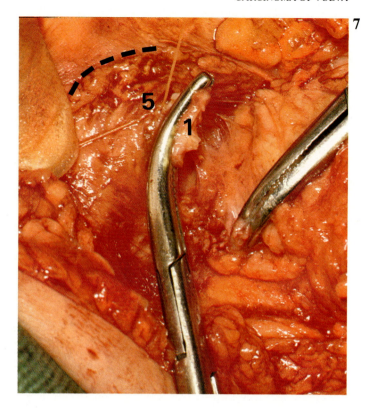

8

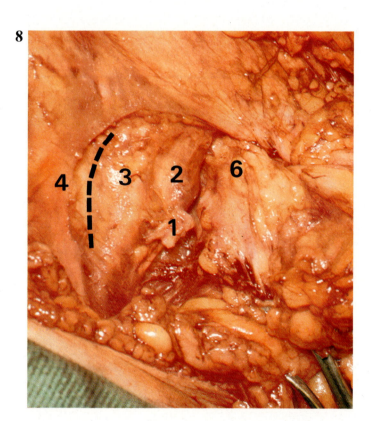

6 to 8 Removal of segment of great saphenous vein – securing upper end of vein (right)

In Figure 6 the vein is displayed (1) on the forceps just where it joins the femoral vein (2) and the femoral artery is lateral (3) with the edge of the femoral triangle at (4). In Figure 7 the vein has been doubly clamped and divided and the proximal end transfixed and is being ligated (5). Figure 8 shows the femoral triangle now quite empty following dissection. The ligated great saphenous vein is seen at (1) and the numerals are as in the other illustrations. The entrance to the femoral canal is at (6). The grid reference is VIII and IX.

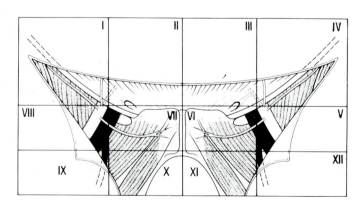

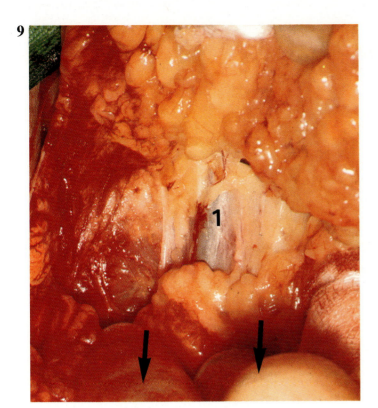

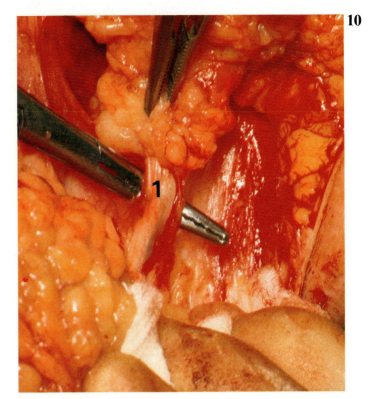

10

9 to 11 Removal of segment of great saphenous vein – securing lower end of vein

In Figure 9 the skin edges are retracted in the direction of the arrows to expose the great saphenous vein (1) as it ascends the thigh surrounded by fat and lymph glands. In Figure 10 it is defined as it lies on the forceps preparatory to division. In Figure 11 the segment has been doubly clamped and divided. The lower end of the segment for removal is held in forceps (2) while the upper end of the trunk from the thigh is held in forceps (3) and is being transfixed before ligation. The grid reference is IX.

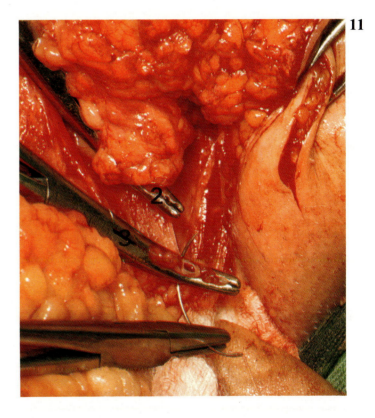

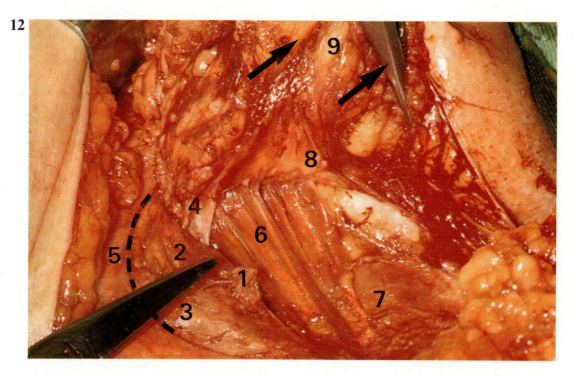

11

12 Completion of dissection of superficial glands
The femoral triangle has been completely cleared of fat, fascia and glands to expose the muscles, and the laterally freed triangle of tissue is held medially in the direction of the arrows. The various structures are indicated on diagram 8. The grid reference is VII and VIII.

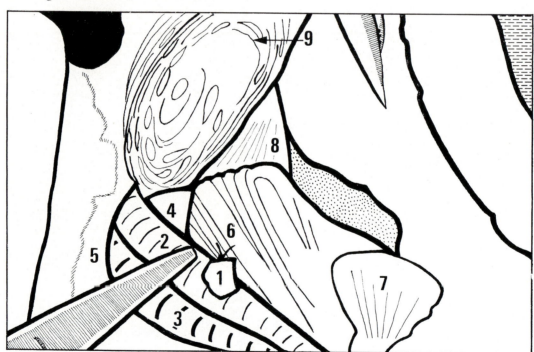

Diagram 8

1 Stump of great saphenous vein
2 Femoral vein
3 Femoral artery
4 Femoral canal
5 Edge of femoral triangle (sartorius muscle)

6 Exposed pectineus muscle
7 Exposed adductor longus muscle
8 Pubic bone
9 Mass of fat and glands

Stage 2: Deep gland dissection

13
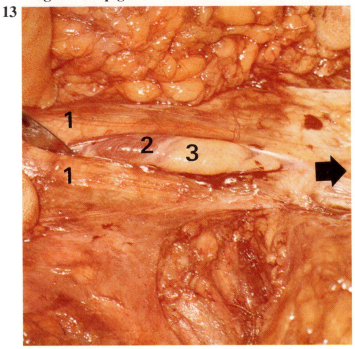

14
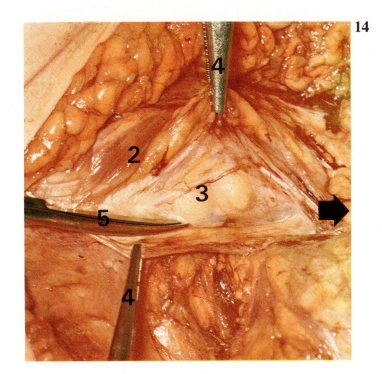

15
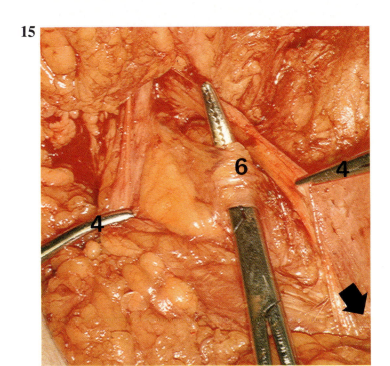

16
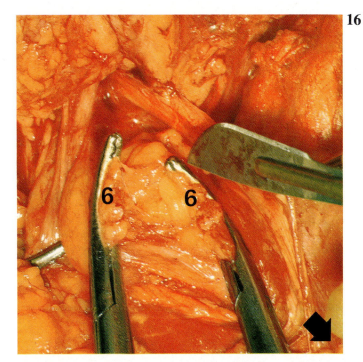
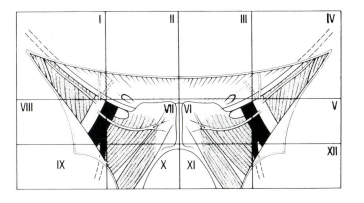

13 to 16 Opening inguinal canal and securing deep epigastric vessels (right side)

In Figure 13 the scalpel is seen splitting the external oblique aponeurosis (1) to expose the conjoint tendon of the internal oblique (2) and the transversalis fascia (3). In Figure 14 the edges of the external oblique are held apart by forceps (4) and (4) while the scissors (5) divide the transversalis fascia. In Figure 15 the underlying deep epigastric vessels (6) are displayed on the forceps, and in Figure 16 they are divided between clamps and await ligation (6) and (6). The broad arrow points towards the symphysis pubis in this and succeeding photographs. The grid reference is I and VII.

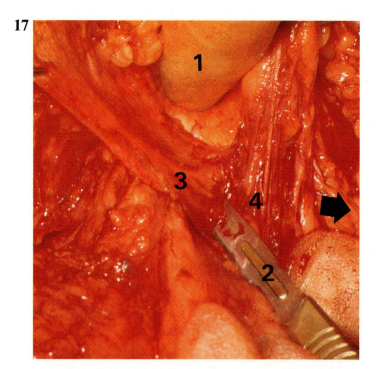

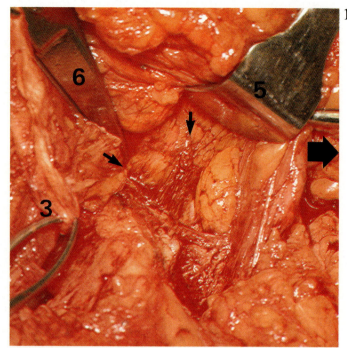

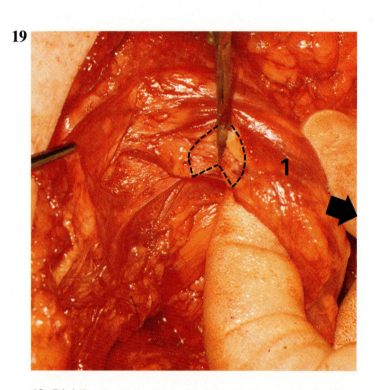

17 and 18 Detaching inguinal ligament from pubis (right)
The inguinal ligament is detached from the pubic bone with a plaque of periosteum and this has to be done with the scalpel. If the inguinal ligament is cut at any other point in its length the ends quickly become frayed and repair is exceedingly difficult. With a base-plate of strong tissue, i.e. periosteum, as described, it is easy to suture back in place later. In Figure 17 the finger (1) retracts the structures while the scalpel (2) detaches the inguinal ligament (3) from the pubic bone (4) as described. In Figure 18 the medial end of the detached inguinal ligament is held in forceps (3) and with a retractor (5) and scissors (6) the femoral canal is being opened widely, where arrowed. The grid reference is VII.

19 Dividing lower border of internal oblique muscle (right)
This step is not absolutely necessary but it gives greatly increased access to the glands without the need for strong retraction. The muscle (1) is held between finger and thumb and divided with a scalpel to a depth of 1.5 cm. The cut edge is outlined. The grid reference is I.

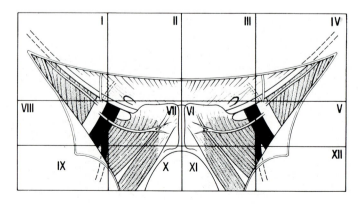

20

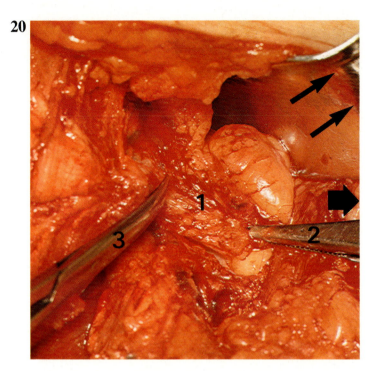

21

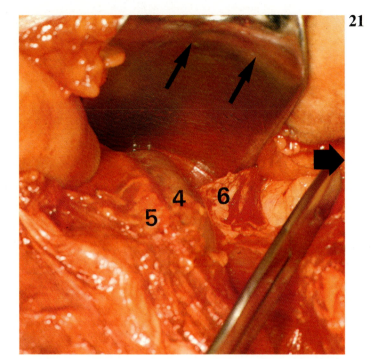

20 to 22 Removal of deep (extra-peritoneal) glands (right) (i)

Commencing at the femoral canal in Figure 20 the mass of fat and glands (1) is steadied with the dissection forceps (2) while the scissors (3) strip it off the femoral vessels. The femoral vein (4) and the femoral artery (5) with the adjacent femoral canal medially (6) are obvious in Figure 21. Dissection proceeds upwards into the pelvis in Figure 22 and the scissors at (7) are detaching a medially placed gland. In all three photographs the retractor draws the upper wound edge and peritoneum clear of the operative field in the direction of the arrows. The grid reference is VII.

22

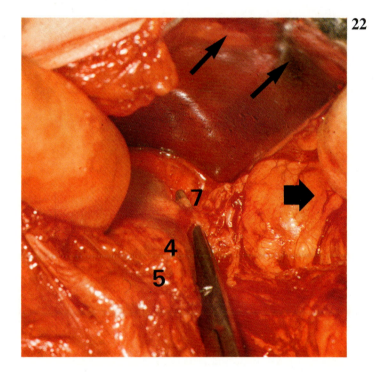

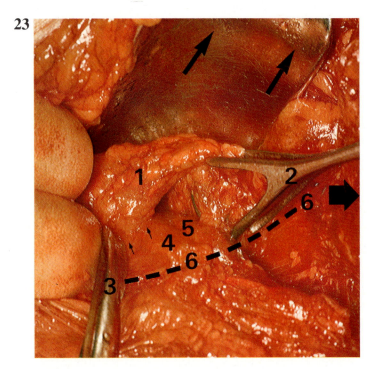

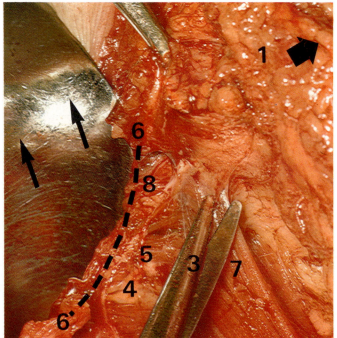

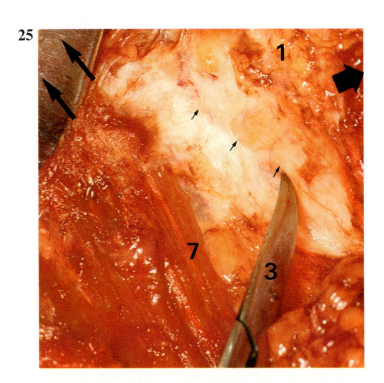

23 to 25 Removal of deep (extra-peritoneal) glands (right) (ii)

The glands lying extra-peritoneally on the iliac vessels are gradually stripped up as far as possible and at least as far as the bifurcation of the common iliac artery. The retractor draws the peritoneum and pelvic viscera clear of the external iliac vessels to give access to the glands. In Figure 23 the glands (1) are held in gland-holding forceps (2) while scissors (3) gently separate them from the external iliac artery (4) and vein (5) in a cephalad direction; the plane of separation is arrowed. The general line of the inguinal ligament is indicated by the broken line, the detached end and its base is at (6) and (6). The separated iliac glands are in continuity with the deep femoral glands in the femoral canal. In Figure 24 the gland mass has been delivered medially (1) and attention is focused on the femoral canal (8) which is now clear; the scissors (3) are freeing the elevated tissues from the surface of the adductor longus muscle. The femoral artery (4) and the femoral vein (5) are seen on the pectineal border of the pubis. The divided ends of the inguinal ligament are at (6) and (6). In Figure 25 the fat and glands are dissected medially on to the anterior aspect of the pubic bone and a plane of cleavage has been found where arrowed. The bare adductor longus muscle is at (7). The grid reference in these photographs is VII.

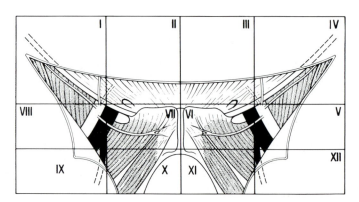

26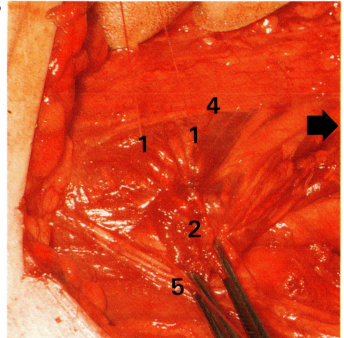

27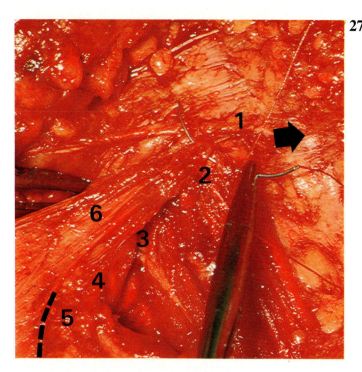

26 Reconstitution of internal oblique muscle

Two figure-of-eight stitches of PGA No. 0 material are used to repair the cut in the muscle. One stitch is in place but untied at (1) and another is less obvious where it overlies the forceps at (2). The upper and lower leaves of the external oblique aponeurosis are at (4) and (5).

27 Re-attachment of inguinal ligament

The fascial end plate which was removed with the scalpel is re-attached by two figure-of-eight stitches. In the photograph, the first stitch is completed at (1) and the second is being placed at (2). The femoral canal (3), the femoral vein (4), and the femoral artery (5) are visible. The lateral border of the femoral triangle is shown by the dotted line and the inguinal ligament is at (6).

28 Obliteration of femoral canal

To attach the inguinal ligament firmly and to obviate femoral herniation, the canal is closed by two sutures which attach the inferior surface of the medial end of the inguinal ligament to the pectineal fascia on the upper border of the pubis. In the photograph, the pectineal fascia has already been transfixed in the area (2) and the needle is now traversing the inferior border of the inguinal ligament at (2) with the curved arrows indicating the line of the stitch. The inguinal ligament (6) is reattached to the pubis at (1) and the triangular area outlined by the broken line is the femoral canal (3). The femoral vein (4) and artery (5) are largely hidden by the needle holder. The grid reference for the three photographs is VII.

28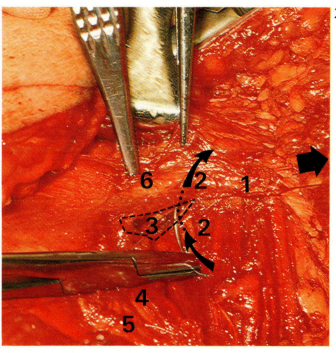

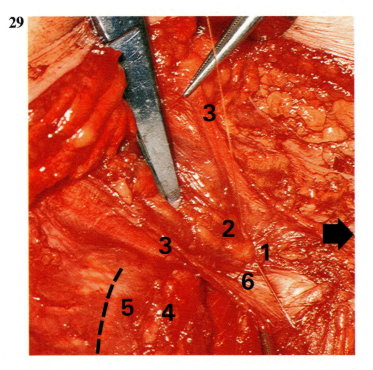

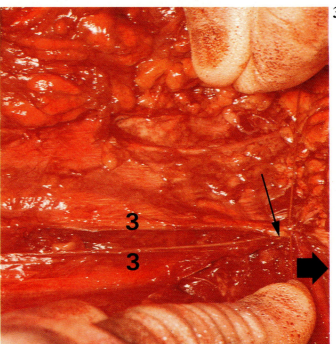

29 Attachment of conjoint tendon to inguinal ligament

The conjoint tendon is now attached to the inguinal ligament and pectineal fascia, to strengthen the posterior wall of the inguinal canal. Two or three stitches are required and the

first is seen being tied at (1). The edges of the external oblique aponeurosis are at (3) and (3). The conjoint tendon is at (2), the inner surface of the inguinal ligament (6) and the femoral vein and artery (4) and (5).

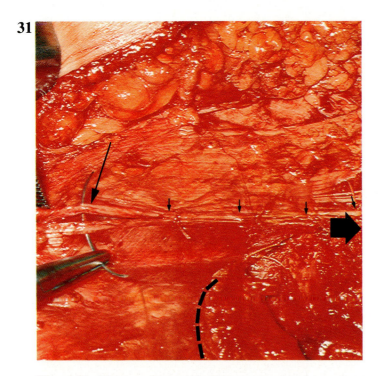

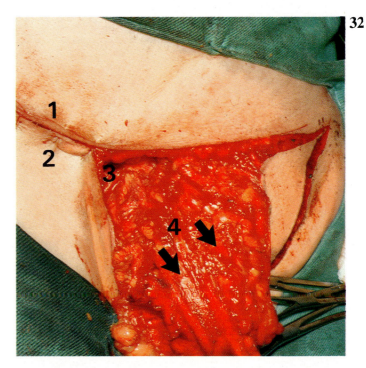

30 and 31 Closure of external oblique aponeurosis

A series of interrupted PGA No. 0 sutures is used. The first is being tied medially (arrowed) in Figure 30 and the final one inserted laterally (arrowed) in Figure 31. The grid reference for the three photographs is VII.

32 Skin closure completed on right side

The upper and lower skin edges (1) and (2) have been approximated by a series of carefully placed vertical mattress sutures as far medially as the pubic tubercle (3). The mass containing the dissected lymph glands is reflected medially and distally (4) and the outline incisions on the left side can be seen.

33

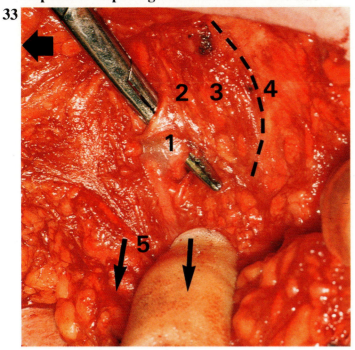

34

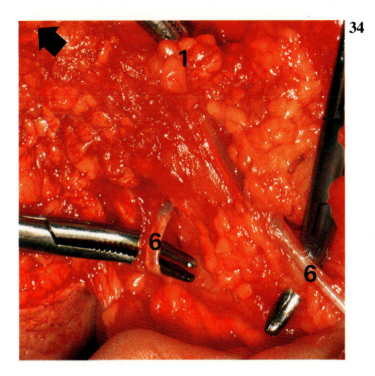

33 Definition of left great saphenous vein (i)

The great saphenous vein (1) is displayed on the forceps where it joins the femoral vein (2). The femoral artery is at (3) and the outline of the femoral triangle is at (4). The block of gland tissue (5) is retracted distally with the fingers in the direction of the arrows.

34 Definition of left great saphenous vein (ii)

This illustrates the situation where a single great saphenous trunk is replaced by two tributaries from the thigh. The proximal end of the segment for removal is (1) as in Figure 33. The two tributaries (6) and (6) which, in this case, replace a single trunk are displayed on the forceps.

35

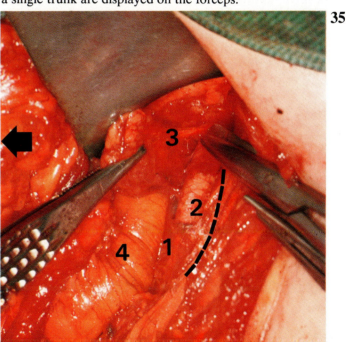

The grid references are: Figure 33 – VIII, Figure 34 – IX, Figure 35 – II.

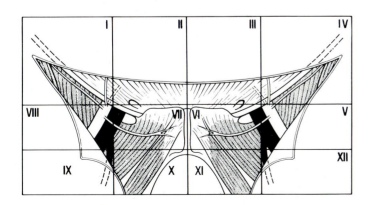

35 Deep gland dissection – left side

This gives a clear view of the gland chain being separated upwards off the external iliac vessels. The vein is at (1), the artery at (2), and the gland mass at (3). The peritoneum (4) has escaped from under the retractor (5) and is pushing into the wound and partially covering the vein.

Stage 3: Vulvectomy

With the inguinal incisions closed and the abdominal skin flap fixed in the region of the symphysis pubis, the patient is ready to be placed in the lithotomy position and suitably draped for vulvectomy. As mentioned previously, this change of position should be made very slowly in order to avoid shock. It is not always possible to cover the raw and infected area of a large fungating growth with a dressing because it may impede access in vulvectomy. In such circumstances, it is best to use the tissue forceps on the lateral skin edges as levers to turn these edges medially towards each other and to some degree exclude the open growth from the operative field.

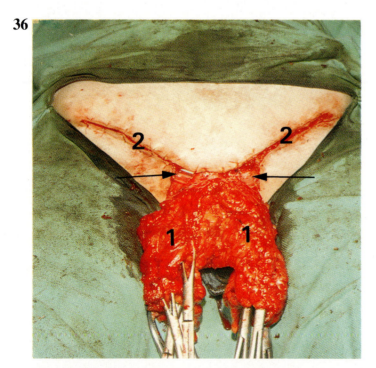

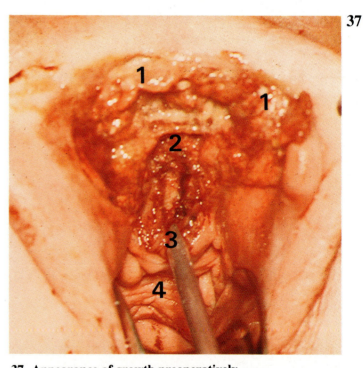

36 Appearance at commencement of vulvectomy
The dissected gland mass (1) is held distally by a series of tissue forceps. The closed inguinal incisions (2) and (2) are clearly seen and a series of stitches fixes the abdominal flap to the symphysis pubis and the pubic crest. Corrugated drains are already in place (arrowed).

37 Appearance of growth preoperatively
It is obvious that the growth is an advanced one which involves the region of the clitoris. The edges (1) and (1) are typically rolled and vascular and the base (2) is necrotic. The external urethral orifice is indicated by the indwelling catheter (3) and it will be seen that the growth involves the whole circumference of that structure. The vagina (4) is clear of growth as far as can be seen. The actual vulvectomy is done very much as previously described (page 54) but it is modified to meet the special circumstances of this case.

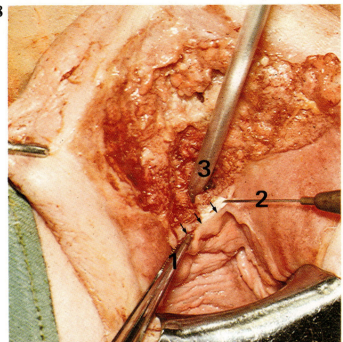

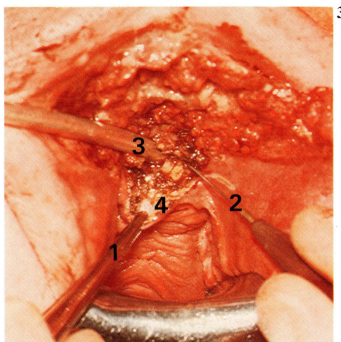

38 and 39 Inner vulvectomy skin incision (i)

The procedure described in this case has to take account of involvement of the external urethral orifice by the growth. Instead of commencing the anterior part of the incision below the orifice, it must be placed posteriorly and above it if the actual growth is to be avoided. In Figure 38 a fold of redundant and healthy vaginal skin is held in forceps (1) while the diathermy point (2) makes a skin-deep incision just clear of the growth. The line of this incision is arrowed. The catheter (3) is in the urethra. In Figure 39 the healthy skin edge has been dissected off the underlying tissues of the lower vaginal wall to form a shallow flap (4). The incision is at least 1.5 cm from the tumour edge, although it appears less in the photograph. The higher in the vagina the incision is made, the less the support given to the terminal urethra and the greater likelihood of urinary incontinence. The authors are not as sanguine as most regarding removal of the terminal urethra and find that a degree of incontinence is the rule. The use of a shallow flap to bolster and support the terminal urethra can be very effective and is described in Volume 4 of the Atlas.

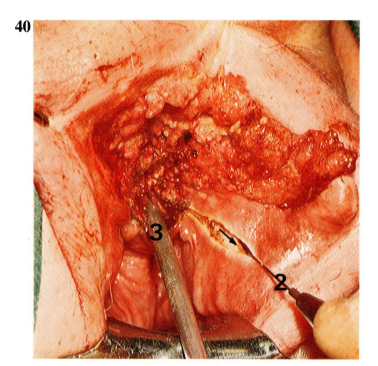

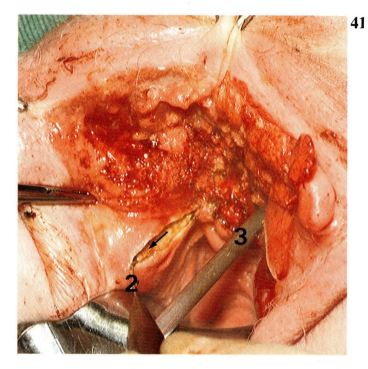

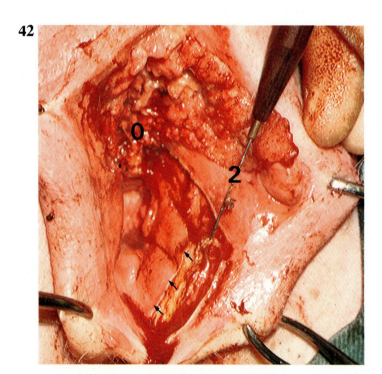

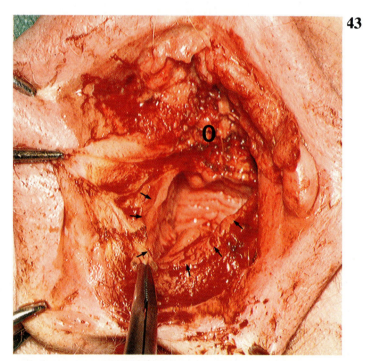

40 to 43 Inner vulvectomy skin incision (ii)
The incision is carried posteriorly at full skin depth, first on the left side in Figure 40 and then on the right side in Figure 41. The direction of these incisions is indicated by arrows and the catheter in the urethra orientates the picture. In

Figure 42 the incision is carried posteriorly on the left side and the lower edge of vaginal skin is indicated by small arrows. In Figure 43 the complete inner incision has been made and the lower vaginal edges on both sides are arrowed. The urethral orifice is at (0) in Figures 42 and 43.

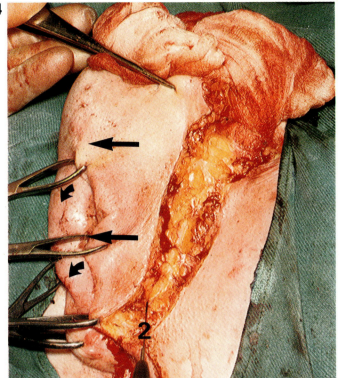

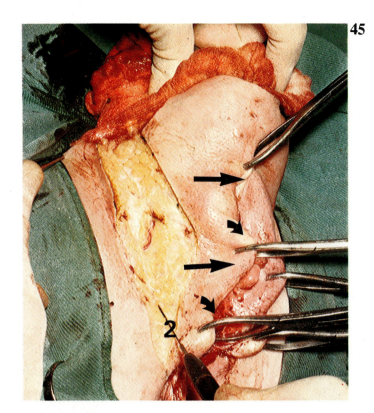

44 to 46 Outer vulvectomy skin incision

The left-sided skin incision is made in the line of the labio-crural fold in Figure 44 and on the right side in Figure 45. The labia are held to the opposite side by tissue forceps in each case in the direction of the arrows and it will be seen that the growth is partially concealed by rolling the lateral sets of forceps medially, as previously mentioned. In Figure 46 a radial incision is being made postero-laterally with the diathermy needle on the left side to allow better access and elevation of the two labial flaps separately. The lower edge of vaginal skin is seen in the introitus (arrowed) and the radial incision is outlined by the dotted line.

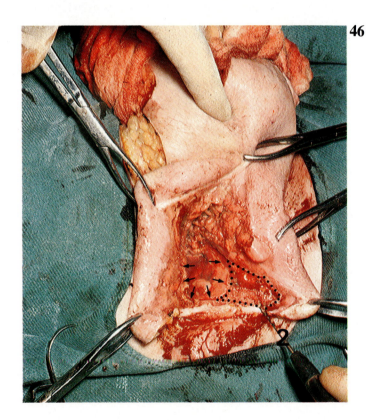

46

47 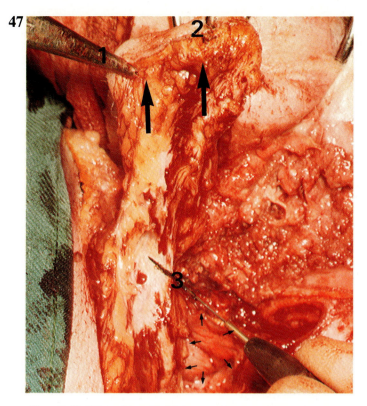 48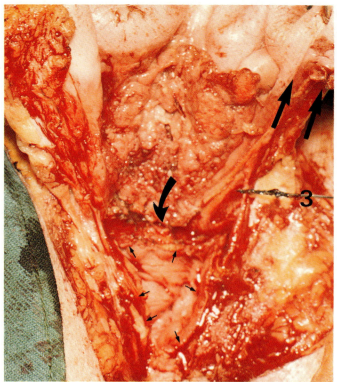

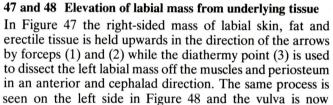

47 and 48 Elevation of labial mass from underlying tissue

In Figure 47 the right-sided mass of labial skin, fat and erectile tissue is held upwards in the direction of the arrows by forceps (1) and (2) while the diathermy point (3) is used to dissect the left labial mass off the muscles and periosteum in an anterior and cephalad direction. The same process is seen on the left side in Figure 48 and the vulva is now detached, except where the growth involves the urethra and in the region of the clitoris. The entrance to the urethra is indicated by the curved arrow. The next step is to cut across the lower urethra and remove the distal part of that structure. The vaginal skin edge is indicated by fine arrows in each photograph to aid orientation.

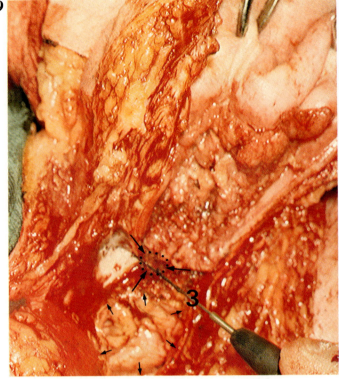

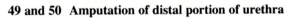

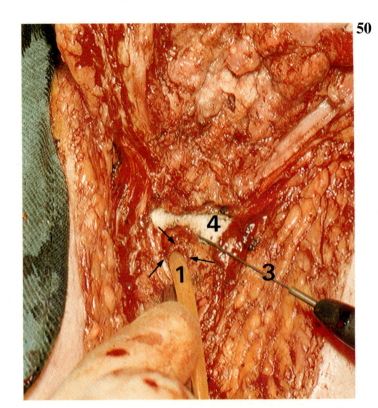

49 and 50 Amputation of distal portion of urethra

In Figure 49 the diathermy point (3) is cutting across the urethra at a distance of 1.5 cm from the external orifice and the lumen is visible with the cut ends of the urethral tube shown by arrows. In Figure 50 a Foley catheter has been re-inserted and the cut end of the urethral tube is clearly seen. The diathermy needle (3) continues the upward dissection of the vulvar growth from the anterior aspect of the pubes in the general direction of the clitoris. A plane of separation is sought and followed directly on the surface of the periosteum. This is seen as a white area at (4).

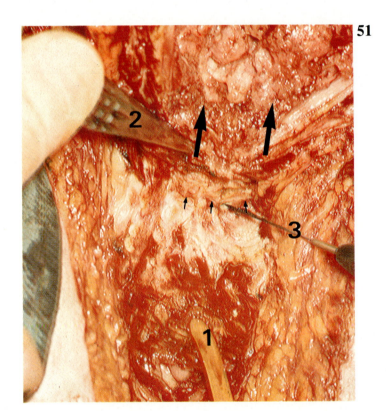

51 Elevation of growth from anterior aspect of pubes

The area of the growth is steadied by the dissecting forceps (2) while the diathermy needle (3) continues the upwards separation in the plane of cleavage and in the direction of the arrows. The level is now well above the urethral orifice shown by the catheter (1). The clitoral vessels and ligaments will be encountered at this level and some spouting blood vessels may be troublesome and require to be underrun with a stitch.

52

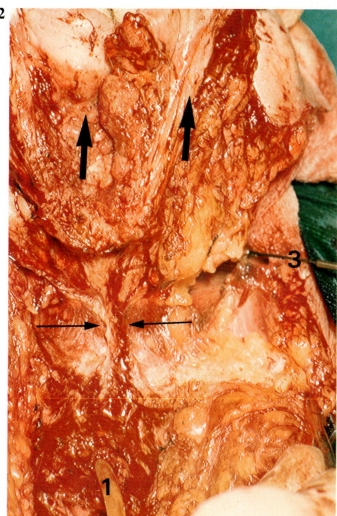

52 Completing removal of vulva and growth (i)
The whole vulvar mass, including the growth, is held upwards in the direction of the arrows and separation proceeds with the diathermy needle (3) on the left side. The location of the clitoral vessels and attachments is indicated by fine arrows and haemostasis has already been secured.

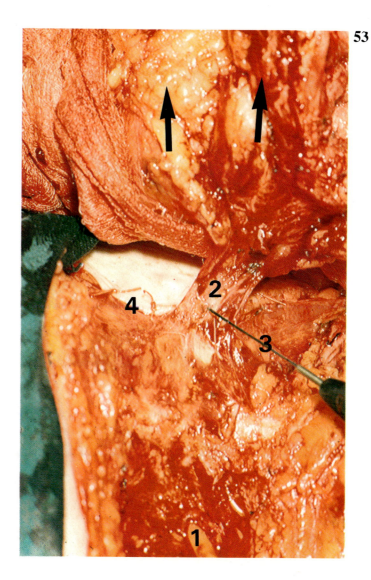

53

53 Completing removal of vulva and growth (ii)
The last strands of tissue attaching the vulva to the pubes (2) are being divided with the diathermy needle (3) and removal of the vulva and growth is now complete. The stitches anchoring the abdominal skin flap at the pubic crest are seen at (4).

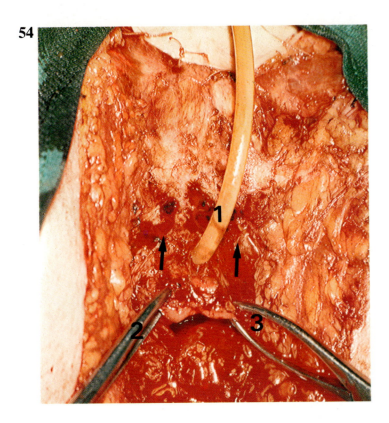

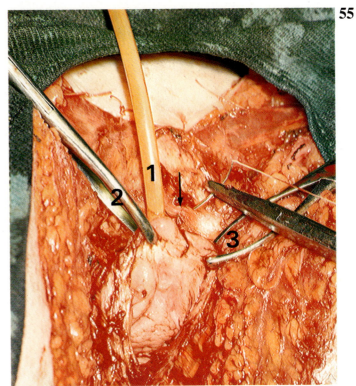

54 to 56 Supporting terminal urethra with vaginal skin flap

In Figure 54 the bare area following removal of the vulva is demonstrated and a Foley catheter (1) is in the urethra. The shallow flap of vaginal skin is held in the two pairs of forceps (2) and (3) and will be brought forwards and upwards in the direction of the arrows to support or buttress the shortened urethra. In Figure 55 the flap is held in place with the tissue forceps (3) while the left side is about to be sutured to the periosteum of the pubic bone which is seen being picked up by the needle, where arrowed. In Figure 56 that part of the flap held by forceps (2) is similarly anchored on the right side. This step may not be mandatory but it does prevent traction of the urethra under the pubic arch and also provides badly needed support for the structure.

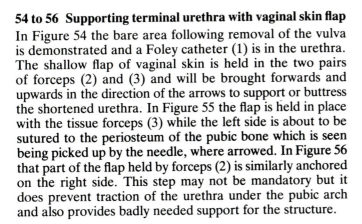

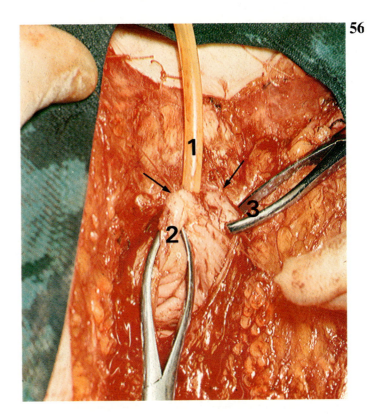

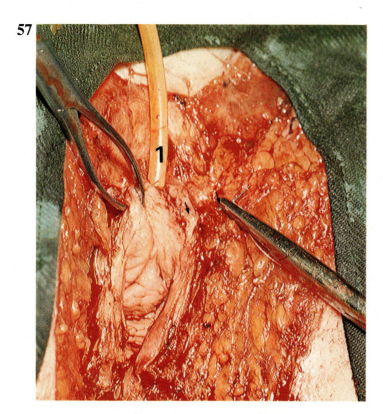

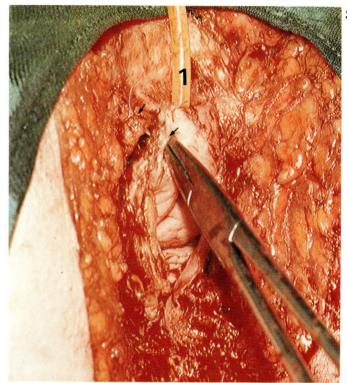

57 to 59 Anchoring lower edge of vaginal skin

A few fine sutures are inserted around the introitus to attach the free border of the vaginal skin to the adjacent structures and prevent retraction into the vagina. These sutures are also used for haemostasis where required. Two such stitches are being placed and are arrowed in Figures 57 and 58. Figure 59 shows the denuded area now quite dry. It can either be left completely open, as seen here, or partially closed posteriorly to accelerate healing.

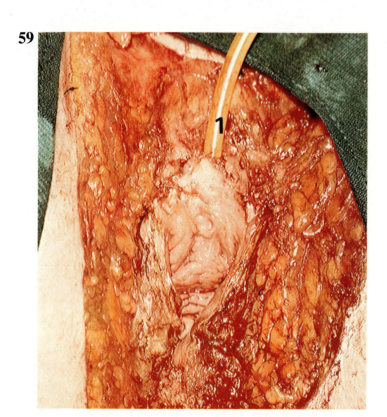

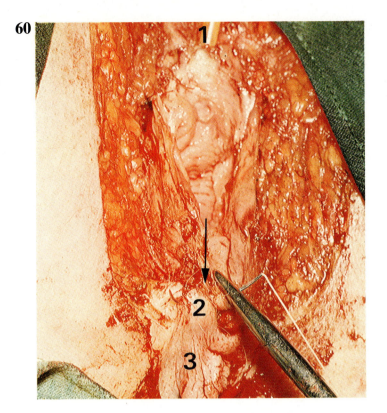

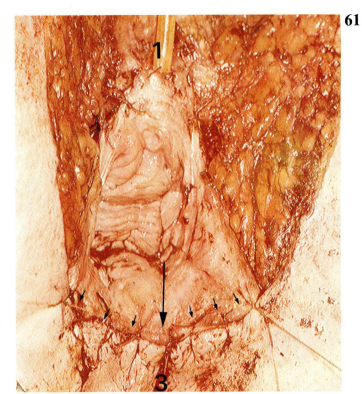

60 to 62 Limited closure of vulvar wound posteriorly

Since the growth was so obviously anterior in origin it was felt safe to cover the perineum and the immediately adjacent postero-lateral areas by inserting a few sutures as previously discussed (page 61). The first of these stitches is being placed at (2) just at the midline in Figure 60. The urethra is at (1) and the anus is at (3). This central stitch and three lateral stitches on each side are seen in Figure 61 and are arrowed. The suture being placed (4) in Figure 62 is merely to anchor an un-attached portion of vaginal skin while leaving the wound open. It is emphasised again that there is no attempt at a primary closure; these seven posterior stitches are to prevent soiling from the bowel and at the same time expedite healing.

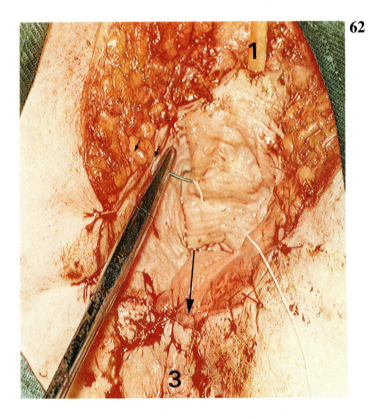

63

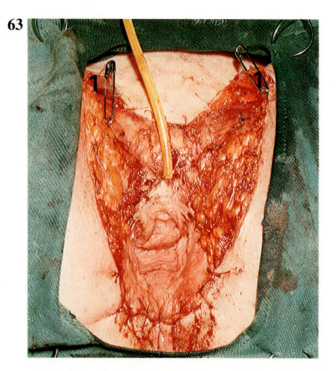

64

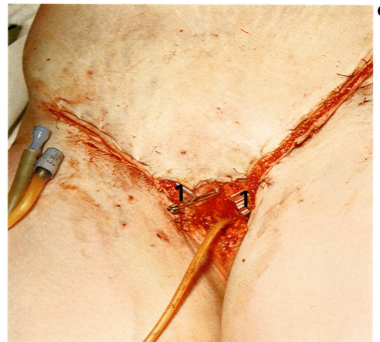

63 and 64 Vulvectomy completed

Figure 63 shows the completed operation with the patient still in the lithotomy position. Corrugated drains (1) and (1) are in position (see page 61) and a Foley catheter *in situ*. Figure 64 shows the appearances with the patient supine and it is seen that the wounds are not under any tension.

65

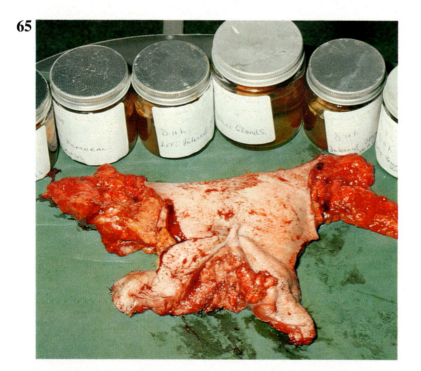

66

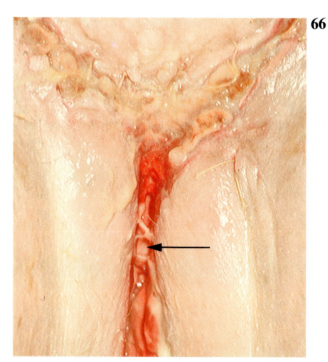

65 Specimen

The main mass of the vulva and growth is shown with the superficial and some of the deep glands still attached. Although the upper deep lymphatic system was removed in a continuous chain, each group of glands was defined and labelled separately in the containers shown, preparatory to sending them for histological examination.

66 Appearance of vulva 10–12 weeks following operation

Healing from the lateral edges proceeds satisfactorily despite the large raw area. After 11 weeks it is seen that the whole area is epithelialised although the skin is not yet strong and there is some initial scarring. Some muco-purulent exudate persists: the site of the urethral orifice is arrowed.

Radical vulvectomy with pelvic lymphadenectomy – without division of inguinal ligaments

The principal reason for division of the inguinal ligament in radical vulvectomy and pelvic lymphadenectomy is to gain maximum access to the extra-peritoneal glands. Other reasons given for doing so are that it opens up the femoral canal to allow removal of lymph glands and vessels, and especially of Cloquet's gland under direct vision while, at the same time, keeping the lymph chain unbroken during removal. The first reason is sound if the patient is obese with a deep pelvis, but good access is obtainable in many cases without division, especially if the pelvis is shallow and the patient is thin. The second reasons are hardly valid. The importance, and even existence of Cloquet's gland is in doubt and glands encountered in the femoral canal probably represent the lower nodes of the external iliac group. It is quite simple to check with the forefinger that the femoral canal is cleared of gland tissue. The concept of keeping deep and superficial glands as an intact chain is a vain one and, unless there is definite need or indication for dividing the ligaments, time and trauma can be saved by following the description given below. The authors emphasise that in dealing with vulvar cancer, the operations should be tailored to the needs and general condition of the patient. The only proviso is that the growth be completely removed.

Stage 1: Exploration of inguinal canal

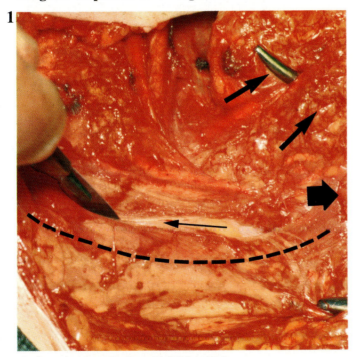

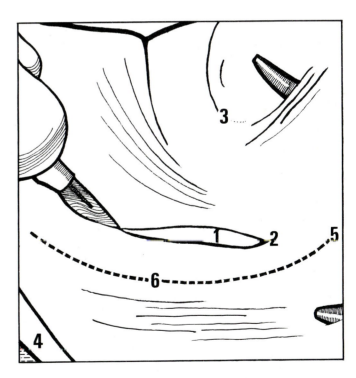

1 Opening inguinal canal (right side)

The scalpel splits open the external oblique aponeurosis in the line of its fibres from the external inguinal ring to the level of the junction of the lateral and middle thirds of the inguinal ligament. The mass of skin, superficial glands and fat is held medially in the direction of the arrows. The broken line overlies the inguinal ligament and, as previously, a very broad arrow points to the symphysis pubis. The grid reference is I and VII (see inset, page 88).

Diagram 9

1 Incision in external oblique aponeurosis
2 Site of external inguinal ring
3 Skin, fat and superficial gland mass
4 Lower skin edge retracted by forceps
5 Pubic tubercle
6 Inguinal ligament (broken line)

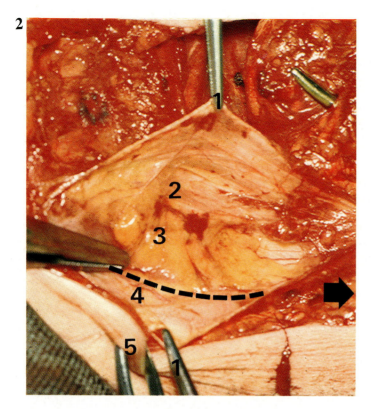

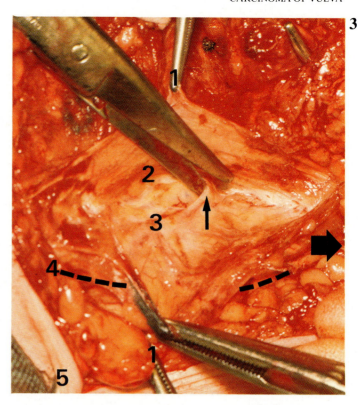

2 Identification of structures in inguinal canal

The cut edges of the external oblique aponeurosis are held apart by the small forceps (1) and (1) to expose the conjoint tendon (2) and the transversalis fascia (3). The point of the scissors is retracting the deeper tissues to show the line of the inguinal ligament (4). The lower skin edge (5) is retracted with tissue forceps.

3 Incisions of transversalis fascia

The point of the scissors picks up and incises a fold of transversalis fascia where arrowed. This incision is made carefully because the peritoneal cavity and, particularly, the deep epigastric vessels are just underneath it and could be injured. (The various structures are numbered as in Diagram 2, page 39.) The grid reference is I and VII.

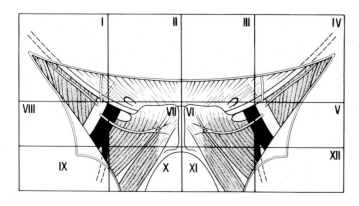

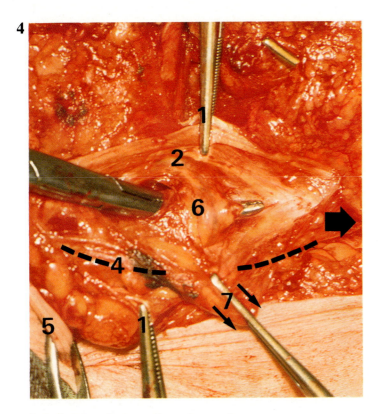

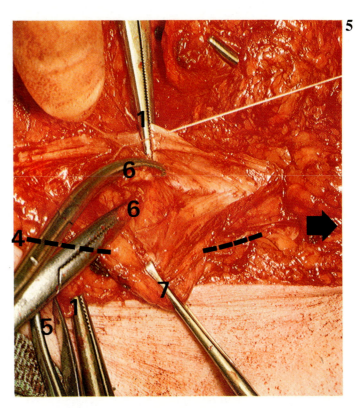

4 Definition of deep epigastric vessels

The definition and ligation of these vessels is an important landmark in the operation. The artery is a branch of the external iliac just as it becomes the femoral artery under the inguinal ligament, so that location is easy. The photograph shows the artery and accompanying veins (6) supported on a Phillips forceps, ready to be doubly clamped, cut and tied. The incised transversalis fascia is retracted in the direction of the arrows by tissue forceps (7). (The other structures are numbered as previously.)

5 Ligation of divided deep epigastric vessels

The vessels have been divided and are held in forceps (6) and (6). The ligature has been placed under the distal end and is in the process of being tied. (The other structures are numbered as in Diagram 2, page 39.) The grid reference is I.

Stage 2: Exploration of femoral canal

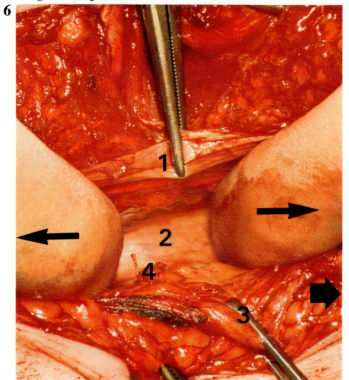

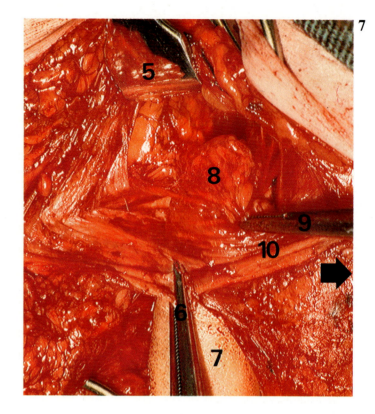

6 to 8 Opening and exploring femoral canal (right)

In Figure 6 the forefingers are inserted in the opening in the transversalis fascia and pull in the direction of the arrows to reveal the peritoneum (2). The fascia is held distally in forceps (3) and the upper external oblique edge is at (1). The ligature on the proximal end of the deep epigastric artery is seen at (4). In Figure 7 the inner aspect of the femoral canal is exposed between the retractor (5) and the forceps on the inner end of the inguinal ligament (6); the forefinger (7) is inserted upwards into the canal. An enlarged gland lying in the canal (8) is being displaced upwards by the finger and is held by dissecting forceps (9). This probably represents the gland of Cloquet. In Figure 8 the gland (8) is held up clear of the finger by the forceps and the canal is now seen to be quite empty of further glands. The inguinal ligament is at (10) in Figures 7 and 8. The grid reference is VII.

Stage 3: Deep gland dissection

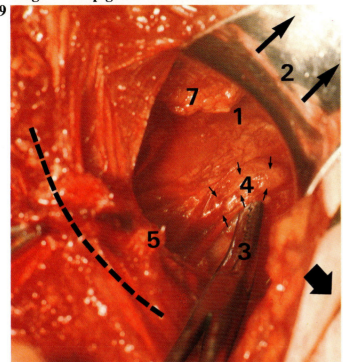

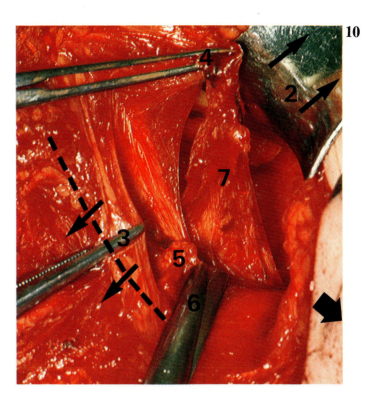

9 Reflection of peritoneum to expose extra-peritoneal space (right side)

Once the femoral canal is known to be clear the dissection proceeds upwards along the external iliac vessels. The first step is to displace the peritoneum (1) medially and in a cephalad direction, with the retractor (2) in the direction of the arrows. The femoral canal is immediately beneath the handle of the forceps (3) which is used to display the right ureter (4) lying extra-peritoneally and outlined as it lies on the tip of the forceps. The proximal ligated end of the deep epigastrics is at (5) and indicates the area of the junction of the external iliac and femoral vessels. Enlarged glands are already visible at (7) being displaced medially with the peritoneum.

10 Commencing dissection of deep glands

With the retractor still at (2) and the lower edge of the inguinal ligament retracted at (3), the lower end of the lymph chain is held in tissue forceps (4) while the scissors (6) commence upward separation from the anterior and medial surfaces of the external iliac vessels. This dissection is best done carefully with scissors under direct vision as digital separation is liable to tear the smaller veins and cause troublesome haemorrhage. The angle of photography was altered for better demonstration: the broad arrow pointing to the symphysis pubis, and the broken line over the inguinal ligament restore perspective. The grid reference is VII.

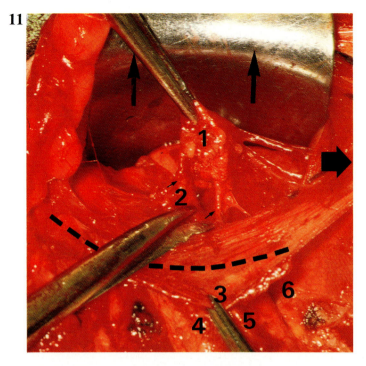

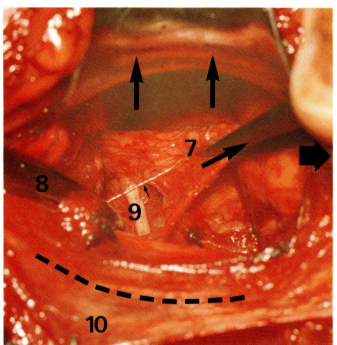

11 and 12 Further dissection of deep glands

The process of separation of the glands from the vessels continues upwards and along two distinct paths. The lateral is along the anterior aspect of the external iliac vessels towards the common iliacs and this generally produces a narrow and continuous chain of lymphatics and glands.

The other path lies more medially between the external iliac vein and the internal iliac artery. The gland tissue here is in the form of a shorter and thicker chain and represents the hypogastric or internal glands and the obturator glands with them. This group lies over, and sometimes partially surrounds, the obturator nerve.

Figure 11 shows the separation of the first chain. The lower end of the gland group (1) is held up by dissecting forceps while the scissors dissect it from the vessels beneath

at (2). The lower leaf of the external oblique (3) is held back by forceps and the line and direction of the femoral artery and vein can be followed from where they are indicated by (4) and (5) respectively and just below the inguinal ligament. The femoral canal is immediately adjacent (6). In Figure 12 the internal iliac or hypogastric group (7) (with the obturator glands) is being dissected out. The lower end of this chain is held medially with dissecting forceps in the direction of the arrow, while the scissors (8) dissect the gland tissue clear of the obturator nerve (9) in the depth of the wound. A lymph vessel (arrowed) can be seen crossing over the gland and the obturator nerve. The lower leaf of the external oblique is again held distally at (10). The grid reference is VII.

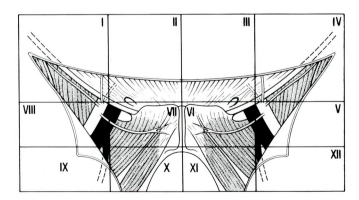

Stage 4: Closure of femoral canal

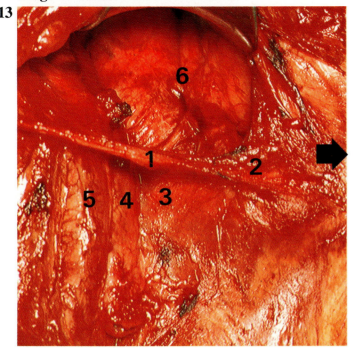

13

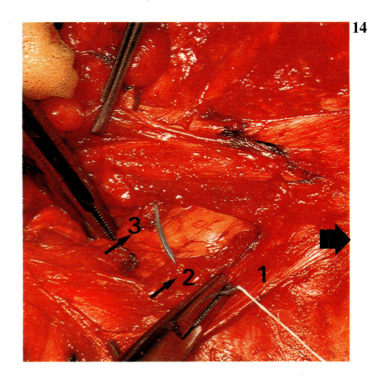

14

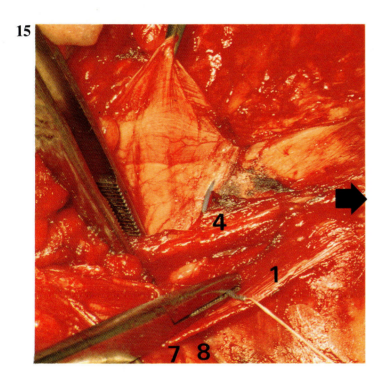

15

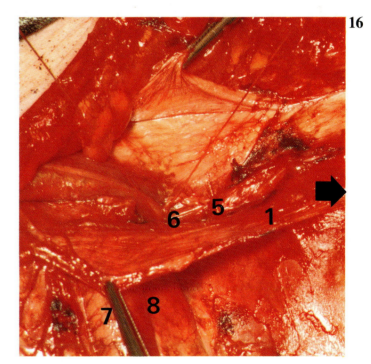

16

13 to 16 Closure of femoral canal

Figure 13 shows the appearances following removal of the glands. The inguinal ligament (1) fans out medially to form Cooper's ligament (2) at its attachment to the pubic tubercle. The femoral canal (3) lies medial to the femoral vein (4) and the femoral artery (5). The peritoneum is at (6). In Figure 14 the needle stitches the lateral curving edge of Cooper's ligament (2) to the pectineal fascia (3) on the posterior edge of the femoral canal to obliterate it. In Figure 15 the needle picks up the lower edge of the conjoint tendon (4) to reinforce the closure. Figure 16 shows this first suture tied at (5) and a second being placed at (6). The femoral artery and vein are seen below the inguinal ligament at (7) and (8) in the latter two illustrations. The grid reference is VII.

Stage 5: Closure of inguinal canal

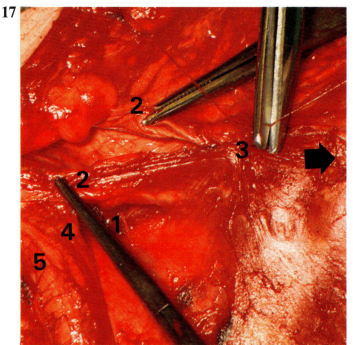

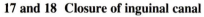

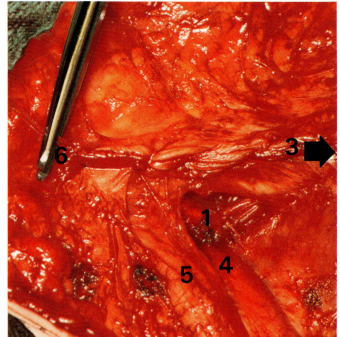

17 and 18 Closure of inguinal canal

In Figure 17 the obliterated femoral canal is at (1) with one of the sutures just visible and the leaves of the external oblique aponeurosis held by forceps (2) and (2). The canal is being closed by a continuous suture which has been anchored at (3) and the end is being cut with scissors. The femoral vein is at (4) and the artery at (5). The canal has been closed in Figure 18 and the stitch is being cut short at (6). The obliterated femoral canal (1), the femoral vein (4) and artery (5) are in the foreground. The grid reference is I and VII.

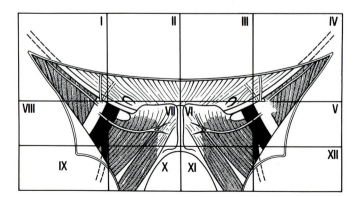

Radical vulvectomy and pelvic lymphadenectomy – with skin grafting

Despite the satisfactory results from non-closure of vulvectomy wounds many surgeons are unable to resist attempts at wound closure. The chief motive is to accelerate healing and cut the hospital stay but there is also a desire to see the wound neatly closed without the need for dressings. The fashioning of skin flaps to cover large areas in radical vulvectomy is unsatisfactory because poor blood supply and haematoma formation lead to sloughing of the skin edges. Either because of trauma or this deficient blood supply, the edges of the skin flaps are particularly liable to recurrences. It is noteworthy and significant that experienced surgeons never attempt such procedures.

The only acceptable form of cover is by split skin grafts which come from completely healthy areas and which are not liable to neoplasia. This permits wide excision of the skin area at risk with replacement by a sheet of healthy tissue which reduces immediate plasma loss and shock. It ensures smooth non-fibrotic healing without contraction and scarring and reduces hospital stay from twelve weeks to four or at the most five weeks.

Split skin grafting has been unfavourably reported on (Way, 1978) mainly because of the low percentage of 'take' obtained, thus giving poor return for time and effort. The actual methods used are scarcely ever detailed and some of the adverse reports relate to skin grafting as a postoperative procedure when the wound is invariably infected and when no real success could be expected. In practice, intermediate skin grafts applied immediately to the vulvar wound by the simple method described here and managed as described will give a consistently high percentage of 'take'. The procedure is simple and readers can be reassured that any operator without plastic surgery experience is capable of cutting a satisfactory graft with a Campbell knife and applying the graft to the bare area. The procedure adds half-an-hour to the operation at a stage when the surgeon's enthusiasm is admittedly waning. It is a small price to pay for the considerable benefits and, with modern anaesthesia, there is minimal additional hazard to the patient.

1 Equipment for cutting and applying split skin graft
1 Campbell modification of Humby knife
2 Fine dissecting forceps
3 Straight scissors
4 Bland skin antiseptic
5 Wide gauze roll to cover donor site
6 Crepe bandage for donor site
7 Normal saline solution to receive the cut skin graft

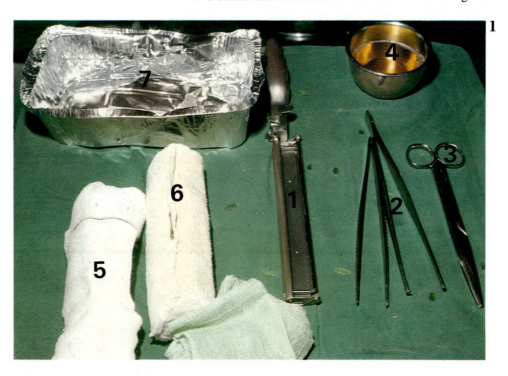

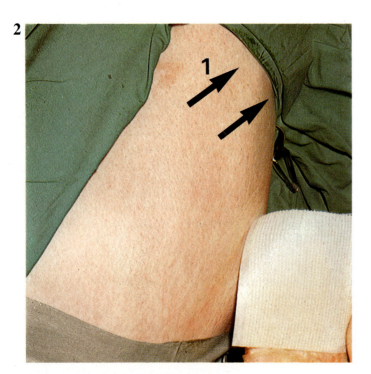

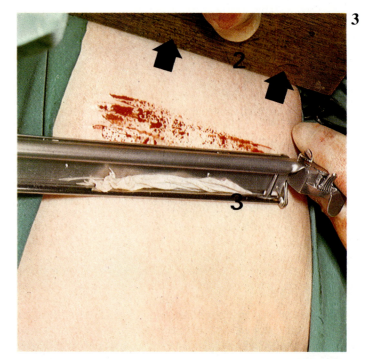

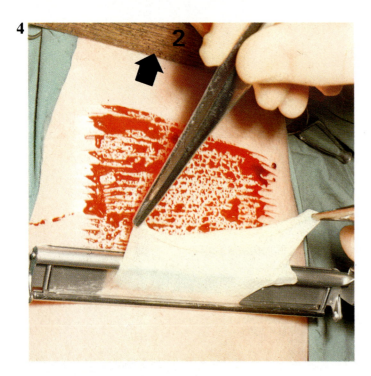

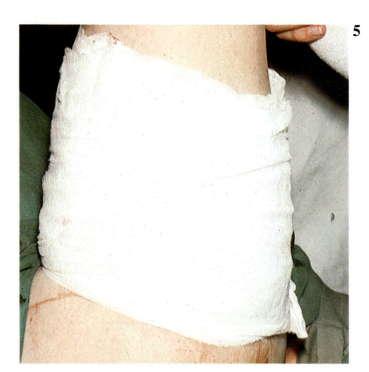

2 to 5 Obtaining split skin graft

The graft is cut just before the patient is put into lithotomy position for vulvectomy: the back of the right thigh is a suitable area. In Figure 2 it has been cleaned and draped and an assistant holding the knee (1) flexes and adducts the right thigh in the direction of the arrows. The skin is smeared with petroleum jelly to reduce friction when cutting and in Figure 3 the left hand keeps the skin quite taut by pressing with a short sterilised wooden board (2) in the direction of the arrows. The graft is cut by to-and-fro strokes

with slow forward advancement of the cutting edge. The adjustable roll guard (3) in advance of the knife edge automatically keeps the graft of uniform thickness. As the graft is cut in Figure 4 it is picked up by the assistant where it emerges between the knife and the guard. When adequate in size it is cut off. In Figure 5 the donor site has been covered by a layer of petroleum jelly gauze and is shown being bound with a wide gauze roll. A crepe bandage is subsequently added.

Since the patient has to be placed in lithotomy position, additional disturbance is avoided if the graft is obtained at this stage. A single sheet of split skin (approximately 10 cm × 8 cm) is ideal and the third notch on the Campbell knife control gives satisfactory graft thickness without danger of cutting through the dermis. The graft is always gently handled with fine forceps and straight 10 cm needles are useful for spreading it out on the recipient site. Raw surface should be applied to raw surface and the surgeon must see that the cut surface of the graft is opposed to the vulvar area.

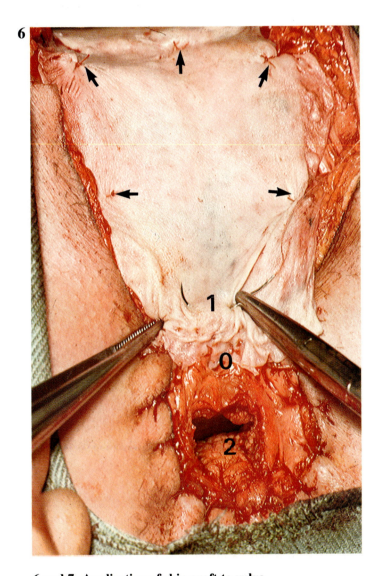

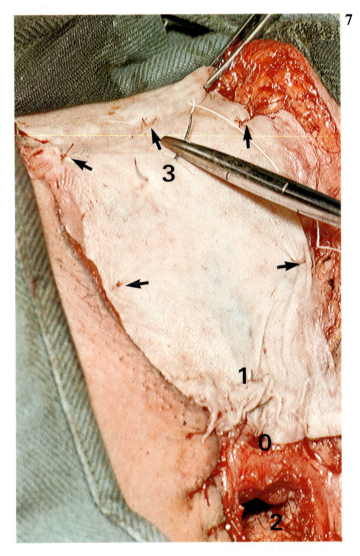

6 and 7 Application of skin graft to vulva

Following vulvectomy and complete haemostasis the skin graft is taken from the bowl of normal saline solution where it was stored and is applied as shown. In Figure 6 it has been attached to the outer edges of the raw area by several retaining sutures which keep it taut on the surface and which are arrowed. The graft is being attached in the region of the clitoris (1) and a PGA No. 00 suture on a fine needle is used. The urethra is designated (0) and the vagina (2). In Figure 7 the first of a series of 'basting' sutures is placed to keep the skin graft in closer apposition with the raw vulvar area and obviate the need for pressure dressings (3). The other sutures are numbered and indicated as previously.

8

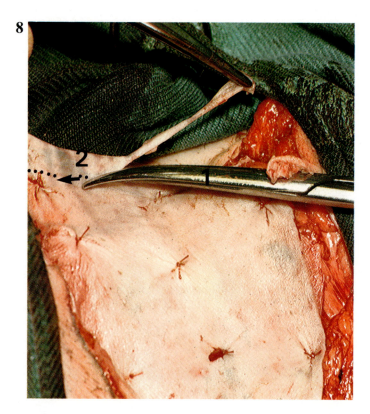

9

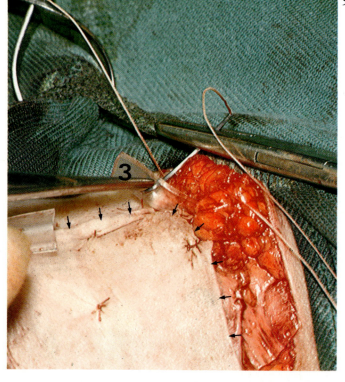

8 to 10 Trimming graft and placing inguinal drains

In Figure 8 excess tissue is cut from the graft so that it fits the area to be covered. This is done with scissors (1) cutting in the direction of the arrow along the line of the pubic crest to remove the excess (2). It is an important step since excess unattached skin quickly becomes necrotic and infects the whole wound. The trimmed upper edge is seen in Figure 9 and the left side of the graft is also seen to be tailored to fit the site. The left inguinal drain (3) is held in dissecting forceps while it is transfixed prior to fixing it to the skin edge. Figure 10 indicates similar points on the right side.

10

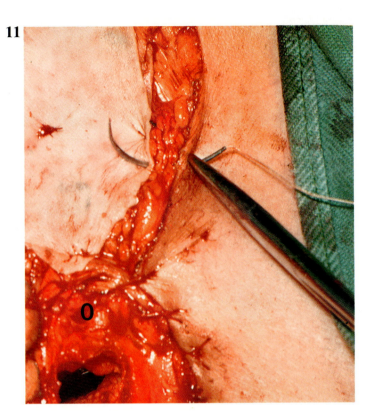

11

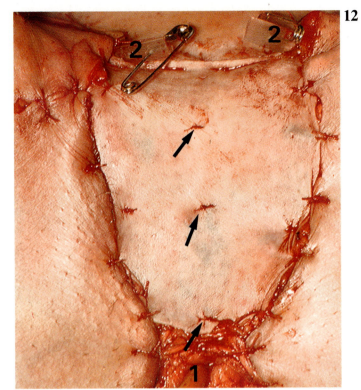

12

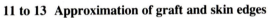

11 to 13 Approximation of graft and skin edges

It is important that there is not a bare area between the graft and the true skin edge, otherwise granulation tissue develops and delays healing. In Figure 11 the first of several such stitches is being placed, and in Figure 12 the whole area has been neatly sutured peripherally. Three central 'basting' sutures are arrowed, a catheter is in the urethra (1) and the drains are numbered (2) and (2). Figure 13 shows the completed operation with the patient in the supine position.

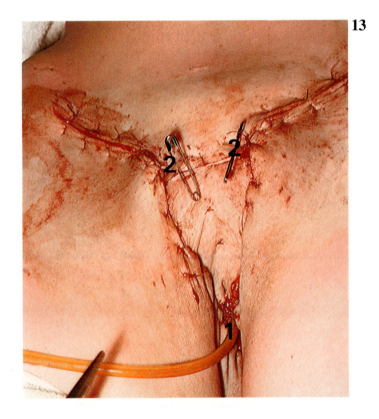

13

14

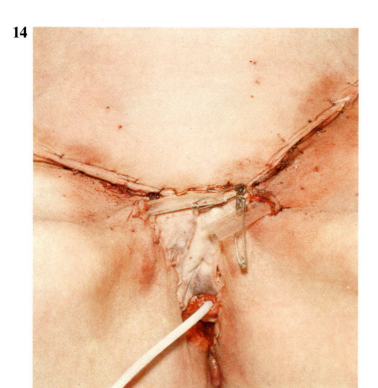

15

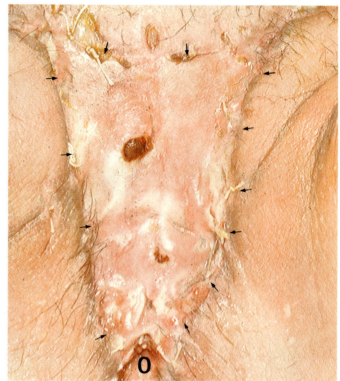

16

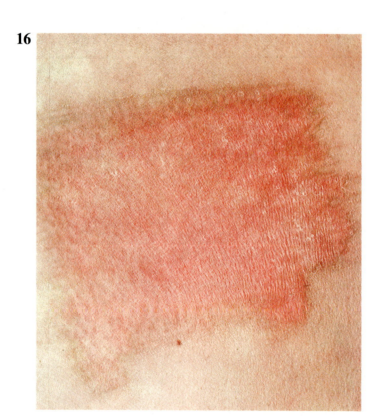

14 to 16 Appearances postoperatively

Figure 14 is a photograph taken five days postoperatively while the catheter and the drains are still *in situ*. It will be seen that the graft is pink and healthy and 'take' is a hundred per cent. Figure 15 is a photograph taken three weeks postoperatively and shows the whole area already covered although the skin is not yet strong. The urethral orifice is at (0) and outlines of the graft are arrowed. The donor site is also shown three weeks postoperatively in Figure 16; healing was rapid and uneventful. As mentioned previously no dressing is applied, the patient being nursed under a cage. Some surgeons will prefer to use prophylactic antibiotic cover; the authors routinely use a combination of 500,000 units Penicillin and 0.5 gm Streptomycin I.M. twice daily for seven days postoperatively.

Surgical management of vulvar recurrence

Recurrence of vulvar cancer can be a great problem. If there is a single recurrence on the skin edge and the growth is well differentiated, wide excision of the recurrence can be expected to give either cure or a long remission. If the growth is poorly differentiated and recurrence takes place soon, the outlook is bleak. We have seen that radiotherapy has little or nothing to offer and chemotherapy in the form of a bleomycin combination is still in its early stages of evaluation. At the present time, surgery is the only way of anticipating the development of a large fungating or ulcerative growth. The case described was of this latter type and the management illustrates the general principles employed in such a situation. Not unexpectedly, there was a subsequent deep recurrence of the growth but the patient had several months' remission of symptoms before dying of another disease.

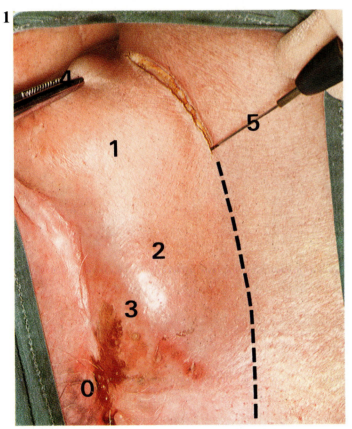

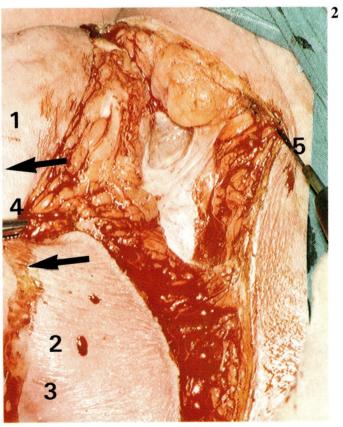

1 and 2 Outlining and excising recurrent growth (i)

The urethral orifice is at (0) in Figure 1 so that the recurrence (2) is over the anterior aspect of the left pubic bone and extending into the sub-pubic angle in the region of (3). The prominent area (1) was largely due to distortion by scarring but malignancy could not be excluded. The area is steadied with the dissecting forceps (4) while the diathermy needle (5) outlines the lateral skin excision line which will be continued along the dotted line. In Figure 2 the skin is held medially in the direction of the arrows by the dissecting forceps (4) and the whole skin, fat and tumour mass is dissected medially off the pubes with the diathermy (5).

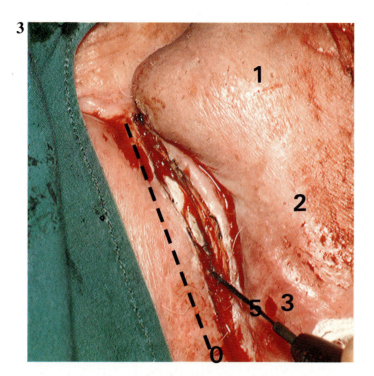

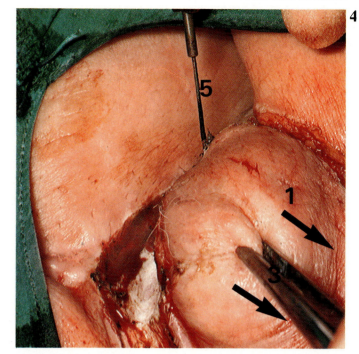

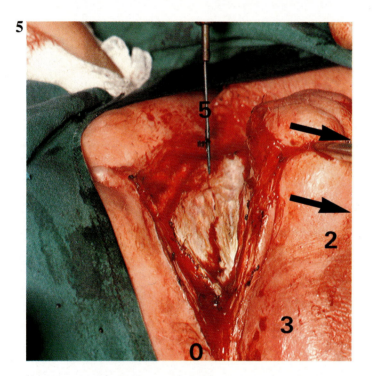

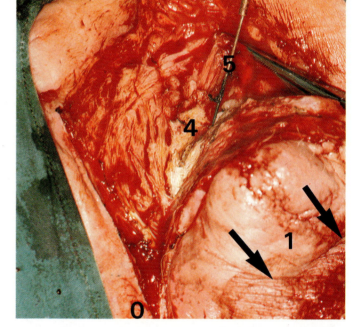

3 to 6 Outlining and excising recurrent growth (ii)

The upper and medial aspects of the growth (2) are outlined. In Figure 3 the diathermy (5) incises to the level of the pubic periosteum on the left of the midline which would underlie the broken line, and the site of the urethral orifice is just below the numeral (0) in the photographs. In Figure 4 the incision is carried laterally above the growth while it is held distally by the dissecting forceps (3), in the direction of the arrows. The incision is deepened to undermine the growth as it is held in the line of the arrows in Figures 5 and 6. It is necessary to incise right on to the pubic periosteum (4) to keep under the actual growth.

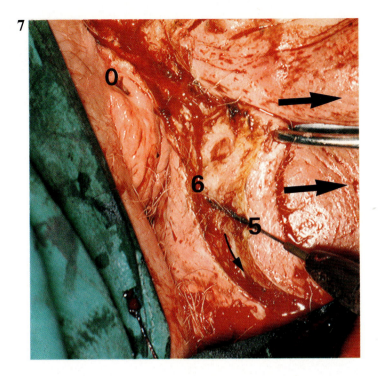

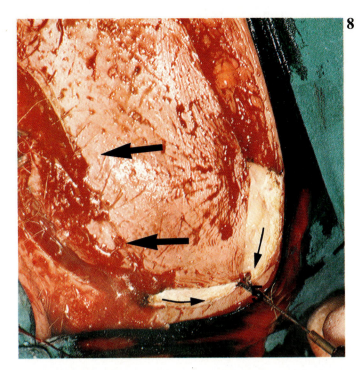

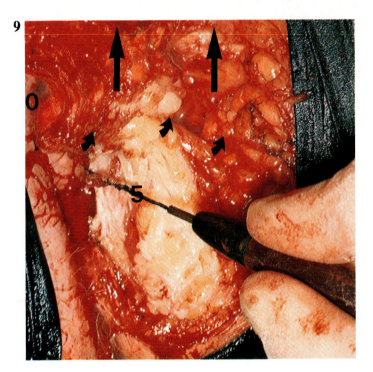

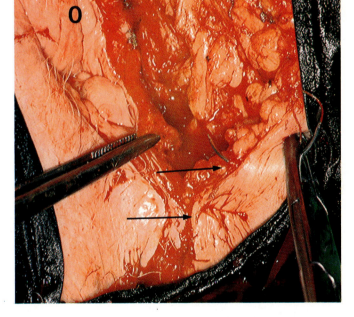

7 to 10 Outlining and excising recurrent growth (iii)

The process continues posteriorly with the growth held laterally by forceps in Figure 7, medially in Figure 8, and proximally in Figure 9, as arrowed. The diathermy (5) makes a deep incision postero-medially just on the introitus (6) in Figure 7 and joins this incision to the lateral one in Figure 8. In Figure 9 the diathermy is cutting deep into the sub-pubic tissues to release and deliver the whole growth upwards in the line of the curved arrows. In Figure 10 the growth is removed and two sutures are being placed (arrowed) posteriorly to prevent contamination from the anus. The recurrence was entirely anterior so that it was considered safe to insert the posterior sutures. Where visible, the urethral orifice is at (0).

11

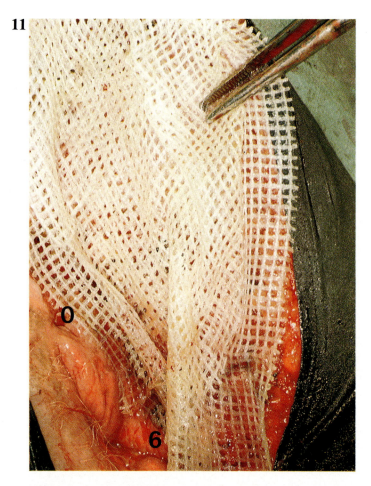

12

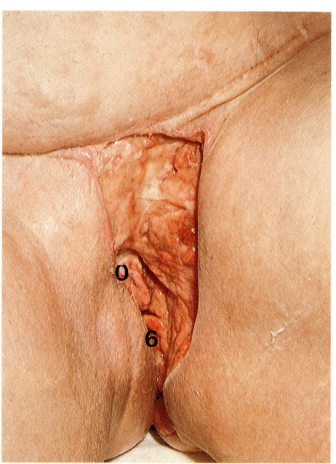

11 Petroleum jelly dressing to open wound

In Figure 11 the rather deep wound is left open except for two posterior stitches and, in this instance, is packed with petroleum jelly gauze to ensure healing from the depth. The gauze is held in position by a pad and bandage and replaced after each daily bath. The urethral orifice (0) and the vagina (6) are seen.

12 Postoperative appearance

The wound has healed from the depth and epithelialised on the surface after a period of nine weeks. Unfortunately, there was a deep recurrence in the sub-pubic angle within a year. The urethra and vagina are at (0) and (6) respectively.

Suggested reading

Parry-Jones, E. (1976). The management of pre-malignant and malignant conditions of the vulva. *Clinics in Obstetrics and Gynaecology*, 2, 2, 217–221.

Plentl, A. A. & Friedman, E. A. (1971). *Lymphatic Systems in the Female Genitalia*. W. B. Saunders, Philadelphia.

Way, S. (1977). The lymphatics of the pelvis. *Scientific Foundations in Obstetrics and Gynaecology*. Second edition, 118–126, edited by E. E. Philip, J. Barnes & M. Newton. Heinemann (William) Medical Books, London.

Way, S. (1978). The surgery of vulval carcinoma: an appraisal. *Clinics in Obstetrics and Gynaecology*, 5, 1, 623–628.

3: Cervical carcinoma

During the past 25 years important developments in the diagnosis of cervical cancer have greatly influenced its management. The advent of cytological screening has resulted in a situation where the gynaecologist now has to deal with two very different forms of the disease, i.e. the clinical and preclinical. The former group comprises those malignant lesions which have the easily recognisable features of an epithelial tumour; they frequently present in a form where effective curative treatment is impossible. The preclinical lesions are unrecognisable by the usual clinical methods of detection, i.e. inspection and/or palpation. The surgeon's rôle is equally important in treating both groups. In this chapter it is proposed to deal separately with the management of both forms of the disease.

Preclinical cervical carcinoma

All cancers must exist in a premalignant or non-invasive stage before they invade surrounding tissue. The existence of such stages in the cervical epithelium has been known for many years. Histologically they are well recognised and fall into three groups; dysplasia, carcinoma *in situ* and early invasive carcinoma. All are preclinical and are initially detected either by exfoliative cytology and/or colposcopy and confirmed by biopsy – either a punch biopsy taken under colposcopic monitoring, or a more formal cone biopsy.

Dysplasia is a term used to describe an epithelium in which distinct cellular abnormalities, such as an increase in the nuclear-cytoplasmic ratio, hyperchromatism, and occasional mitoses occur and are associated with disordered growth. There is still some differentiation present in the epithelium. It has been traditional to divide the dysplastic lesions into three subgroups of mild, moderate and severe, on the basis of the epithelial architecture and cellularity. Figure 1 shows a moderate dysplastic epithelium with increased cellularity associated with lack of differentiation in the lower four-fifths (1); flattened and differentiated layers of cells exist at (2). The basement membrane is intact at (3).

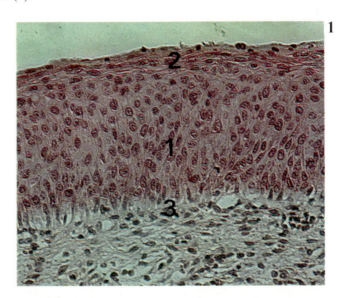

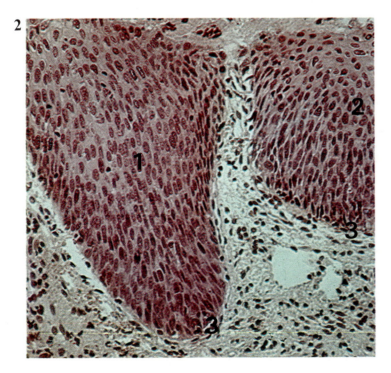

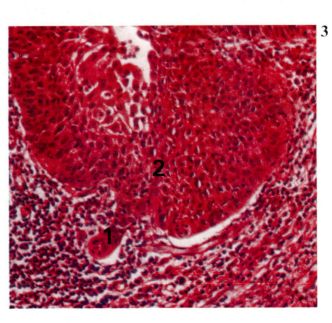

Carcinoma in situ is defined as an epithelium which, in the absence of invasion, has a full thickness loss of differentiation. A typical example can be seen at (1) in Figure 2; the adjacent epithelium at (2) is occupied by a severe dysplasia. The basement membrane at (3) is intact.

Many authors have proposed the abolition of the terms dysplasia and carcinoma *in situ* and their replacement by *cervical intraepithelial neoplasia* (CIN). There are three subdivisions in this classification with CIN I representing mild dysplasia, CIN II moderate dysplasia, and CIN III severe dysplasia and carcinoma *in situ*. This new terminology reflects the current biological evidence that there is *one* process of carcinogenesis leading to invasive squamous carcinoma and not two, as suggested by the dual system of diagnosing dysplasia or carcinoma *in situ*.

The malignant potential of the CIN lesions, i.e. their conversion to invasion, is estimated at 10–40 per cent. CIN I lesions have a high rate of regression, estimated at 20–40 per cent, while CIN III lesions are more likely to progress to invasion. The former occur in women in their early twenties while the latter have a peak incidence in the late twenties and early thirties. There is no way, at present, of predicting which will progress, so all are regarded as premalignant. However, since the most common age for detection of invasive cancer is in the forties, it is obvious that a degree of conservation can be considered when dealing with young women, especially those with CIN I and II lesions who are in their early/mid-twenties.

Preclinical invasive carcinoma includes cases in which the intraepithelial lesion breaks through the basement membrane of the epithelium and infiltrates the cervical stroma. If the infiltration is 3–5 mm the term micro-invasive carcinoma is applied; beyond these limits the term occult invasive carcinoma is used. In Figure 3 a small finger-like projection of microinvasion (1) from a CIN III lesion into the underlying stroma (2) is seen clearly. F.I.G.O. classifies both these lesions as stage Ia carcinoma of the cervix; in comparison, clinical cancer which is confined to the cervix is stage Ib. The pelvic lymph node involvement in the former is reckoned to be below 1 per cent compared with 16–22 per cent in the latter. Coppleson (1976) has recently reviewed the subject in detail.

Detection of preclinical cervical carcinoma

As the lesions of CIN are preclinical, the cervix containing them appears normal to the naked eye. Occasionally an area of hyperkeratosis (leukoplakia) is noticeable, and with some of the preclinical invasive lesions contact bleeding may be provoked after firm scraping of the lesion with a cytology spatula. The two important diagnostic tools available to the gynaecologist are cervical cytology and colposcopy.

The value of cytology as a screening method is indisputable. It has certain major limitations, however, the most important of which is the problem of the false negative smear. The simultaneous and complementary employment of colposcopy gives the gynaecologist greater accuracy in the detection of these lesions and also allows him to tailor his treatment 'to the lesion and the patient'. It allows definition of the epithelial area containing the CIN and its accurate histological confirmation. With these two parameters available, objective and rational decisions concerning treatment become possible.

Colposcopy allows the cervix to be viewed stereoscopically under illuminated vision at magnifications from ×6 to ×40. The colposcope (a standard model of which is pictured in Figure 4) contains binocular eye pieces (1) and a lens system with a focal length of 125–150 mm. It is a non-invasive technique suitable for outpatient/office patient evaluation. The lithotomy position allows a bivalve speculum (2) (especially the Cusco type) to be inserted easily and, when opened, it exposes both endo and ecto-cervix. In Figure 4 an adjustable magnification drum (×6 to ×40) is at (3) and a camera (4). The authors consider a magnification of ×6 to be adequate for routine examination.

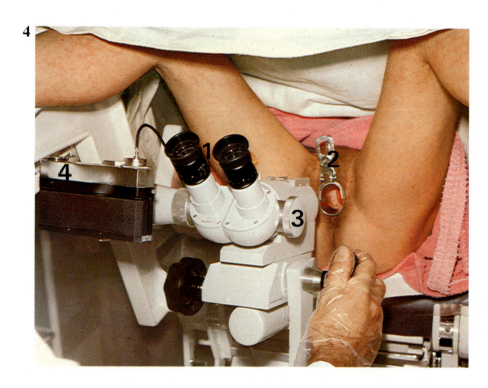

4

5

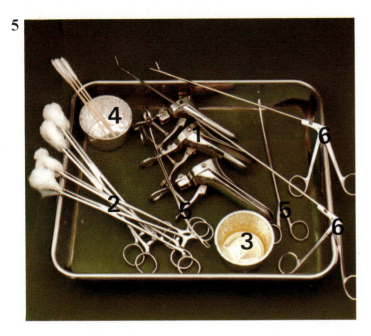

Five per cent acetic acid is gently applied to the cervix and in a few seconds reveals the atypical epithelium in which the premalignant (CIN) lesion resides. This epithelium has distinctive characteristics which allow it to be easily located and biopsied. Figure 5 shows the standard accessories required to make a colposcopic examination. Three bivalve Cusco specula are shown (1) with four sponge-holding forceps with gauze swabs (2). Five per cent acetic acid in a container (3) may be applied to the cervix with gauze swabs, or by fine cotton-tipped swab sticks (4). The extent of any endocervical extension is easily observed with the endocervical specula at (5); the authors use Desjardins gall-stone forceps (5) for this purpose. Biopsies of the cervix are taken by the authors with Patterson colonic biopsy forceps (6) which are extremely effective for this purpose. In Figure 6 they are being used under colposcopic control and their length precludes interference with the magnified field of vision. Figure 7, a colpophotograph (×10) shows a small area of atypical epithelium at (1) (containing a CIN I lesion) about to be biopsied. In Figure 8 two similar areas (1) and (1) on the anterior cervical lip have been accurately biopsied (arrowed); subsequent histological analysis revealed CIN II.

6

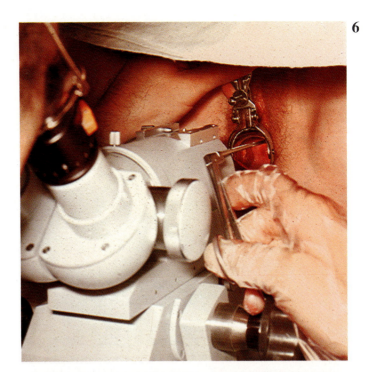

7

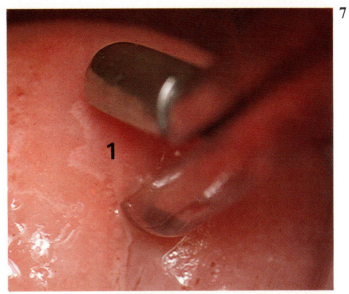

8

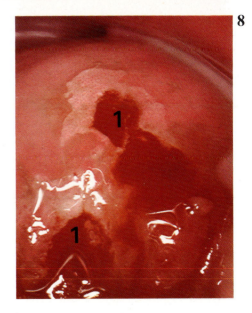

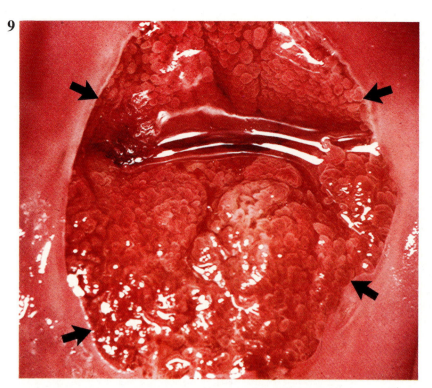

The location of the outer and inner borders of the area in which the premalignant epithelium resides is the most important part of the colposcopic examination. This area or transformation zone has its outer or lateral border marked by the original squamo-columnar junction (a point laid down in foetal life); its inner or medial border consists of the upper extension of the squamous metaplastic process (the new squamo-columnar junction). Squamous metaplasia, an irreversible physiological process, occurs particularly during pregnancy and adolescence and involves the replacement of columnar by squamous epithelium. Figure 9 is a colpophoto-graph (×10) of a cervix showing the original squamo-columnar junction (arrowed) encircling the columnar epithelium which occupies the endo and ectocervix. This columnar epithelium comprises the area of the transforma-tion zone, the area in which squamous metaplasia will occur.

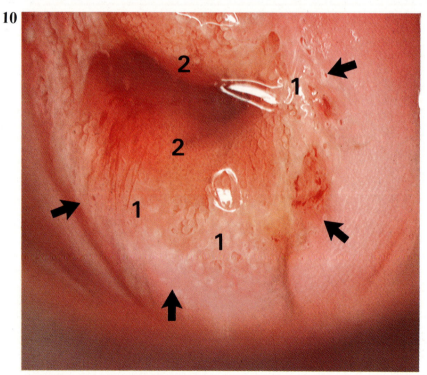

In Figure 10, a colpophotograph (×14), this metaplastic process (1) has occurred within the squamo-columnar junction (arrowed); endocervical columnar epithelium is seen at (2).

It is during metaplasia that mutagenesis occurs. Thus the upward extension of the metaplastic process signifies the limits of any transformation, whether it be physiological as in Figure 10, or atypical and, therefore, potentially malign as in Figures 11–14.

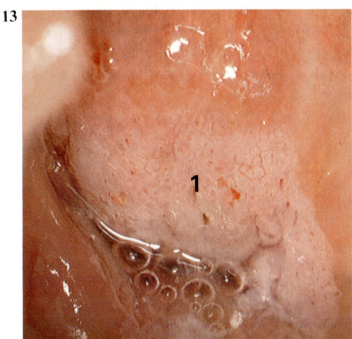

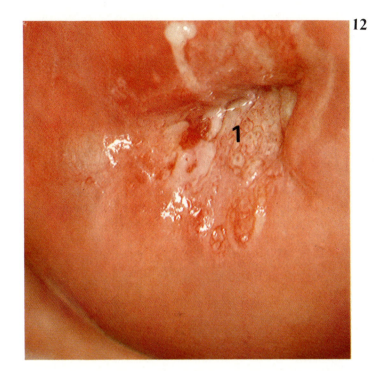

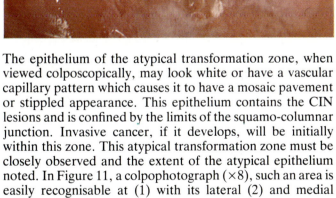

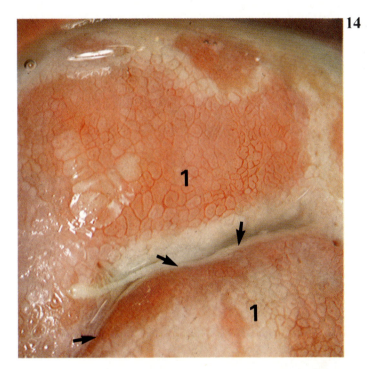

The epithelium of the atypical transformation zone, when viewed colposcopically, may look white or have a vascular capillary pattern which causes it to have a mosaic pavement or stippled appearance. This epithelium contains the CIN lesions and is confined by the limits of the squamo-columnar junction. Invasive cancer, if it develops, will be initially within this zone. This atypical transformation zone must be closely observed and the extent of the atypical epithelium noted. In Figure 11, a colpophotograph (×8), such an area is easily recognisable at (1) with its lateral (2) and medial borders (3) sharply demarcated. In Figures 12 and 13,

colpophotographs (×8), difficulty is encountered in defining the upper or medial limit (new squamo-columnar junction) of the atypical epithelium (1). By using an endocervical speculum these limits were seen and biopsy of both revealed a CIN II lesion. In Figure 14, a colpophotograph (×14), the upper limit of the atypical epithelium (1) could not be seen in the endocervix (arrowed) and the colposcopic examination was classed as unsatisfactory. Such lesions are totally unsuitable for local destructive therapy. Biopsy of this lesion showed it to contain a CIN III epithelium.

Treatment of preclinical cervical cancer

The most suitable method of treating preclinical lesions must take into consideration a number of factors. These include age, parity, a wish for future pregnancies or a desire for sterilisation, and the presence of an associated gynaecological condition such as prolapse or uterine myoma. The nature of the disease, i.e. its histological state and its distribution on the cervix as determined by colposcopy, must be considered. It is only by assessment of all these factors that a rational method of treatment can be determined. The common aim of the different treatment modalities is the eradication of the lesion; some methods are more conservative than others and as such require closer examination.

The three forms of treatment in the majority of preclinical lesions are:
1. Local destructive techniques
2. Cone biopsy
3. Hysterectomy.

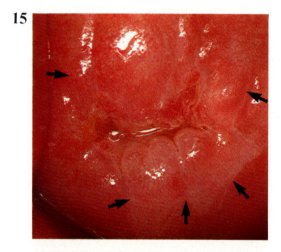

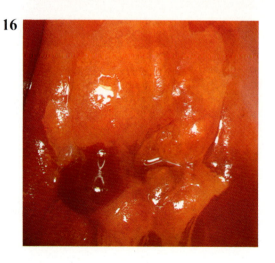

1 Local destructive techniques

These techniques require the simultaneous employment of colposcopy to define the exact limits of the focal lesion. Unless its full extent can be seen, and this implies the visualisation of the columnar epithelium in the endocervical canal above the lesion, these techniques are unsuitable. For example, the atypical areas (histologically proven CIN I, II) seen in Figures 7, 8 and 11 are suitable for local destructive techniques as their full extent can be seen. In Figures 12, 13 and 14, although the lateral extent of the atypical area (i.e. the squamo-columnar junction) is readily visible, its upper or medial border situated in the endocervical canal cannot be seen. Such lesions are not suitable for local therapy and thorough examination of the endocervical canal by cone biopsy is essential. Preoperative visualisation of this area with the modified endocervical speculum ((5) in Figure 5) is helpful. If the colposcope shows a major grade of abnormality, indicating the possible presence of early (preclinical) invasion, it is not suitable for such conservative therapy.

With these provisos, local destruction is clearly the optimal method of treatment, especially in young women desirous of future pregnancies. Its economic advantage is obvious.

Three methods are available: cryotherapy, electro-coagulation diathermy under general anaesthesia, and laser therapy. Electrocautery is suitable for very small and minor lesions, but its inability to destroy tissue beyond a depth of 2–3 mm without unacceptable discomfort to the patient, precludes its general use.

Prior to employing these techniques the atypical area is defined by colposcopy and the Schiller iodine staining test. Iodine is not taken up by the glycogen-deficient epithelium which contains the CIN lesions and consequently this epithelium appears pale when iodine is applied. In Figure 15 the outline of the atypical epithelium is just visible (arrowed) after the application of acetic acid for colposcopy. In Figure 16 the area becomes sharply demarcated by the application of iodine and any local destructive procedure must encompass all the iodine negative area. The physiological squamous epithelium of the ectocervix and vaginal vault has taken up the dark brown iodine stain.

Cryosurgery (without anaesthesia)

This increasingly popular technique involves the freezing of tissue by using either carbon dioxide or nitrous oxide. The resultant tissue destruction is enhanced when freezing is rapid and thawing is slow. Because of its anatomical configuration and accessibility, the cervix is an ideal organ for cryotherapy. Its use in the treatment of benign cervical disease is detailed in Volume 1. The cryogens are usually delivered directly on to the cervix via a gun type of appliance ((1) in Figure 17) with interchangeable probe tips of variable shape ((2) in Figure 17). These have been designed to approximate to the surface area of the atypical epithelium. The probe tip is coated with a thin film of lubricating jelly ((3) in Figure 17) which facilitates a more rapid freeze which is essential in achieving efficient tissue destruction. Once the tip has been positioned on the cervix, the refrigerant is circulated until the edge of the ice ball extends at least 5 mm on to normal tissue. The tip is defrosted and the cervix examined colposcopically to ensure that all atypical areas have been treated; any remaining areas obviously will need subsequent freezing. A second freeze after defrosting the area for a few minutes is recommended by some, but

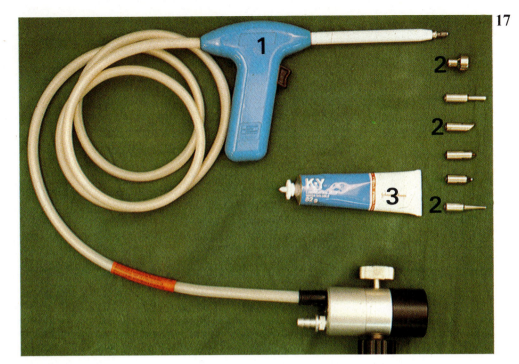

recent reports do not indicate an increase in the success rate over a single freeze procedure. This is particularly so when using liquid nitrogen as the probe tip temperature is reduced to –160°C. With carbon dioxide the reduction is only to –60°C so that a freeze-thaw-freeze technique may be required with this refrigerant.

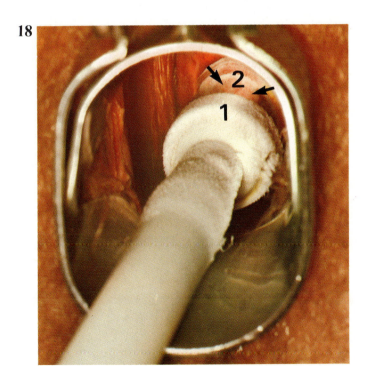

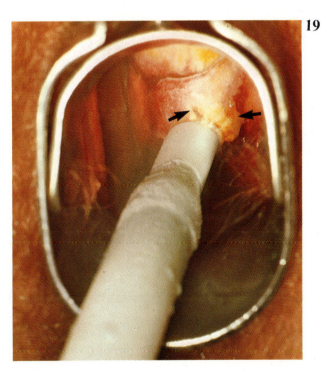

In Figure 18 the probe tip (1) has just been removed from a cervix in which a small circular area of atypical epithelium was present on the anterior and on the posterior cervical lips. The ice ball (2) has extended 5–7 mm lateral to the original site of this lesion (partly arrowed). In Figure 19 a small triangular area (arrowed) of atypical epithelium (histologically confirmed CIN III) is in the process of being

frozen by an appropriately-shaped probe tip. The ice ball is in process of forming around the lesion. These procedures are being performed without anaesthesia and with a Cusco vaginal speculum providing access. A triple sulfa cream is used daily for ten days after treatment to aid healing. The patient is told to expect a watery discharge which may last for ten to fourteen days.

20

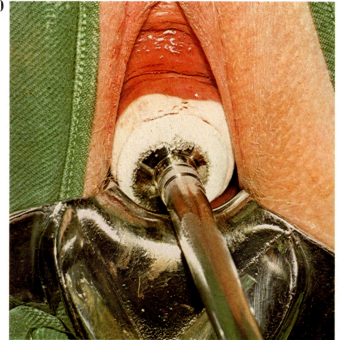

21

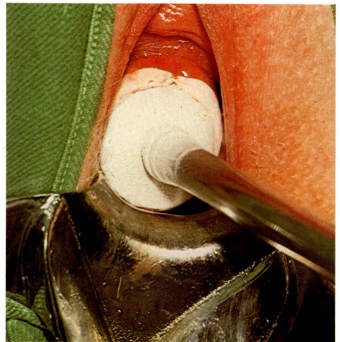

Local destruction of atypical epithelium may be required at the same time as another gynaecological procedure necessitating a general anaesthetic. Such a case is seen in Figures 20–22. The patient was a 35-year-old woman who requested sterilisation and in whom a surprise severely

dyskaryotic cervical smear was obtained. Colposcopy and biopsy in the outpatients department/office revealed the presence of two small ectocervical areas of CIN III. Cryosurgery is seen destroying these areas prior to laparoscopic sterilisation. The ice ball which formed after one-and-a-half

22

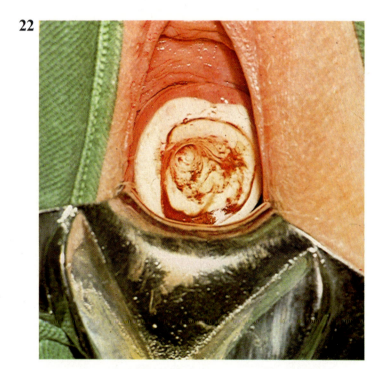

23

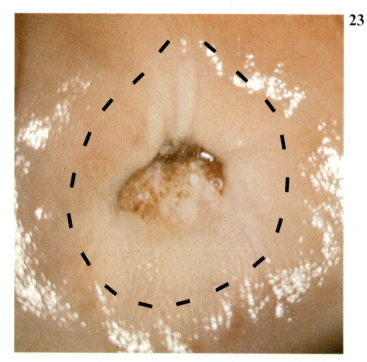

minutes has extended 6–8 mm lateral to the original areas. Recently reported results testify to the efficiency of this technique in properly selected cases. An overall freeze failure rate of 8–12 per cent is reported for the initial freeze; after two freezing sessions the rate is reduced to 3 per cent. It seems that the size of the lesion rather than its histological characteristics determines the success or otherwise of cervical cryosurgery. Other factors which influence success include the tank pressure of the refrigerant (a low tank pressure is associated with a slow inefficient freeze) and poor application of the probe tip to the lesion.

Atypical epithelium should be replaced by mature physiological regenerative squamous epithelium in four to six weeks. This is seen in Figure 23 where regenerative squamous epithelium (outlined) replaces a previous area of atypical epithelium. The new squamo-columnar junction is clearly seen in the endocervix. In cases of regeneration or survival of the original atypical epithelium, repeat refreezing or conisation is required. Follow-up examinations include colposcopy and exfoliative cytology; the first is carried out after four months with two more visits within the first year.

It has been said that where conservative therapy such as cryosurgery, electrocoagulation or even cone biopsy has been used there is a greater risk of eventual malignancy than if hysterectomy had been performed, but this is not proven. The authors and others (as summarised by Coppleson 1976) maintain that, provided the transformation zone has been replaced by mature squamous epithelium, the woman is free of the risk of developing carcinoma within that area.

Electrocoagulation diathermy (under anaesthesia)

This operation destroys the atypical epithelium by heat beyond its colposcopic limits, both ectocervically and in the lower endocervical canal. The aim is to destroy the epithelium and glands to a depth of several millimetres in the stroma. Heat stimulates mucus production and its exudation during the application of the probe shows that the necessary depth of destruction required to destroy the glandular stroma has been achieved. The area to be treated is evaluated and defined by prior colposcopy and biopsy. The diathermy procedure must be done under general anaesthesia, otherwise it is not possible to obtain sufficient depth of tissue destruction.

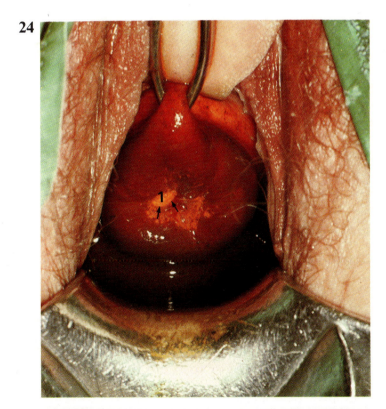

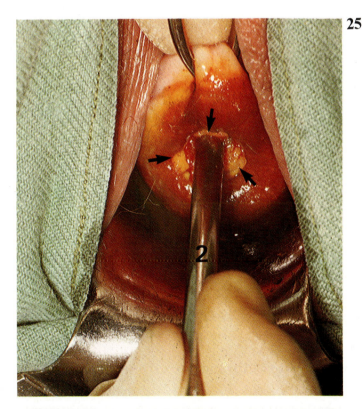

In Figure 24 the limits of a small area of atypical epithelium (1) on the anterior cervical lip of a 19-year-old girl are clearly demarcated after the application of iodine solution. Its upper limits are arrowed. The posterior lip and endocervix are composed of physiological epithelium. This histologically confirmed CIN II lesion can be destroyed simply by local electro-diathermy. Figure 25 shows a more extensive area of atypical epithelium occupying both endo and ectocervix. Its margins are outlined after iodine application and are arrowed. Its upper limit has been clearly visualised by colposcopy when directed biopsy revealed the presence of CIN III. Preliminary dilatation (2) to Hegar No. 9 is shown in Figure 25.

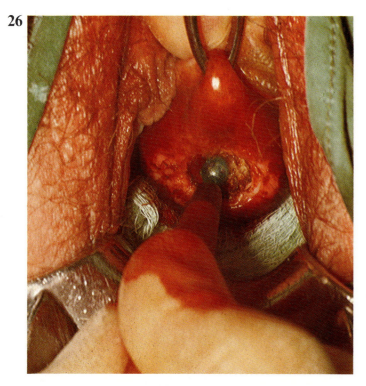

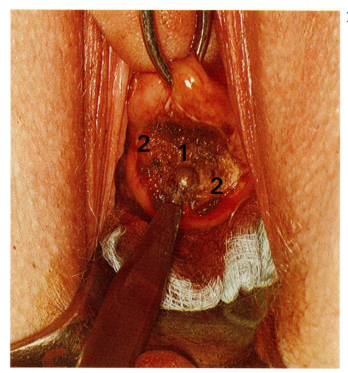

In Figure 26 a ball and pen device is used to coagulate the atypical epithelium by electrodiathermy. In Figure 27, the endocervix (1) with a margin of at least 10 mm beyond the lateral extent of the lesion, has been treated (2). In lesions containing obvious cervical glands or nabothian follicles, a diathermy needle probe is first introduced into the depth of the structures and followed by application of the ball electrode as illustrated.

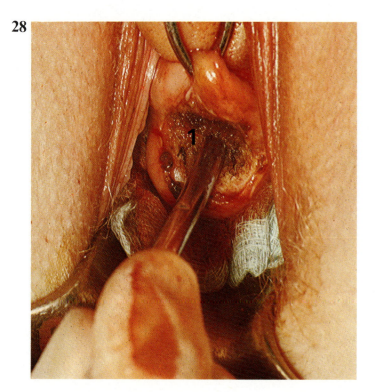

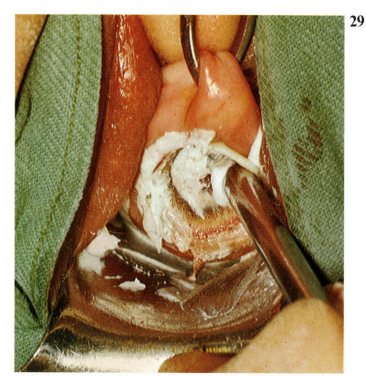

The treated area (1) is shown in Figure 28 and a dilator (Hegar 9) is being reinserted to discourage postoperative stenosis of the reformed cervical os. In Figure 29 triple-sulfa cream is being inserted to aid healing which should be complete in four to six weeks. A heavy vaginal discharge persists for about two weeks but other complications are minimal. It might be thought that cervical physiology would be adversely affected by deep diathermy, particularly if the lesion were extensive, but this does not appear to be so. The cure rate is excellent and following one application of electrocoagulation diathermy, a number of studies reported an average success rate of over 95 per cent.

Laser destruction of atypical epithelium

Laser (or light amplification by stimulated emission of radiation) is a new and expensive technique currently being used and evaluated in the treatment of preclinical cervical cancer. Preliminary results suggest that it may be the optimal technique for the local destruction of such lesions. Jordan and his associates have recently confirmed a 95 per cent initial treatment cure rate of CIN lesions treated by laser therapy. There is less surrounding tissue reaction than in the other techniques described (cryo and diathermy) and a more accurate destruction of the atypical epithelium can be obtained.

The CO_2 laser emits electromagnetic radiation of high intensity by controlled discharge of CO_2, nitrogen and helium. This energy appears in the infra red area of the electromagnetic spectrum and, with this energy, vaporisation is achieved in all biological tissues with little difficulty. The intensity of the heat, with intracellular temperatures of around 100°C, coagulates vessels with resultant minimal blood loss. The area to be destroyed is precisely monitored so that a healthy border of undamaged tissue remains.

Oedema in the healing tissue is rare and the squamous regeneration is rapid within twelve to fourteen days. Recent modifications by changing the fixed time-controlled laser beam exposure to a continuous beam exposure have increased substantially the success rate of this technique.

Figure 30 shows a carbon dioxide laser (1). It is connected to a colposcope (2) through which the operator views the cervix and directs the laser beam. The finder beam of visible light indicates the precise point where destruction is required and the visible spot seen through the colposcope indicates where the invisible laser beam will strike. By means of a manipulator attachment (3) the spot can be moved and this allows precise and selective destruction of pathological tissue. The depth of destruction can be adjusted by altering the power output of the laser. A suction device (4) removes fumes created by tissue vaporisation. Plastic tubing (5) connects the suction apparatus to a specially designed, disposable plastic speculum; plastic material reduced the hazard posed by deflection of the laser beam. In Figure 30, observer tubes (6) are connected to the colposcope; the laser power unit with its stored gases is at (7).

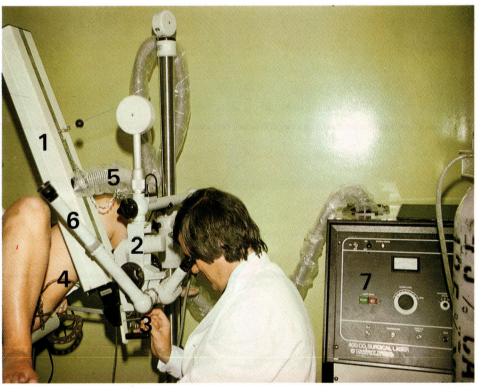

30

31

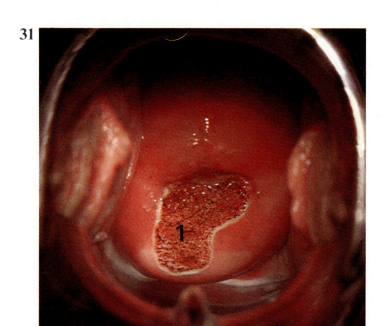

32

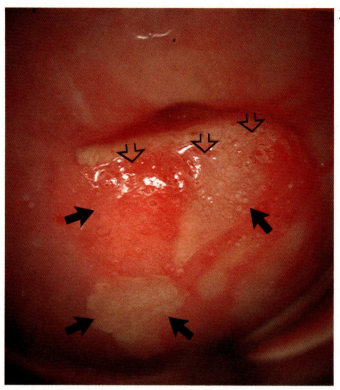

Figure 31 shows a view of the posterior cervical lip imme- diately following laser destruction (1) of a CIN lesion in this area. The sharply defined borders and the dark carbon pigments within the destroyed area are characteristic.

Figure 32 shows the same cervix as in Figure 3 six weeks after laser therapy. An area of mature squamous (closed arrows) has replaced the previous atypical epithelium. The new squamo-columnar junction (open arrows) is just within the endocervix; physiological and undamaged columnar epithelium can be seen above this line.

Summary of indications for local destructive techniques

1 The atypical transformation zone must be visual- ised in its entirety by colposcopy and special attention paid to the new squamo-columnar junction (i.e. its medial or upper border). If this cannot be done a cone biopsy is obligatory.

2 Colposcopic observations must be consistent with a CIN lesion; any suggestion of preclinical invasion contraindicates local destructive therapy and cone biopsy is required.

3 If colposcopically direct biopsy fails to explain a positive cytological smear (e.g. there is any sug- gestion of invasive disease), such therapy is contra- indicated.

4 The patient must be responsible and willing to return for follow-up examinations (colposcopy and cytology). This is particularly important in the first year after treatment.

2 Cone biopsy

This is the most common form of treatment for preclinical cervical carcinoma. The safety of this technique can be seen by the excellent long-term follow up results of women treated by cone biopsy. Coppleson (1976) recently summarised the outcome of 3764 conisation and cervical amputations reported by 23 units between 1958–1975. In only nine cases subsequent overt invasive cancer developed; in most of these, a pre-existing preclinical invasive lesion probably was present. Conisation is a safe treatment in the following conditions:

Focal lesions when the exact limits can be seen colposcopically;

Lesions extending for an unknown distance into the cervical canal and when the upper sections of the cone are histologically free of cancer.

If these criteria are maintained, there is no logical reason for performing a more radical procedure such as a hysterectomy, simply because the patient is over 40 or 50 years of age.

The cone should be sufficiently radical to remove the lesion completely and the cone can be tailored accurately if prior colposcopy has been performed. The operation is done as an inpatient procedure under general anaesthesia; the aim is to remove a cone of cervical tissue, the base of which lies outside any area shown by Schiller's iodine to be suspect (see Figures 15 and 16 on page 112). The apex of the cone is above the level of the atypical epithelium. This ensures that the epithelium, plus a cone of cervical stromal tissue, is available for histological examination. Uterine curettage is carried out immediately the cone has been obtained. It is unfortunate that this comparatively minor operation is sometimes followed by secondary haemorrhage with the patient requiring re-admission to hospital and possibly blood transfusion. Since using PGA suture material and the technique described below, there has been a significant reduction in this complication.

1 Preoperative appearance of cervix

With the patient in the lithotomy position and draped, an Auvard and a Sims' speculum jointly expose the cervix. There is a wide transformation zone and without the application of Schiller's iodine it would be difficult to decide on the line of incision on the ectocervix. Schiller's iodine is therefore applied to the cervix and upper vagina.

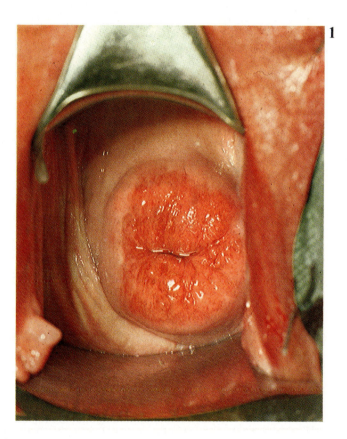

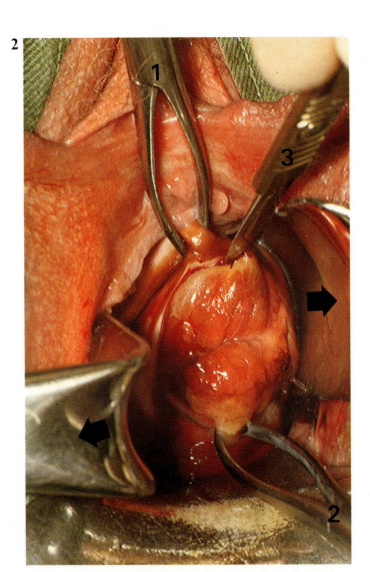

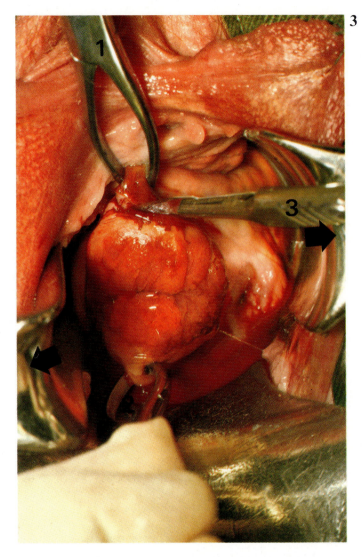

2 and 3 Excision of cone – anterior incision

The Schiller's test shows a large area of atypical epithelium over the ectocervix emphasising the need for a widely-based cone. In Figure 2 the anterior aspect of the cervix is held by tissue forceps (1) which are applied on the healthy brown-staining skin. Another pair of tissue forceps is applied posteriorly (2), also on a brown-staining area. The incision is being made with the scalpel (3) clear of the suspect area and it is held at an angle that will ensure that the apex of the cone is above the atypical epithelium. It will be seen that the epithelium on the area for biopsy is not held with forceps or traumatised in any way. In Figure 3 the anterior incision is deepened and extended in the direction described and making circular sweeps to form the body of a cone with its apex in this case at about the level of the internal os. It is essential to have a good view of the cervix when doing this operation and Sim's specula are used to retract the vaginal walls laterally in the direction of the broad arrows.

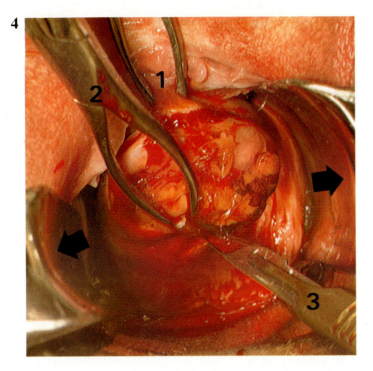

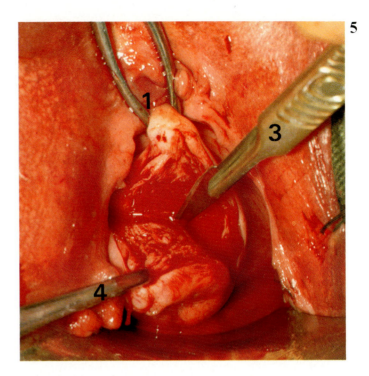

4 and 5 Excision of cone – posterior and lateral incisions

In Figure 4 the tissue forceps (2) are pulled to the right while the scalpel (3) makes a left postero-lateral incision well outside the non-stained area. In Figure 5 the incision is deepened and brought forward to join the previous anterior incision thus freeing the cone on the left side. The dissecting forceps (4) are steadying the cone but are applied to the cut muscular surface and not to the epithelium.

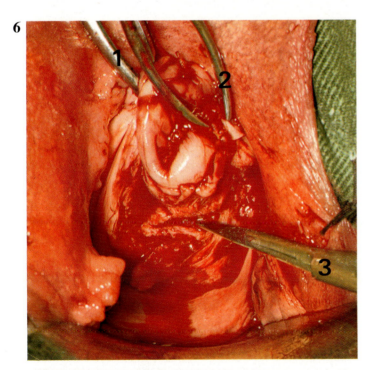

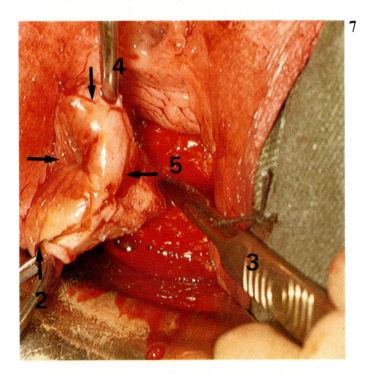

6 and 7 Excision of cone – complete removal

In Figure 6 the scalpel continues to free the cone posteriorly with the line of incision towards its apex. In Figure 7 a left lateral view shows the cone being separated from the uterus at (5). A tissue forceps (4) has replaced the dissecting forceps in supporting the cone anteriorly and the extent of the biopsy is now obvious (arrowed).

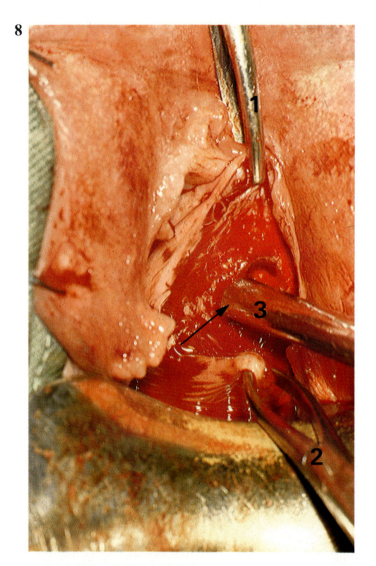

8

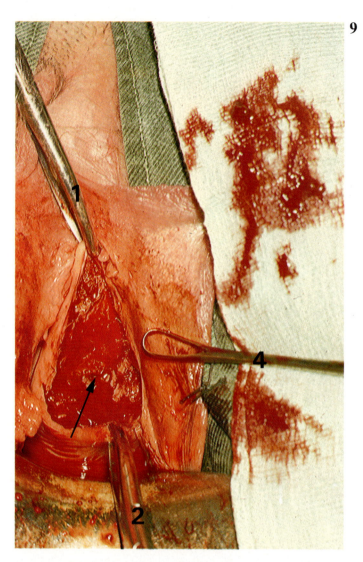

9

8 and 9 Dilatation and curettage

With the cone removed there is no danger of traumatising the cervical epithelium and the anterior lip of the cervix is grasped firmly with tissue forceps (1) and also steadied posteriorly by tissue forceps (2). Dilatation to at least No. 12

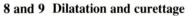

Hegar is carried out (3) in Figure 8. In Figure 9 curettage has been done with a medium-sized curette (4) and the curettings are seen on the gauze swab to the left of the introitus. The position of the internal cervical os is indicated by an arrow in each photograph.

3 Hysterectomy in the treatment of preclinical cervical cancer

This alternative is seldom indicated for CIN unless there is some other reason for hysterectomy; with preclinical invasion the operation is more frequently indicated. In the latter group there has been a recent but distinct trend towards hysterectomy, especially in the younger woman where prior conisation or punch biopsy under colposcopic vision has revealed histological evidence of microinvasive carcinoma. Coppleson (1976) and other authors present convincing evidence of the excellent results obtainable in the treatment of preclinical invasive disease by hysterectomy or even cone biopsy.

The presence of a surprise positive cytological smear in association with other gynaecological conditions such as dysfunctional uterine bleeding, prolapse or fibroids and which would normally require hysterectomy, needs a full colposcopic assessment prior to surgery. If the whole lesion is visible and the colposcopic appearance does not suggest preclinical invasion and where columnar epithelium is present above the lesion in the endocervix, preliminary conisation is unnecessary. The criticism that invasive cancer has not been satisfactorily excluded and might be under-treated does not arise if colposcopy has been employed in preoperative assessment.

Although many authors prefer the vaginal to the abdominal route in such cases, there is an important place for the latter. This is especially so if there is associated intra-pelvic pathology such as large fibroids, endometriosis, or the frequent presence in this group of chronic inflammatory disease. There is some controversy as to the value of removing a cuff of vagina at hysterectomy. The ectocervix must be completely excised but the authors do not believe that special efforts need be taken to remove vaginal skin since the atypical transformation zone extends on to the vaginal fornix in only about 3–4 per cent of cases. On the other hand, Figures 1 and 2 show the atypical area (1) outlined (arrowed) by the Schiller iodine stain extending on to the vaginal fornix. This area certainly must be removed and this is shown being done in the course of the operation. Failure to eradicate such an area results in the appearance of so-called recurrent CIN at the vaginal vault and could well explain some of the rare recurrent invasive cancers which have been reported in this site following hysterectomy.

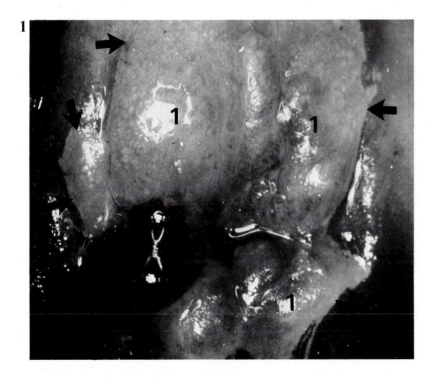
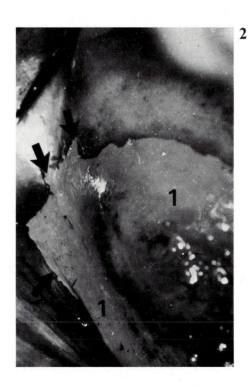

Stage 1: Securing upper uterine attachments

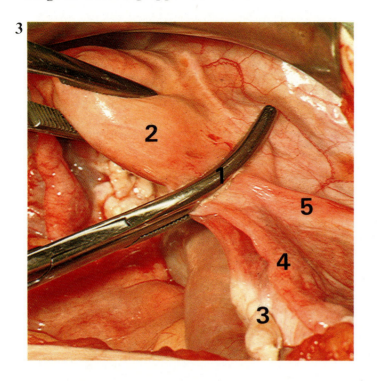

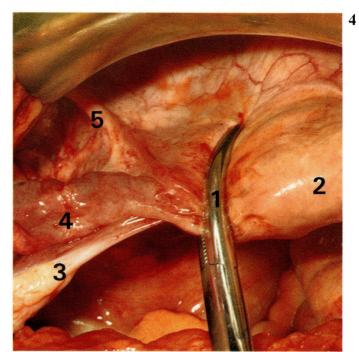

3 and 4 Clamping broad ligament
A curved Oschner forceps (1) is applied to the right broad ligament in Figure 3 and to the left broad ligament in Figure 4. The uterus and corresponding ovary, tube and round ligament are at (2), (3), (4) and (5) in each case.

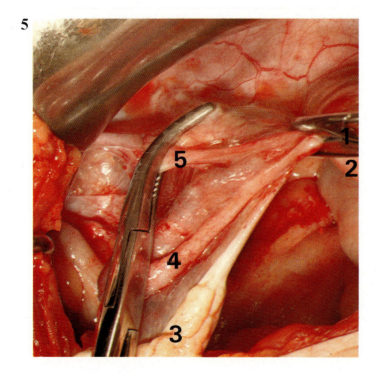

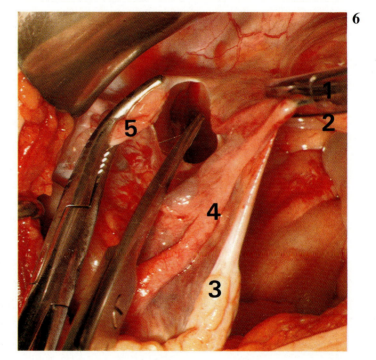

5 and 6 Detaching left round ligament
The left round ligament (5) is held in Phillip's forceps in Figure 5 and has been detached with the scissors in Figure 6.

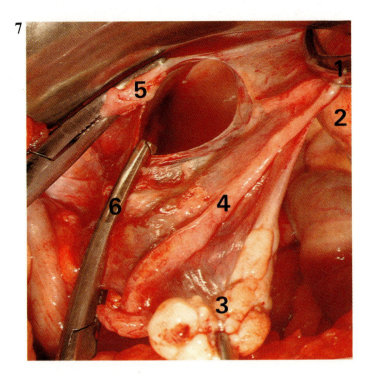

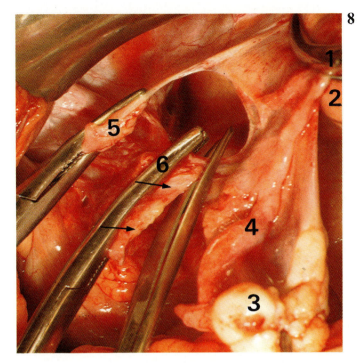

7 and 8 Securing left ovarian pedicle

The left ovarian pedicle is clamped with forceps (6) in Figure 7 and the appendages are detached just distal to it but leaving about 0.5 cm cuff of tissue in Figure 8 (arrowed).

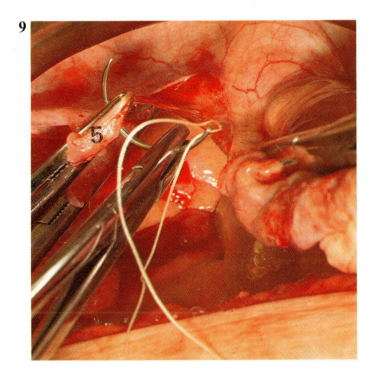

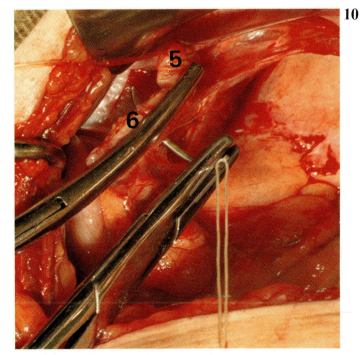

9 and 10 Ligating left round ligament and ovarian pedicles

A round-bodied needle carrying a PGA No. 1 suture transfixes the left round ligament pedicle (5) prior to ligation in Figure 9. The left ovarian pedicle (6) is similarly transfixed in Figure 10 and the ligated round ligament pedicle is seen (5).

Stage 2: Opening broad ligament and defining uterine vessels

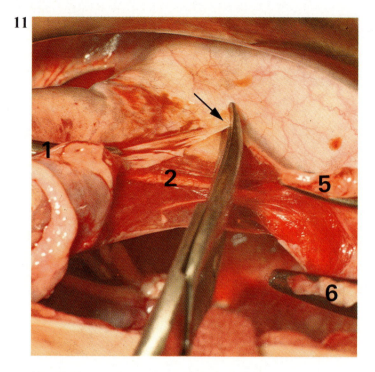

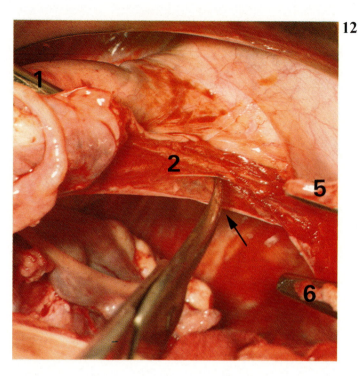

11 and 12 Opening up right broad ligament

In Figure 11 the anterior layer of the right broad ligament is opened up with scissors where arrowed, and in Figure 12 the posterior layer is similarly opened where arrowed. The broad ligament forceps is at (1) and the still untied right round ligament and ovarian pedicles at (5) and (6) respectively. The uterine vessels are seen at (2) in both photographs.

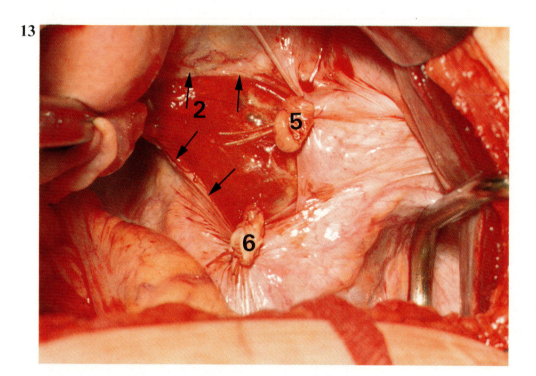

13 Right round ligament and ovarian pedicles ligated

The pedicles are at (5) and (6) and the anterior and posterior edges of the opened broad ligament are arrowed. The uterine vessels are still visible at (2). The same procedure is now carried out on the left side.

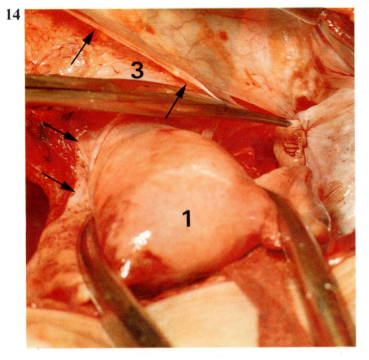

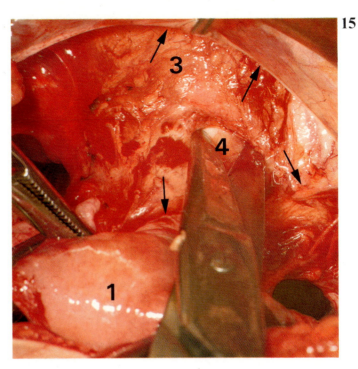

14 and 15 Opening utero-vesical pouch

In Figure 14 the uterus (1) is held up by the broad ligament forceps while the scissors divide the peritoneum over the utero-vesical pouch to expose the bladder (3). The edges of the cut peritoneum are arrowed. In Figure 15 the scissors separate the bladder off the front of the uterus and cervix where a good plane of separation has been found at (4). The peritoneal edges are again arrowed.

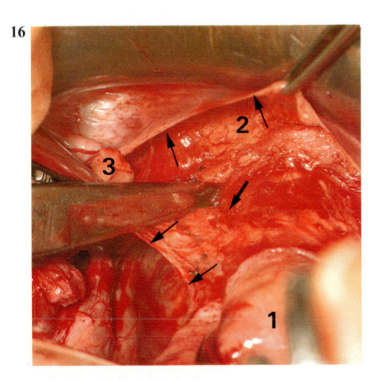

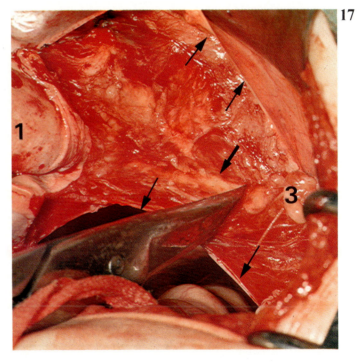

16 and 17 Defining uterine vessels

The scissors define the uterine vessels by blunt dissection on the left side in Figure 16 and on the right side in Figure 17. Other structures in the photograph are: uterus (1), bladder (2), round ligament pedicles (3); the uterine vessels are indicated by arrows.

Stage 3: Securing lower uterine attachments

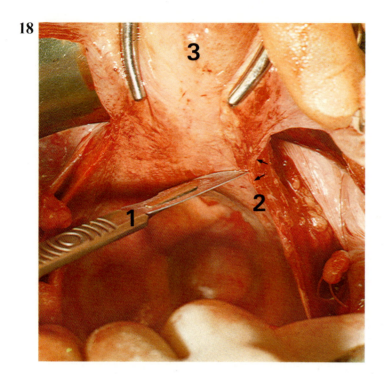

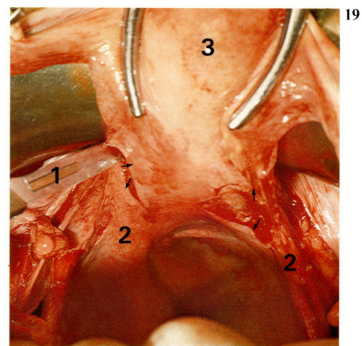

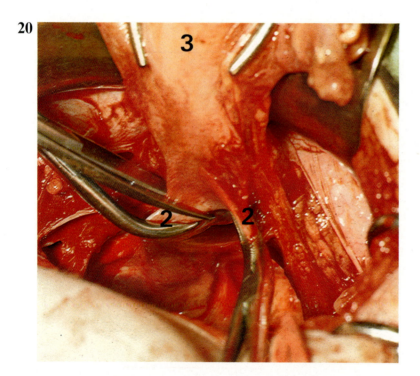

18 to 20 Defining and clamping utero-sacral ligaments

In Figure 18 the scalpel (1) divides the posterior layer of the right broad ligament where arrowed to expose the right utero-sacral ligament (2) at its attachment to the uterus (3). In Figure 19 the same procedure is carried out on the opposite side and the same numbers are used. In Figure 20 each utero-sacral ligament has been secured by forceps and the scissors are about to detach the left ligament from the uterus.

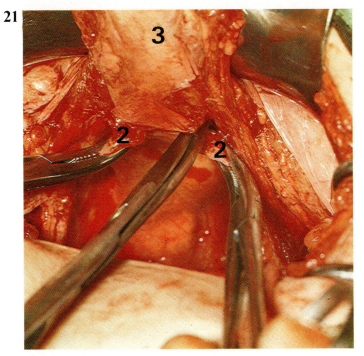

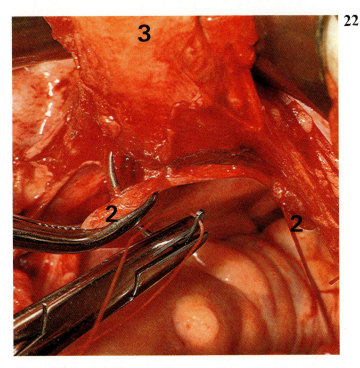

21 and 22 Detaching and ligating utero-sacral ligaments

In Figure 21 the scissors have divided the left ligament from the uterus and are doing the same on the right side. In

Figure 22 the right ligament has been ligated and the sutures left long (2) and the other utero-sacral pedicle is being transfixed prior to ligation.

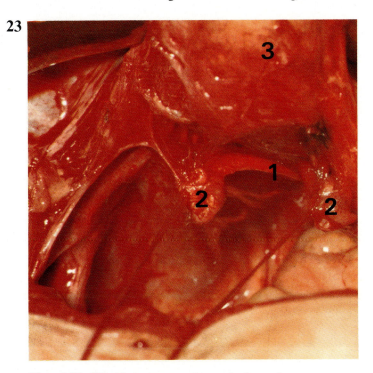

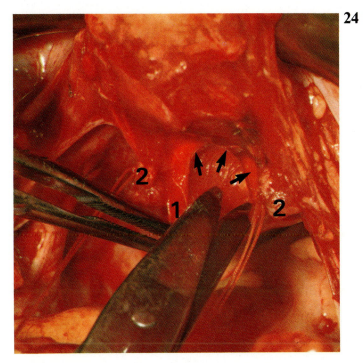

23 and 24 Opening upper recto-vaginal pouch

It is important that a liberal cuff of upper vagina be removed in this case and the utero-sacral pedicles with the intervening parietal peritoneum are stripped off the posterior vaginal wall in the region of the posterior fornix to free the

vaginal skin in that area. The ligated pedicles (2) and (2) with the intervening peritoneal edge (1) are displayed by traction on the uncut sutures in Figure 23 and the scissors open the upper part of the recto-vaginal space (arrowed) where it overlies the posterior vaginal fornix in Figure 24.

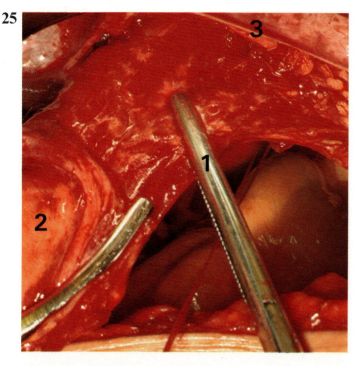

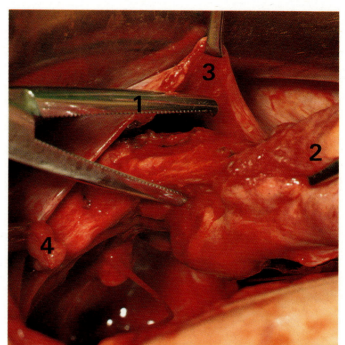

25 and 26 Clamping uterine pedicles

The straight Oschner forceps (1) clamps the previously defined right uterine vessels in Figure 25 and the same is being done on the left side in Figure 26. The uterus is at (2), the bladder (3) and the round ligament pedicle (4).

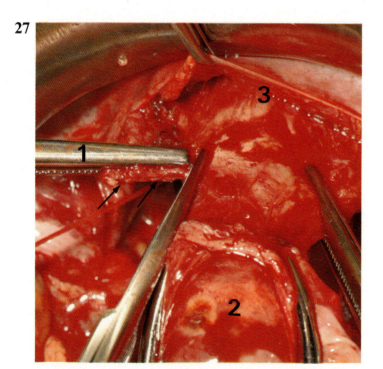

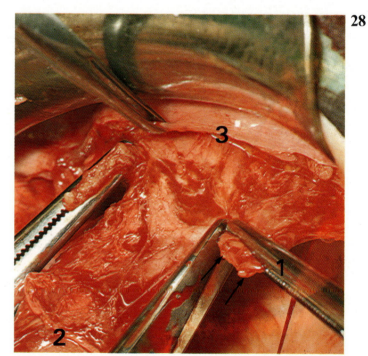

27 and 28 Detaching uterine pedicles from uterus

The left uterine vessels are detached with scissors distal to the forceps leaving a cuff of tissue and ensuring that the pedicle is sufficiently freed to allow secure ligation. The same is done on the right side in Figure 28. The pedicle is arrowed on each side.

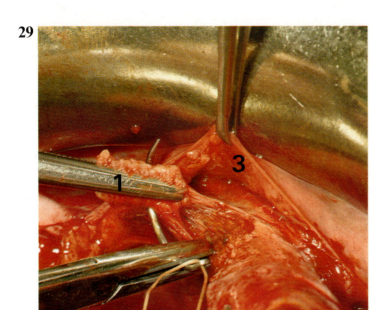

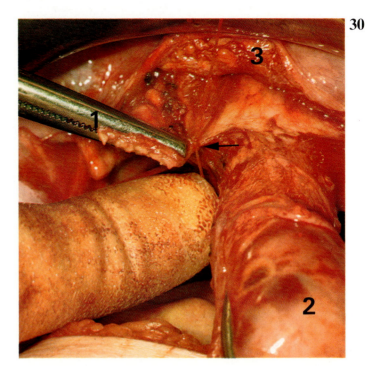

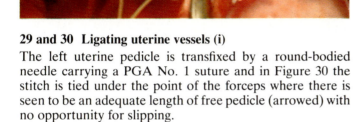

30

29 and 30 Ligating uterine vessels (i)

The left uterine pedicle is transfixed by a round-bodied needle carrying a PGA No. 1 suture and in Figure 30 the stitch is tied under the point of the forceps where there is seen to be an adequate length of free pedicle (arrowed) with no opportunity for slipping.

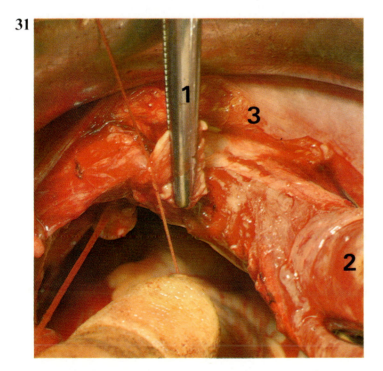

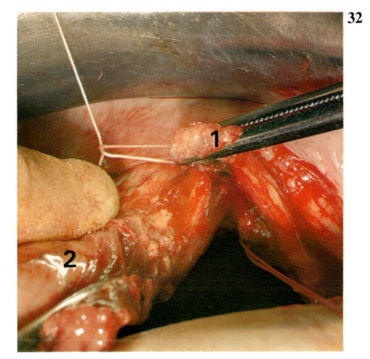

31 and 32 Ligating uterine vessels (ii)

The ligature is now taken under the heel of the forceps in Figure 31 and there is adequate tissue beyond it to prevent any slipping. These pedicles are always double-tied and in Figure 32 the forceps have been reapplied at (1) and the second ligature is being placed.

Stage 4: Removal of uterus

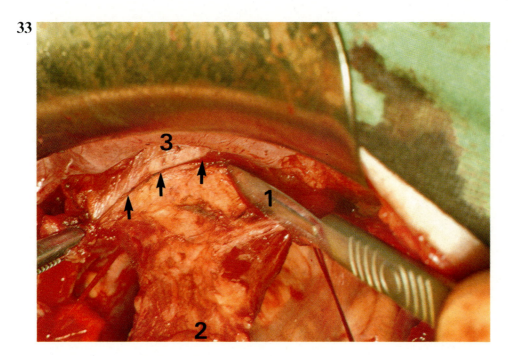

33 Separation of bladder from uterus (i)

When it is important, as in this case, to remove a generous cuff of upper vaginal skin, the surgeon must completely separate the bladder downwards off the cervix to free the vagina in the region of the anterior fornix. In the photo-graph, the scalpel (1) is being stroked across the upper part of the vagina to divide any remaining fibres of the pubo-cervical fascia and the bladder (3) is then pushed away from the uterus (2) along the line of the arrows.

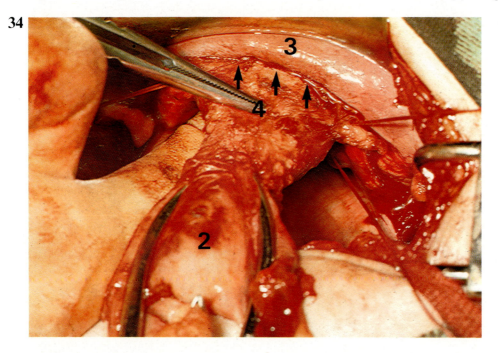

34 Separation of bladder from uterus (ii)

This more general view shows the uterus (2) pulled upwards with the bladder (3) stripped off the vagina as far as the arrowed edge. The point of the dissecting forceps (4) indicates the level of the external cervical os so that the incision line into the vagina must be distal to it.

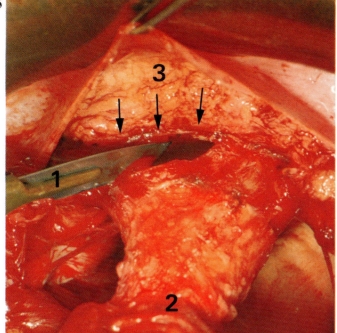

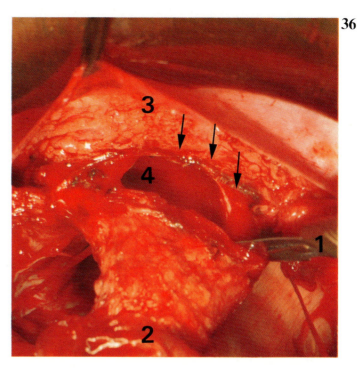

36

35 and 36 Opening into vagina anteriorly

The application of forceps to the vaginal angles before opening into the canal limits the amount of anterior vaginal wall skin that can be removed. In a case like this, the scalpel (1) is used to cut boldly into the anterior vaginal fornix just clear of the bladder edge (arrowed) and remove the maximum amount of vaginal skin anteriorly. The incision is taken towards the left in the first instance. The edge of the bladder is clearly seen so that there is little danger of injuring it. In Figure 36 the anterior fornix is opened towards the right side and the cavity of the vagina (4) is clearly seen.

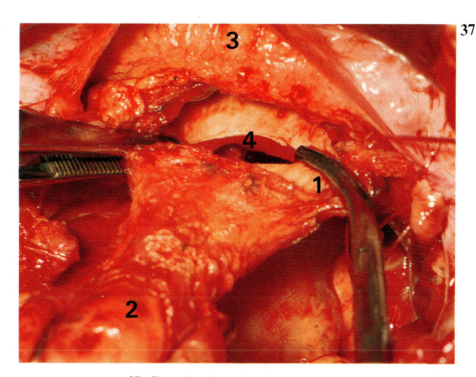

37 Clamping the vaginal angles

There is much more skin available posteriorly and the vaginal arteries reach the vaginal wall postero-laterally so that it is appropriate to apply clamps in that area. This is seen being done on the right side (1) with one limb of the forceps within the vagina and the other external to it.

38

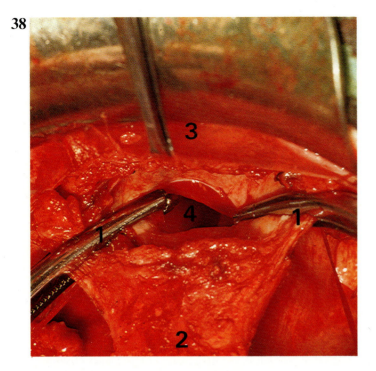

39

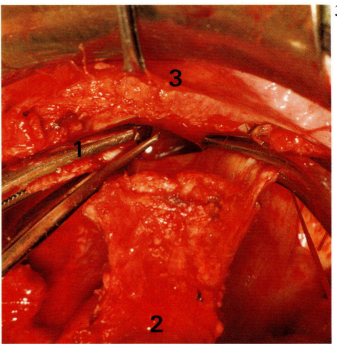

38 to 40 Opening the vagina posteriorly

In Figure 38 a second forceps (1) clamps the left side to match that on the right (1) and in Figure 39 the scissors detach the uterus on the left side by cutting through the posterior vaginal wall distal to the forceps (1). The same has been done on the right side in Figure 40 (1) and the uterus (2) is now free.

40

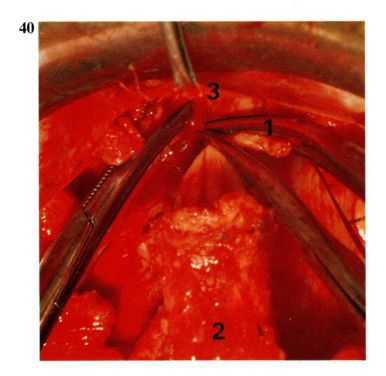

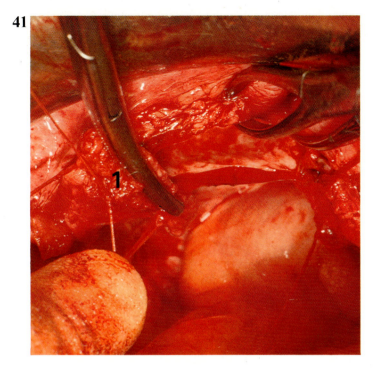
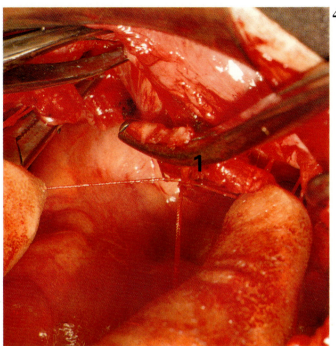

41 and 42 Ligation of vaginal angles

Secure ligatures (1) and (1) are applied to the vaginal angles on the left in Figure 41 and on the right in Figure 42. When forceps are applied with one leg external to, and the other within the vaginal canal, the pedicle consists of a single rather than a double layer of vaginal wall and it is therefore more easily ligated. It is possible to place a first tie under the point of the forceps before carrying it round the heel to complete ligation.

Stage 5: Closure of vaginal vault

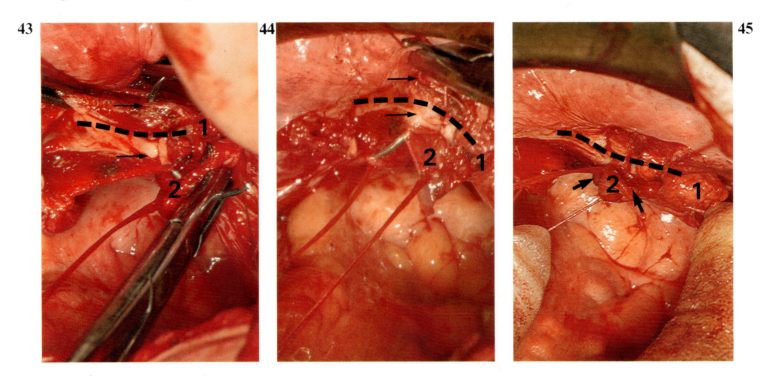

43 to 45 Incorporation of right utero-sacral ligament in vault closure

The left vaginal angle is ligated at (1) in all three photographs. The needle carrying the mattress suture transfixes the right utero-sacral ligament pedicle (2) and both edges of the vaginal wall (arrowed) in Figure 43. It returns through the same structures in the reverse direction in Figure 44 (arrowed) and is tied off in Figure 45 to embrace the utero-sacral ligament which is thereby fixed to the right posterior wall of the vaginal vault, where indicated by short arrows.

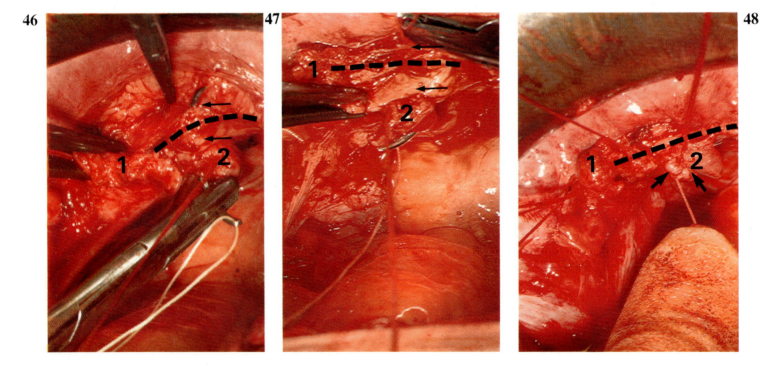

46 to 48 Incorporation of left utero-sacral ligament in vault closure

Exactly the same procedure is carried out on the left side and the same numbers and indicators are used.

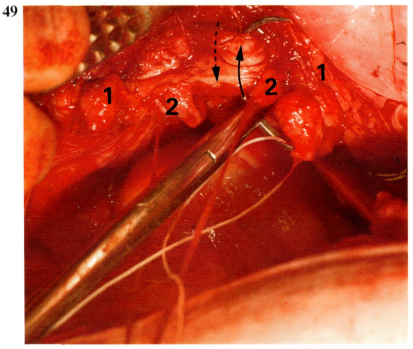

49 Central mattress stitch to vaginal vault

The suture-carrying needle transfixes both walls of the vagina postero-anteriorly and returns in the opposite direction (as arrowed) to complete the central mattress suture. The vaginal angle pedicles are at (1) and (1) and the utero-sacral pedicles are now incorporated in the vault (2) and (2).

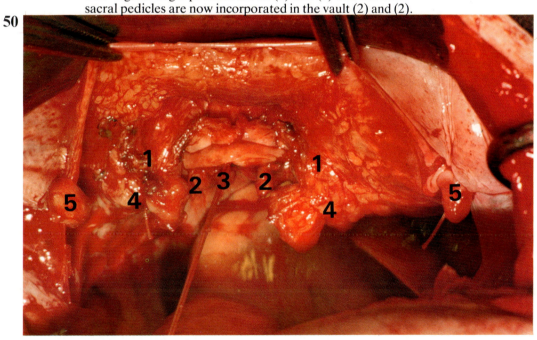

50 Closure of vaginal vault completed

The central mattress suture (3) is still uncut and used as a tractor. The various pedicles are numbered thus: vaginal angles (1), utero-sacral ligaments (2), uterine pedicles (4), round ligament pedicles (5).

Stage 6: Reperitonisation

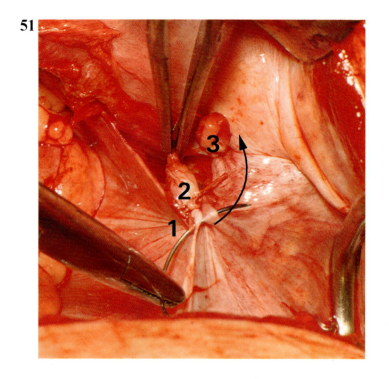

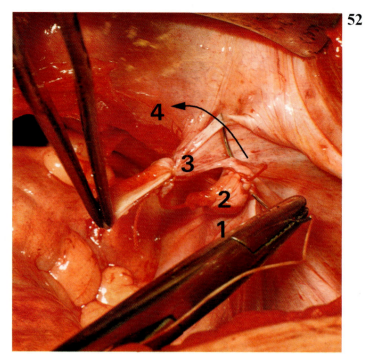

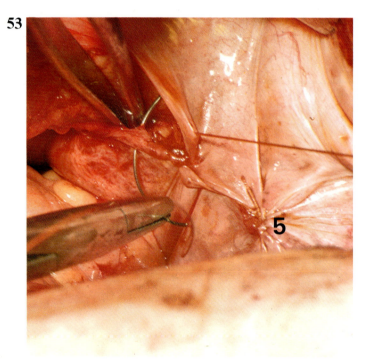

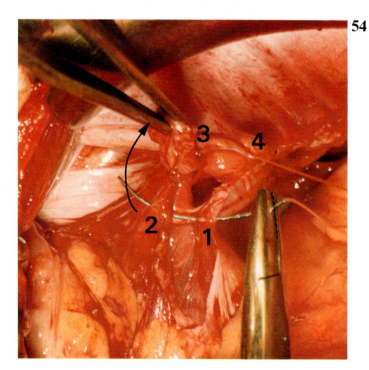

51 to 54 Steps in closure of pelvic peritoneum

The round-bodied needle carrying a PGA No. 00 suture commences the half purse string stitch from the posterior layer of the broad ligament (1) round the right ovarian pedicle (2) and right round ligament pedicle (3) in the direction of the arrow. In Figure 52 it picks up the peritoneum over the round ligament and will then include the anterior edge of the broad ligament at (4). In Figure 53 the half purse string suture has been tied off at (5) to cover the pedicles and the stitch proceeds across the pelvis. In Figure 54 a similar half purse string stitch is commencing on the left side and the numbers of structures involved are the same as on the right side.

55

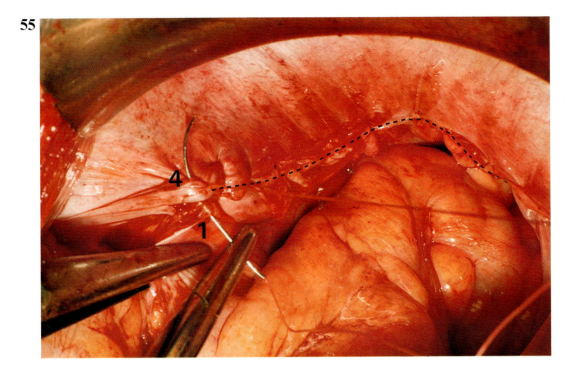

55 Closure of pelvic peritoneum completed

The needle is seen transfixing the posterior (1) and the
anterior (4) edges of the broad ligament and the left ovarian
and round ligament pedicles are already hidden from view.
When the stitch is finally tied they are completely extra-
peritoneal. The dotted line indicates the transverse peritoneal closure.

56

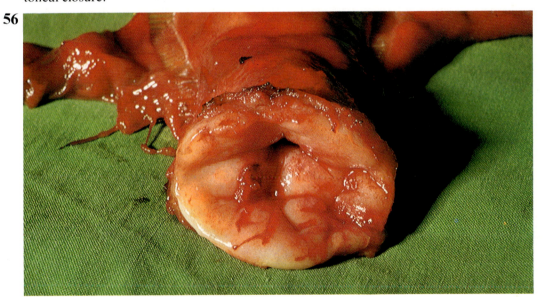

56 Specimen

The uterus is seen to have a very generous cuff of vagina
attached to it and this is obviously important in such a case as
the preoperative assessment showed the area of atypical
epithelium to extend on to the vaginal vault.

Clinical cervical carcinoma

General considerations in treatment

Established or invasive cervical cancer may be treated in either of two ways. One is by a combination of internal solid radiation sources and external irradiation; the other is by radical surgery. On the basis of clinical staging there is little to choose between the five-year cure rate obtained by good surgery and by radiotherapy. Unless there are exceptional circumstances, radiotherapy is in the hands of specialist radiotherapists; a brief description is given in Chapter 7 of the methods and techniques used in this centre. Surgical treatment is described below and takes the form of the Wertheim radical hysterectomy. Its only possible rival is the Schauta vaginal procedure which, in the authors' view, has the inadmissible disadvantage of not including pelvic lymphadenectomy.

Since the Wertheim operation is a formidable one for surgeon as well as patient, readers will wish to know in what circumstances they ought to use radical surgery and, since radiotherapy has given comparable results, whether they need to use it at all.

It is easier to start by saying where it should not be used. Stage 3 and Stage 4 growths are beyond the scope of surgery and only an expert would be persuaded by special indications to do the operation in Stage 2b cases.

There are cases where it might seem that the advantage lies with surgery. These are in clinical stages 1b and 2a where the growth is well, or even moderately well, differentiated. Fractionally higher five-year and especially ten-year cure rates have been reported with surgery but it must be remembered that in many of these cases radiotherapy is employed in an ancillary rôle and could claim some of the credit. Surgery avoids radiation burns and it is satisfying to the patient to know that the growth has been extirpated. Most women still have a fear and distrust of radiotherapy which it is difficult to overcome.

Surgery also has its disadvantages. There is a mortality rate of around one per cent, bladder symptoms can be very troublesome and the joint incidence of uretero- and vesico-vaginal fistulae is about 5 per cent. The vagina is shortened and dyspareunia may result. Even with meticulous selection the growth may be found at operation to involve the outer parametrium or the bladder. Bleeding from the pelvic side wall or from internal iliac vessels can make controlled lymphadenectomy impossible: then, even in the hands of an expert, the operation becomes incomplete.

Cancer of the cervix at the various stages of pregnancy presents additional problems in treatment. These will be fully discussed in Volume 6 of the Atlas but there is general agreement that surgery is to be preferred in the early stages of pregnancy.

There are cases where there is virtually no choice and surgery must be looked on as the correct method:

1 Growths of adenomatous type which usually involve the cervical canal. Such tumours respond poorly to radiotherapy.

2 Growths where the radiotherapist has histological evidence that there is little response to initial treatment. Surgical treatment should be substituted without delay.

3 Severe previous pelvic inflammatory disease is almost certain to be reactivated by radiotherapy and this risk should be avoided.

4 Large uterine fibroids or ovarian cysts distort the anatomy and make accurate positioning of internal radiation sources impossible. Such tumours are themselves liable to irradiation necrosis with resultant severe intra-abdominal complications.

5 Cases where congenital, traumatic or postoperative narrowing of the vaginal vault prevents satisfactory placement of internal radiation sources.

6 Cases of cervical cancer in early pregnancy.

7 Some patients will not countenance radiotherapy and ask specifically for surgical treatment.

Operation is indicated in one group of cases and contra-indicated in another. In a third group, the gynaecologist can choose with propriety either radiation or surgery as the primary treatment. It is not in any way reprehensible that he should elect to treat some of this latter group surgically to ensure that he become sufficiently skilled in radical operations to offer an adequate standard of surgery to all his patients. The authors believe that this is the policy adopted by most young surgeons.

Results of treatment of cervical carcinoma

The Annual Report (1976) gives the five-year survival rates for each of the four stages of cervical cancer for the period 1964–1968. These are compiled from 61,146 patients treated in 109 Institutions (Table 1). There is, of course, considerable variation in treatment ranging from radiotherapy alone to surgery alone and with many combinations of these two methods. The figures are set out in Table 1 below and they give an overall estimate of what can be expected from a combination of all types of therapy. The results from radical surgical treatment will be considered later.

Table 1

Five-year survival rate (all methods of treatment) for each of the 4 stages for the years 1964–1968

	Number of patients treated	Alive at 5 Years	Survival rate (%)
Stage 1	18,440	14,829	80.4
Stage 2	22,482	13,231	58.9
Stage 3	17,290	5,668	32.8
Stage 4	2,934	208	7.1
Total	61,146	33,936	55.5

Examination, staging and biopsy

The initial management of clinical carcinoma of the cervix is so important that the gynaecologist should have a clear-cut plan of action which he can apply to each case.

The first requirement is to confirm the diagnosis by biopsy and the second is to establish by clinical, histological and other available methods the extent of the disease and the cell behaviour of the tumour. Then an appropriate treatment can be chosen, a prognosis be given and the result of therapy eventually assessed. The F.I.G.O. classification was introduced to correlate the extent and severity of the disease with the treatment given; the results obtained and the benefits from its universal application are enormous.

The gynaecologist first sees the patient in clinic or office. The diagnosis is usually obvious and the patient is admitted to hospital for biopsy and investigation. In very advanced cases patients are sometimes referred directly to a radiotherapist with a request for palliative treatment. This is inadvisable because the case is primarily a gynaecological one and should be assessed as such. In addition, the radiotherapist is being used as a technician and is denied the opportunity of acting in a proper and equal consultative capacity. Surgeon and radiotherapist should work in close liaison and jointly decide on the best method of treatment but, in our opinion, the patient should retain the personal support of the gynaecologist, as the doctor in charge of her case.

The patient is admitted to hospital without delay and her general condition is investigated in routine fashion. She is informed that a preliminary examination under anaesthetic is necessary before deciding on the appropriate treatment. This examination is described in the text and conveniently combines several procedures. A detailed and careful bimanual vaginal examination is made to 'stage' the growth according to the F.I.G.O. classification and digital rectal examination forms an essential part. Biopsies of the cervix are taken from representative areas and the cervical canal is dilated and curettings taken separately from the cervical canal and from the cavity of the uterus. The bladder is examined by cystoscopy and there is increasing interest in laparoscopy as a method of obtaining maximum information. The various investigations may be done in whatever sequence is thought likely to cause the least amount of bleeding and contamination of healthy structures; this is considered in the text.

Once the growth has been 'staged' and the histological report is available, the situation can be explained to the patient and the suggested line of treatment discussed. The method of treatment has to take into consideration her general medical condition which, also, might be discussed with the patient.

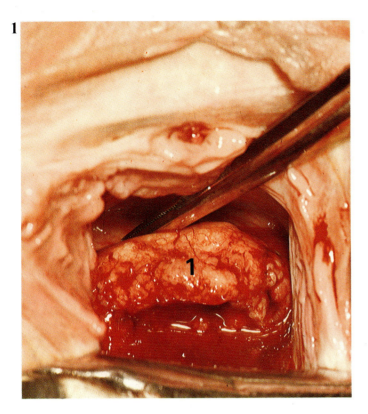

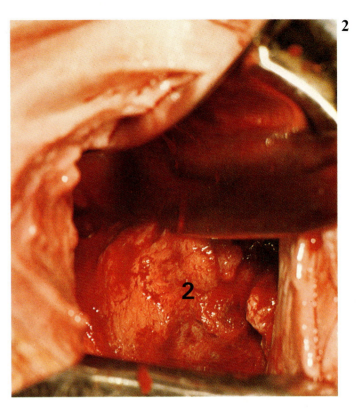

1 and 2 Speculum examination

The carcinoma illustrated is of exophytic type, involving the whole circumference of the cervix but limited to the upper third of the vagina. In Figure 1 the Auvard speculum exposes the upper vagina and the sponge-holding forceps displaces the anterior wall to show the anterior lip of the cervix. The appearances are typical of clinical carcinoma of the cervix. In Figure 2 an anterior retractor lifts the anterior vaginal wall and lower uterus forward to expose the posterior lip of the cervix. The friable and necrotic growth is clearly seen. The anterior lip of the cervix is at (1); the posterior lip (2).

3 Bimanual vaginal examination

The size, position, consistency and mobility of the uterus and appendages are estimated as accurately as possible. Particular attention is paid to outward spread of the growth from the cervix. The degree to which the parametrium is involved is all-important in 'staging' and prognosis, and it is essential to gain a clear impression of whether or not such spread has reached the side wall of the pelvis. To do so, the surgeon feels carefully with the forefinger to determine whether there is a soft area or space between the growth medially and the pelvic wall laterally on each side. Spread along the utero-sacral ligaments is also estimated vaginally, although it can be done more accurately by rectal examination as described subsequently.

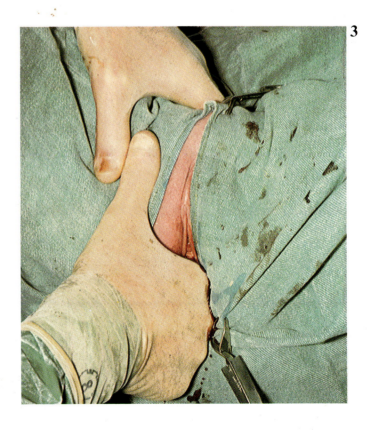

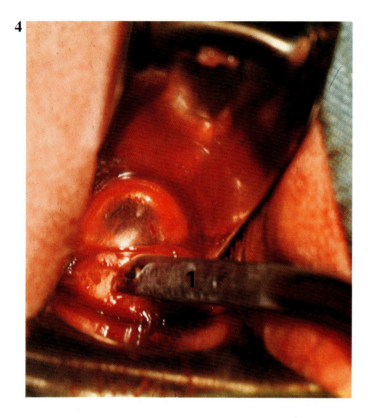

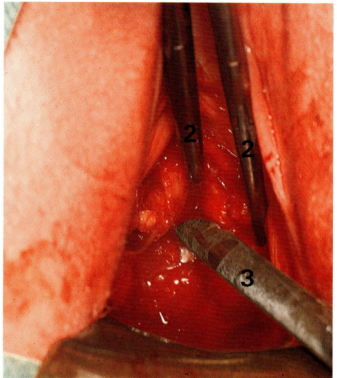

4 Biopsy of cervix

Biopsies are taken with punch forceps (1) from representative areas of the growth. Although the whole cervix is

vascular the growth is necrotic and bleeding is minimal so that stitches are not required: they should be avoided if possible.

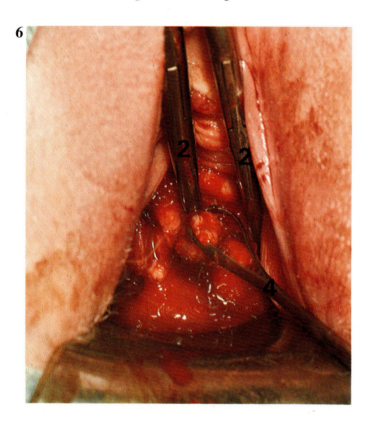

5 and 6 Dilatation and curettage

It is important to know whether there is spread to the cervical canal and whether there is any intra-uterine growth. D. and C., therefore, is essential. The cervix is seen being dilated in Figure 5. The external os may be difficult to find and care should be exercised in using fine uterine dilators and the uterine sound, because it is easy to make a false passage in the soft tissue and cause bleeding and infection. We recommend the use of a bladder sound as very useful and safe in locating the external os. Curettings are seen being obtained in Figure 6 and fractional curettage should be attempted always, so that the epithelium from the cervical canal and from the cavity of the uterus can be examined separately. Tissue forceps on the anterior lip of the cervix are at (2), the cervical dilator (3) and the curette (4).

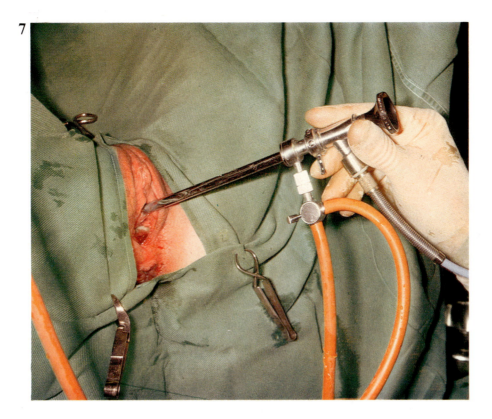

7 Cystoscopy

It is essential to know whether the growth involves the bladder, and the base and posterior wall of that structure are examined with great care. There is nearly always some hyperaemia of the trigone but unless there is visible involvement of the mucosa or severe bullous emphysema and telangectiasis indicating that the subjacent wall is affected, the bladder is unlikely to be involved. Bladder capacity, ureteric orifice efflux and any bladder lesion or abnormality are carefully observed.

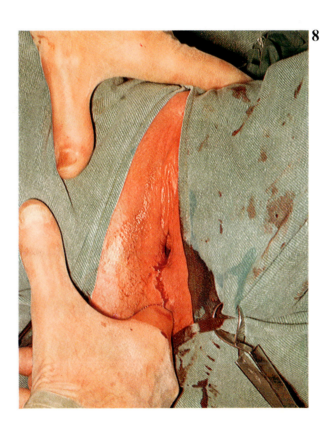

8 Rectal examination

This important examination should be made last to avoid soiling the raw vascular area of the cervix and upper vagina. The most important point to establish is whether there is spread postero-laterally along the utero-sacral ligaments and, if so, to what extent. The degree to which surgery can be successful depends very much on the extent of such spread. Extension of the growth in the recto-vaginal space should be excluded and this can be done by rectal examination. Some surgeons make the rectal examination with the middle finger and with the forefinger of the same hand in the vagina, but we find no particular advantage in so doing.

Radical hysterectomy with pelvic lymphadenectomy (Wertheim's hysterectomy)

The primary object of the Wertheim operation is to remove the uterus and its appendages, the upper third or half of the vagina, the parametrial tissue and the pelvic lymph glands as far as the brim of the pelvis. An important consideration is to do so with minimal tissue trauma and to avoid damage to ureters, bladder and large blood vessels.

There have been many modifications of the operation as first described and not all are improvements on Wertheim's technique. Teachers naturally develop and promote their own preferences and the importance of variations in technique can be over-emphasised. This can confuse the less experienced who are primarily interested in learning how to do the operation adequately and with minimal danger to the patient. The procedure described here meets these requirements and has produced results which are extremely satisfactory.

General anaesthesia with controlled hypotension afforded by epidural or spinal anaesthesia, provides additional advantages both during and after the operation. A transverse abdominal incision gives adequate exposure and heals strongly and it is immensely more comfortable postoperatively. A fairly steep Trendelenberg position aids visualisation.

As practised by Victor Bonney, the operation is done in two stages – firstly, removing the uterus and appendages and then removing the glands. The most frequently described method at the present time is to remove the glands from the side wall of the pelvis before completing the hysterectomy. One reason for doing so is to make a block dissection of the glands, with the theoretical advantage of preventing dissemination of malignant cells into the blood stream. This reason would be difficult to substantiate. It is claimed, also, that the uterine artery is easily defined during the dissection of the glands and can be secured well lateral to the uterus at an early stage in the operation. This might be a valid point

except that the uterine veins are the vessels usually responsible for bleeding. They form an ill-defined plexus of vessels quite unsuitable for definitive ligation in this position and need to be secured properly at a later stage in the operation. In considering the incidence of uretero-vaginal fistulae (page 151), it will be seen that several authorities avoid ligation of the uterine artery lateral to the ureter since branches to the latter structure may be divided and lead to necrosis from impoverished blood supply.

The authors feel that, as it is impossible to know what difficulties will be encountered in a Wertheim operation, it is much more satisfactory to concentrate on removing the uterus initially. If an unexpectedly extensive spread of growth is encountered, the operation can be curtailed and lymphadenectomy abandoned in favour of radiotherapy before surgical intervention has gone beyond a point of no return. With the glands already dissected from the side walls of the pelvis before the true extent of the parametrial spread is recognised, the surgeon still has to embark on the most dangerous stage of the operation which, in the circumstances, will be incomplete. The operation may have occupied over an hour already and the patient lost considerable blood and fluid. Haemorrhage is most likely to occur when removing the pelvic glands and, if this happens, it is easier to deal with when the uterus has been removed from the pelvis and there is adequate access to control the bleeding. In an obese patient with an advanced growth this can be very important. We take the view that in all respects the Bonney procedure is a simple and safe operation with no loss of effectiveness in comparison with other methods. It is recommended for routine use to all who are not experienced cancer surgeons.

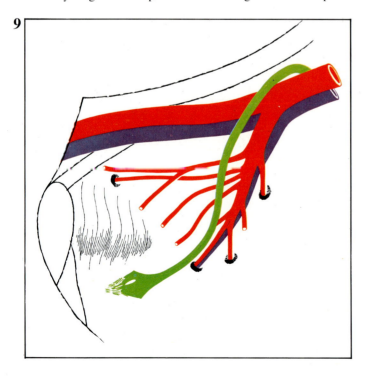

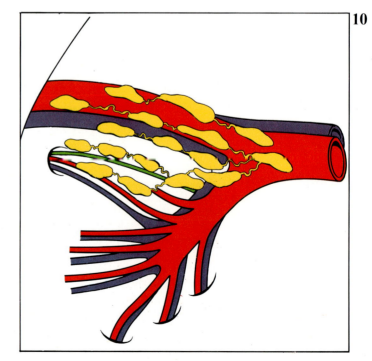

The vault of the vagina is closed as a routine, and extra-peritoneal Redivac drains are placed across the vault of the shortened vagina. Some surgeons prefer to leave the vault open and this is equally satisfactory, providing haemostasis is secured. An indwelling Foley catheter with bag drainage is used for five days postoperatively and it is the authors' routine to administer prophylactic antibiotics. Early ambulation is prescribed and subcutaneous heparin is being used increasingly as prophylaxis against venous thrombosis, remembering the increased risk of patients with gynaecological malignancy developing such complications.

Revision of surgical anatomy

The lymph drainage of the pelvis is shown diagramatically in Figure 10. The main line of lymph drainage from the cervix is by the internal iliac and the medial chain of the external iliac glands via the common iliac group to the para-aortic glands. Lymphography can be of assistance, as the dye stains the glands green and the radio-opaque material produces an inflammatory gland reaction which enlarges nodes to about twice their normal size. The course of the pelvic ureter in relation to the blood vessels is shown in Figure 9. The points at which the ureter may be damaged during operation have been dealt with in Chapter 1. When shown together, Figures 9 and 10 indicate the part of the ureter at risk when removing any particular group of glands.

The incidence of fistulae following Wertheim hysterectomy

Urinary fistulae are very distressing and so much has been written about their incidence in relation to the Wertheim operation that there is a danger of the surgeon losing perspective in this matter. In the Atlas, the authors have indicated the likely causative factors and possible technical errors and have explained how to anticipate the former and avoid the latter. They appreciate that anxiety persists and there is no doubt that fistulae, nearly all of them ureteric, can occur in apparently favourable surgical circumstances.

The incidence of ureteric fistulae following the Wertheim operation must be very difficult to compute but Mattingley and Borkowf (1978) believe that it has fallen from 8–10 per cent to the 2–3 per cent estimated by Symmonds (1966). The figures are not so frightening when one recognises that they must be influenced greatly by case selection and the extent of the disease.

Apart from operative injuries which should be recognised at the time, the basic factor in the development of ureteric fistulae is necrosis of the terminal ureter following impairment of its blood supply. This has been discussed. Various authors have modified the operation to overcome the problem (Buchsbaum 1978). For example, Burch (1965)

ligates the uterine artery medial to the ureter to preserve any branch to it. Novak (1956) leaves the uterine artery undivided until the end of the operation, when he retains the ureter within the peritoneal cavity to prevent kinking and obstruction to urine flow. Green (1966) suspends the ureter from the superior vesical artery for the same reasons and so that it can obtain an additional blood supply from the pelvic side wall. Ohkawa (1971) goes further and wraps the ureters in peritoneum so that they can develop a new blood supply. Table I, taken from Buchsbaum, shows the incidence of fistulae before and after the adoption of such methods.

Table I
Fistula rate related to change in intraoperative management of the ureters

Author	Years of study	Number of cases	Fistula rate (per cent)
Burch (1965)	1957	56	8.8
	1965	144	1.4
Novak (1969)	1920–1946	372	9.4
	1947–1953	246	11.4
	1954–1968	1,306	2.1
Green (1975)	1962–1966	286	5.6
	1966–1975	225	0.9

From Buchsbaum (1978)

The authors contend that the ureteric blood supply must never be impaired during dissection, for this is by far the most important single factor in causing fistulae. The ureteric mesentery should be preserved always and the technique of dividing the uterine vessels as they lie on the roof of the ureteric tunnel (pages 162–163) achieves what Burch and Novak advise. Using this technique in over 250 cases during the past 15 years, the senior author has not had a single case of ureteric fistula.

The immediate management of ureteric injuries depends upon their extent, and appropriate procedures are described by Mattingley and Borkowf (1978). All but the most severe are within the capacity of the average operator but submucosal re-implantation of the ureter or fashioning a Boari flap would make the presence of a urologist desirable. Subsequent elective closure of a ureteric fistula should be placed in the hands of a urological surgeon from the outset.

The possibility of litigation when a fistula develops is always very real. Without education, the non-medical mind cannot appreciate why the urinary tract should be at risk when removing the uterus and the surgeon must take steps to safeguard himself. It is the authors' policy, when discussing the operation with the patient, to explain that the risks of the operation include possible unavoidable damage to the urinary tract and that this must be accepted.

Wertheim hysterectomy
Stage 1: Vaginal preparation

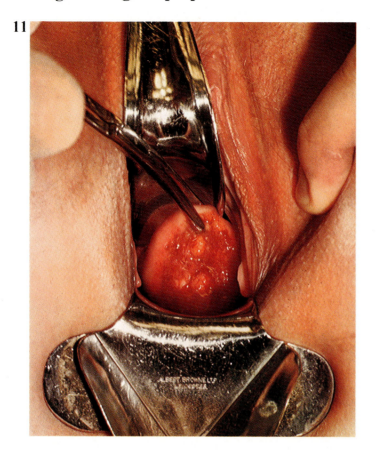

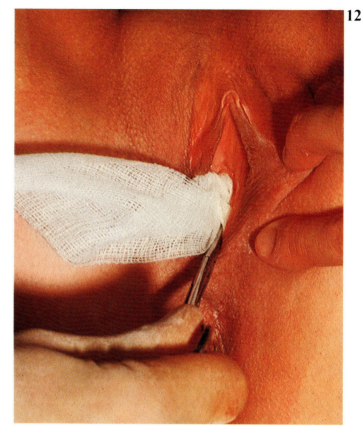

11 and 12 Catheterisation of bladder and packing of vagina

The patient is placed in the lithotomy position. The vagina is gently swabbed with antiseptic solution and the bladder is catheterised. A firm vaginal pack is inserted to elevate the uterus into the pelvis and serve as a central vaginal column which orientates the structures and against which dissection can be directed when defining the lower uterine attachments. In Figure 11 the Auvard's and Sims' specula expose the upper vagina while a tenaculum on the anterior lip of the cervix lifts it forward to give access to the posterior fornix where it is important that the gauze pack be firmly placed. A roll of dry gauze 3 inches wide is used to pack the vagina from the vault downwards and the specula are removed as this is done. Packing is complete in Figure 12 and the remainder of the gauze is strapped to the patient's leg so that it is easily available for removal by a nurse or assistant when dissection is complete. Although not shown in the photograph, it is usual to leave a Foley catheter in the bladder during the operation. If the procedure is prolonged, the bladder fills up with urine and this can be an embarrassment to the surgeon. Doubts about whether the bladder has been injured at any stage can be resolved by checking if there is haematuria.

Stage 2: Opening the abdomen

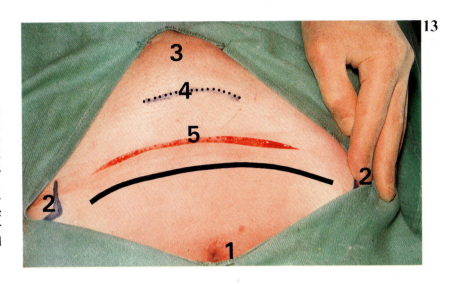

13

13 Skin incision

A transverse abdominal incision is made at the level of the thick black line. It is shown in relation to the usual gynaecological incision to emphasise the fact that the ends can be extended laterally above the anterior superior iliac spines to give whatever width and access is required. Skin markings and numbers are used as references, umbilicus (1), anterior superior iliac spines (2), symphysis pubis (3), low incision for lesser pelvic surgery (4), normal gynaecological incision (5).

14 and 15 Opening rectus sheath for adequate access

In Figure 14 the rectus sheath is opened transversely so that the lateral edges of the muscles are clearly seen. The inferior epigastric vessels lie just laterally (arrowed) and can be definitively secured and divided if the wound is extended. Figure 15 shows the considerable length of access centrally between the recti muscles, and this can easily be increased by further stripping of the rectus sheath from the muscles in the direction of the arrows. This type of transverse incision gives adequate access for a radical hysterectomy.

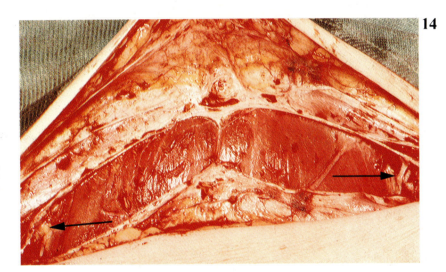

14

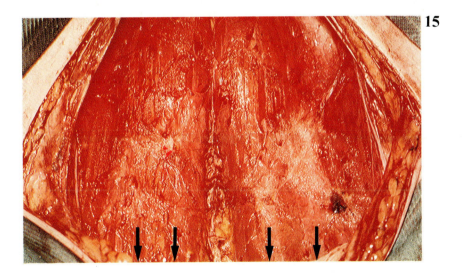

15

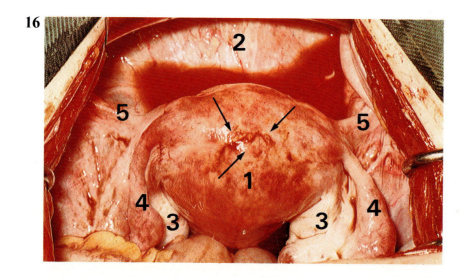

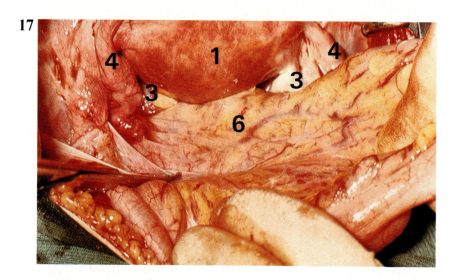

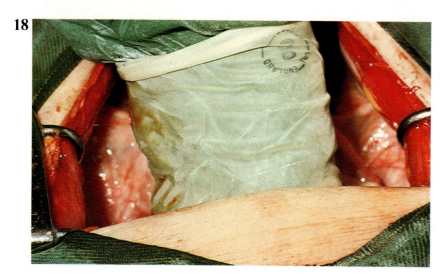

16 to 18 Appearance and findings on opening abdomen

With the peritoneal cavity open and a Balfour retractor in position the general situation can be seen. In Figure 16 the uterus (1) is slightly enlarged with an irregular and vascular fundus (arrowed) and there is some free fluid in the utero-vesical pouch. There are no obvious adhesions. The bladder is at (2), the ovaries (3), the tubes (4) and the round ligaments (5). Figure 17 gives a more posterior view but the omentum (6) occludes the pouch of Douglas which also contained some free fluid. Figure 18 shows manual exploration of the pelvis and upper abdomen in progress. There is no unexpected local extension of the disease and the upper abdominal structures seem normal. Pelvic glands are palpable but not large and not fixed. The case appears to be suitable for radical hysterectomy and pelvic lymphadenectomy.

Stage 3: Securing upper uterine attachments

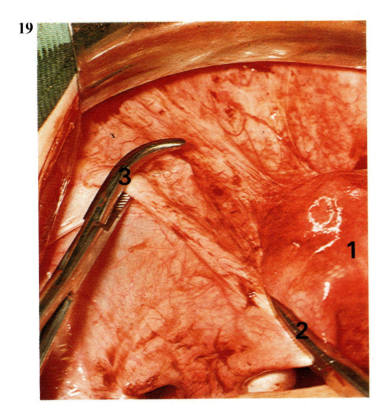

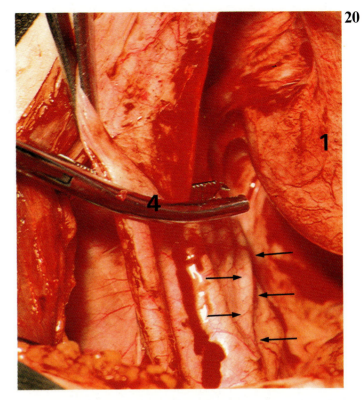

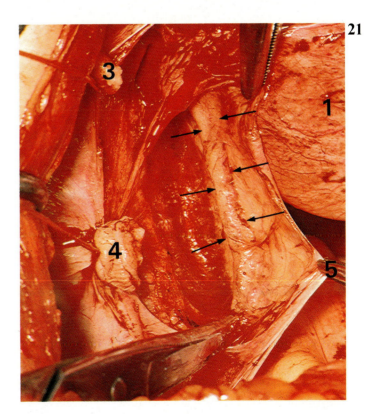

19 to 21 Detaching left round ligament and ovarian pedicles
The uterus is at (1) in each photograph. In Figure 19 the left broad ligament is held in Oschner forceps (2) and the left round ligament is clamped well laterally with Phillip's forceps (3). The ligament was subsequently detached leaving an opening in the anterior layer of the left broad ligament and in Figure 20 the ovarian pedicle (4) is secured by Oschner forceps (4). It is important to avoid the left ureter as it lies in the ovarian fossa and it should always be visualised before closing the forceps. It is well medial and is arrowed in the photograph. In Figure 21 the left round ligament pedicle (3) and the left ovarian pedicle (4) have been ligated and are held laterally by the uncut sutures. The peritoneum of the posterior layer of the broad ligament is held medially by dissecting forceps (5) and the left ureter is clearly seen lying on it extraperitoneally (arrowed).

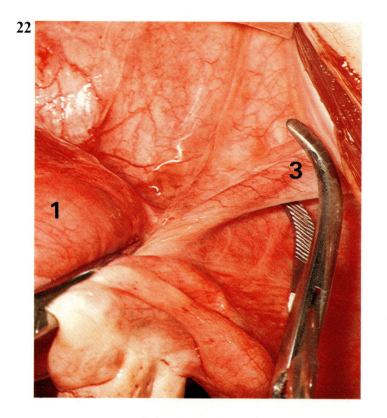

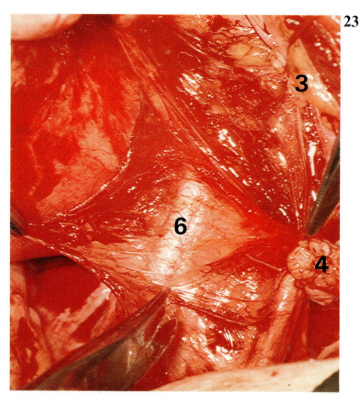

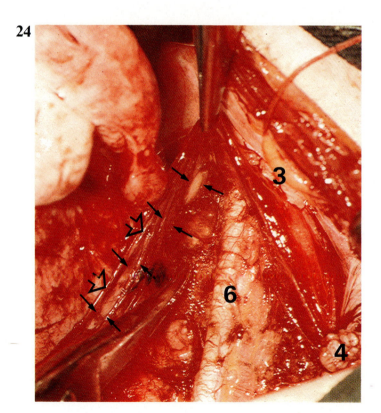

22 to 24 Detaching right round ligament and ovarian pedicles

The same procedure is carried out on the right side and the same numbers are used. The right round ligament (3) is secured well laterally in Figure 22; both it and the right ovarian pedicle (4) have been ligated in Figure 23 and the broad ligament is being opened up by the scissors to show the external iliac artery (6). In Figure 24 dissection has gone a stage further and the points of the scissors indicate the outline of the right ureter lying extraperitoneal to the posterior layer of the broad ligament. The edge of the ligament is indicated by broad arrows: the ureteric outline by fine arrows.

Stage 4: Separation of uterus from bladder

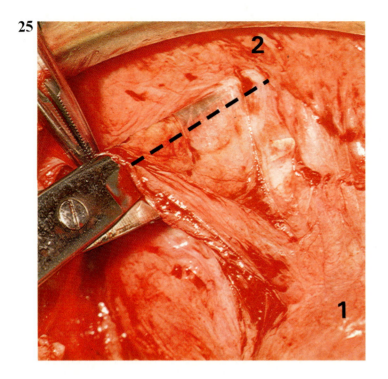

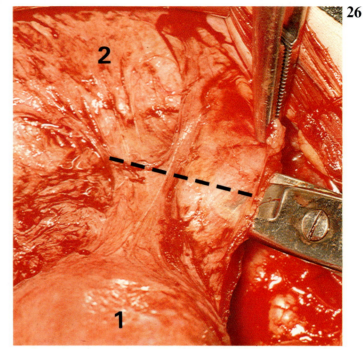

25 to 27 Opening utero-vesical pouch

In Figure 25 the scissors form a tunnel on the left side of the utero-vesical pouch prior to cutting the peritoneum along the dotted line. The process is repeated on the right side in

Figure 26 and in Figure 27 separation of the bladder from the uterus proceeds in the plane of separation which is arrowed. The uterus is at (1) and the bladder (2).

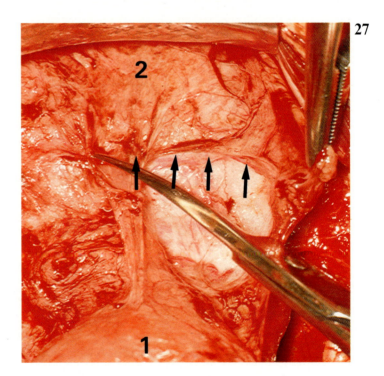

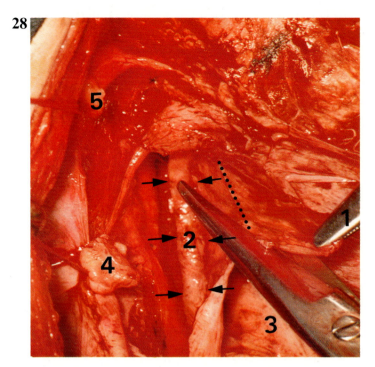

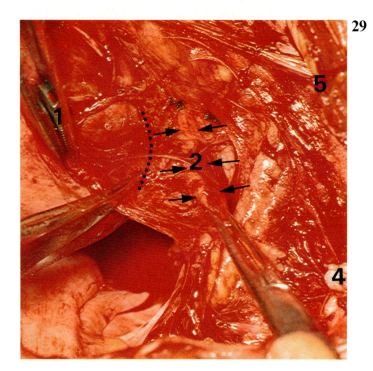

28 and 29 Opening posterior layer of broad ligaments

In Figure 28 the dissecting forceps (1) holds the posterior layer of the left broad ligament while the scissors divide it in the direction of the dotted line and clear of the ureter (2 and arrowed). The uterus is at (3), the ovarian pedicle (4) and the round ligament pedicle (5). The same procedure is followed on the right side in Figure 29 and the same numbers are used.

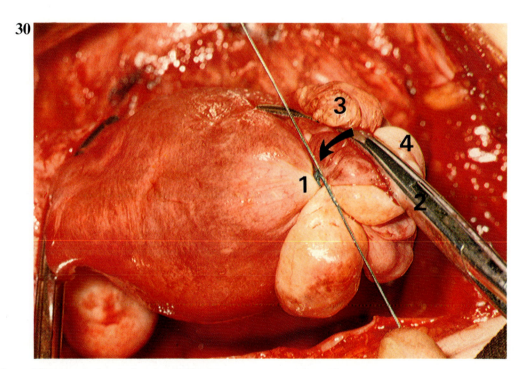

30 Replacing broad ligament clamps by strong ligatures

Replacing the clamps gives a better view of the pelvis and reduces the risk of malignant cell dissemination and spill from pulling on or possibly avulsing the forceps. A strong mersilene ligature secures the appendages at the cornu of the uterus (1) and is tied off. The broad ligament forceps (2) is rotated medially in the direction of the arrow and the ligature embraces the detached ovarian pedicle (3) and tube (4) in a second tier ligature as the forceps is withdrawn. The procedure is repeated on the left side.

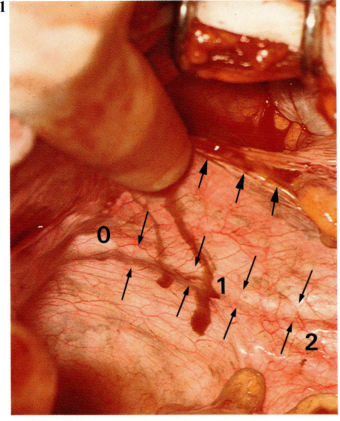

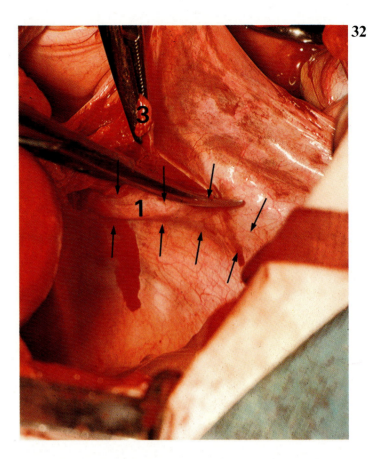

Figures **31–35** are taken from another operation which had slightly different indications. They are used here because the photographs show very clearly the sequence of steps at this very important stage of the Wertheim operation.

31 and 32 Recognition of right ureter

The easiest point at which to locate the ureter is under the posterior layer of the broad ligament on the pelvic floor and about 2.5 cm lateral to the cervix. This was seen in the pre-

ceding photographs (Figures 28 and 29). In Figure 31 this area is at (0) and the broad ligament peritoneal edge is indicated by short fine arrows. The ureter (1 and outlined by long fine arrows) runs downwards on the side wall of the pelvis and crosses the bifurcation of the common iliac artery (2). In Figure 32 the edge of the broad ligament peritoneum is held in dissecting forceps (3) while the scissors commence dissection of the peritoneum over and along the line of the ureter, which is outlined.

33

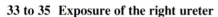

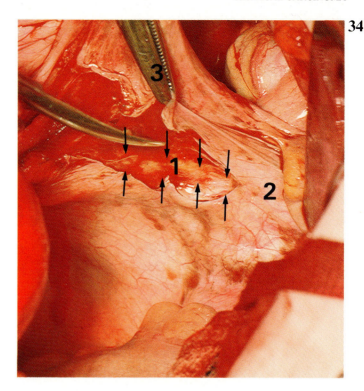

34

33 to 35 Exposure of the right ureter

In Figure 35 the dissecting forceps take a fresh hold on the peritoneal edge (3) and the scissors continue to incise the peritoneum and uncover the ureter (1) as far as the common iliac bifurcation (2). This has been done in Figure 34 and

the points of the scissors are used as blunt dissectors to expose the ureter without disturbing it from its vascular bed. In Figure 35 the pelvic peritoneum is retracted by tissue forceps (4) and (4) and the ureter is exposed from the bifurcation of the common iliac artery to the base of the broad ligament (5). It is outlined by arrows in each photograph.

The same procedure is then carried out on the left side.

35

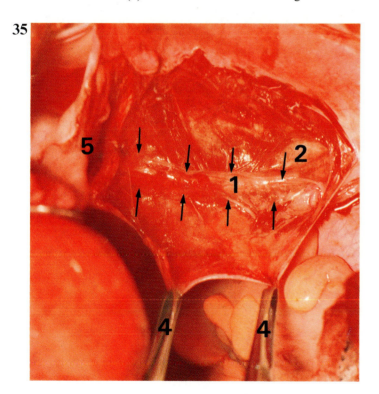

Stage 6: Definition of uretero-vesical junctions

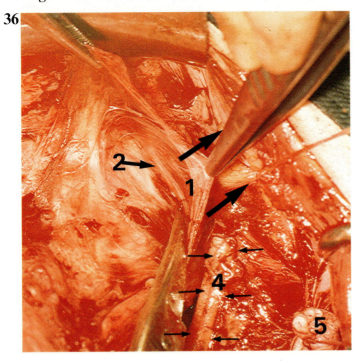

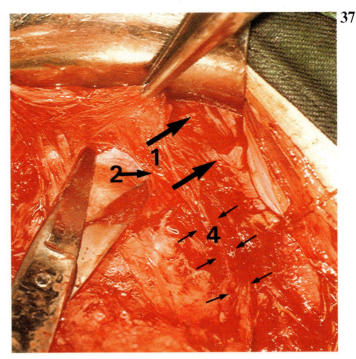

37

36 to 38 Steps in the exposure of right uretero-vesical junction

By blunt dissection in Figure 36 and by scissors snips in Figure 37, the right bladder pillar (1) is freed from the vagina and then pushed laterally and distally in the direction of the arrows to expose the area of the right uretero-vesical junction (2 with attached arrow). In Figure 38 the finger defines the uretero-vesical junction which underlies it at (2). The ureter itself (4) is outlined in each photograph. The ovarian pedicle is at (5).

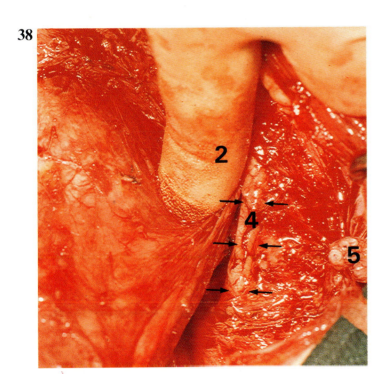

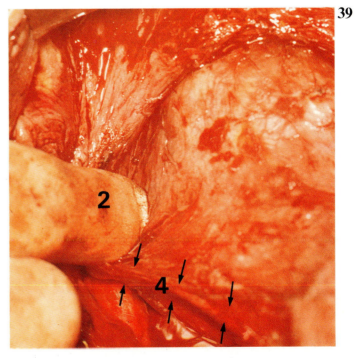

38

39 Exposure of left uretero-vesical junction

The same procedure has been carried out on the left side and the finger is seen displacing the bladder pillar to establish the uretero-vesical junction underlying it at (2). The ureter is outlined running distally towards it.

40

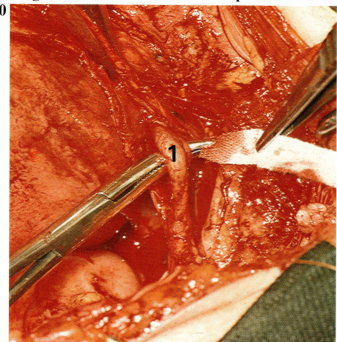

41

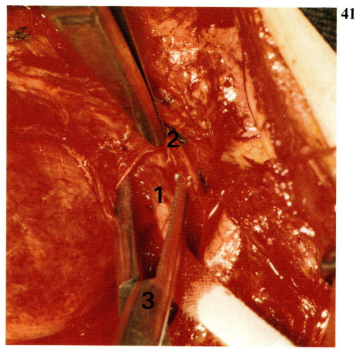

40 to 42 Definition of right ureter in ureteric tunnel

The ureter (1) is underrun by a linen tape in Figure 40 and the roof of the parametrial or ureteric tunnel (2) is held in dissecting forceps in Figure 41 while the Spencer Wells forceps (3), inserted in the line of the ureter, exposes the interior of the tunnel. In Figure 42 the whole roof of the ureteric tunnel with the uterine vessels (arrowed) on its surface is displayed on the closed forceps. The ureter is seen entering the tunnel and the uretero-vesical junction is at (4).

42

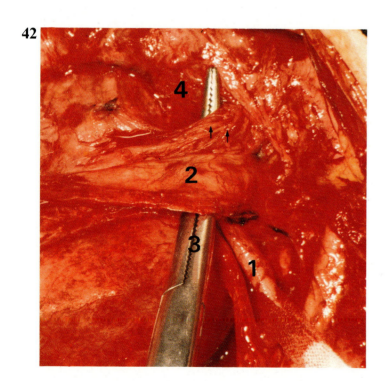

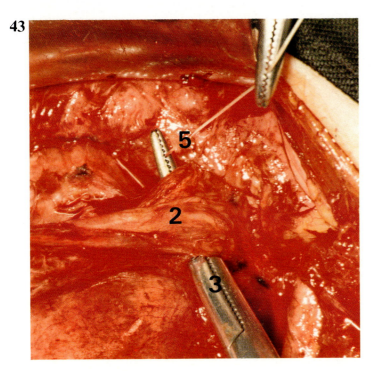

43

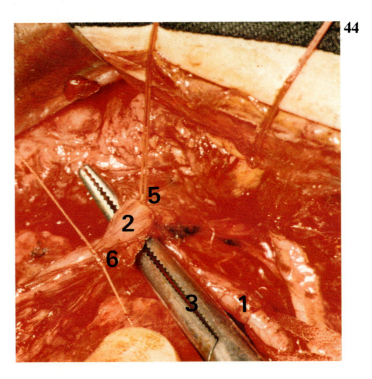

44

43 to 45 Double ligation and opening of right ureteric tunnel

In Figure 43 the Spencer Wells forceps (3) picks up a PGA No. 1 ligature (5) to underrun and ligate the pedicle. In Figure 44 that ligature has been placed and a second one is being tied (6) at a distance of not less than 1 cm from the first.

In Figure 45 the partially opened forceps support the roof of the ureteric tunnel between the two ligatures and it is being divided with the scalpel along the dotted line in such a way as to leave a cuff of tissue beyond each ligature and so that there is no fear of slipping.

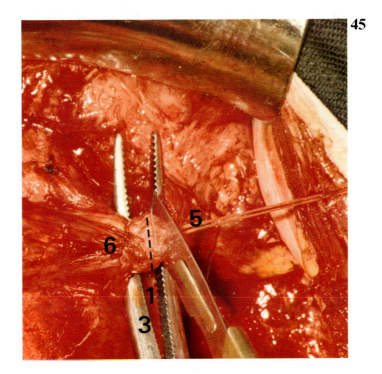

45

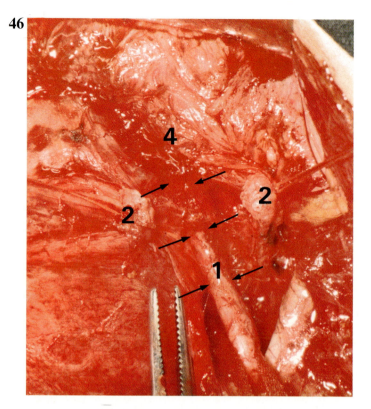

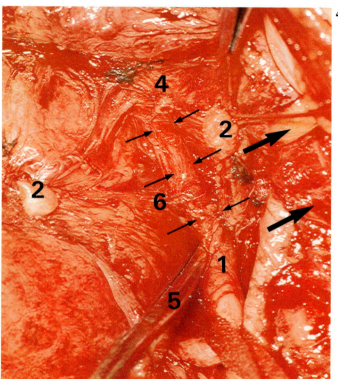

46 and 47 Displacing exposed right ureter laterally

Once the ureter has been exposed in the parametrial tunnel it is displaced laterally so that the parametrium can be divided well away from the uterus and so that at least 2.5 cm width can be removed with the uterus and cervix. In Figure 46 the cut ends of the roof of the ureteric tunnel (2) and (2) with their contained uterine vessels are pulled apart by the

uncut ligatures to show the ureter (1 and arrowed) and the uretero-vesical junction (4). In Figure 47 the ureter is being pushed laterally in the direction of the large arrows by the scissors (5). The ureteric mesentery is clearly seen (6) and can be displaced with the ureter without trauma to leave a sufficient area of parametrium for removal.

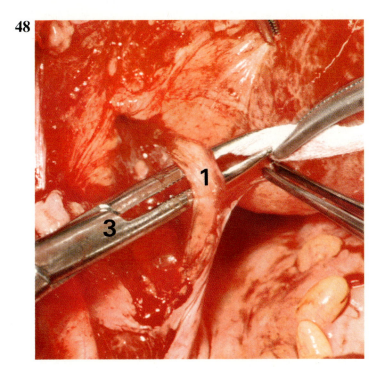

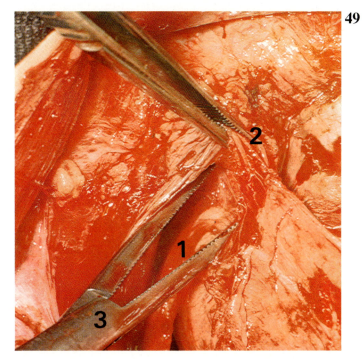

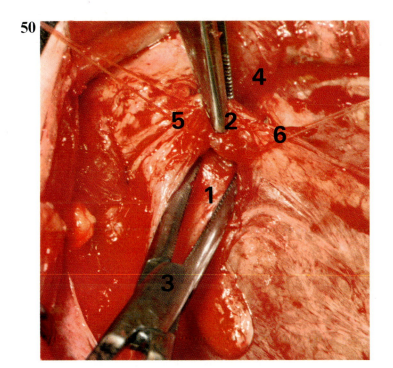

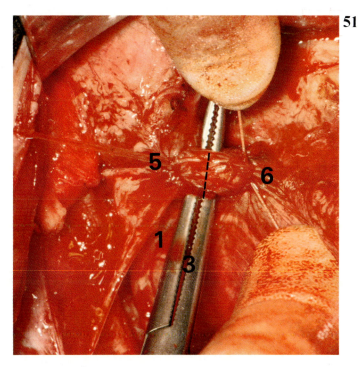

48 to 51 Definition of left ureter and ureteric tunnel
The procedure is exactly as on the right side and the same numbers are used. The ureter is underrun with a tape in Figure 48, the tunnel is defined in Figure 49, double ligatures are in place in Figure 50 and are being tied in Figure 51.

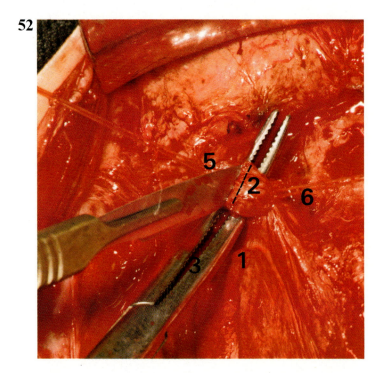

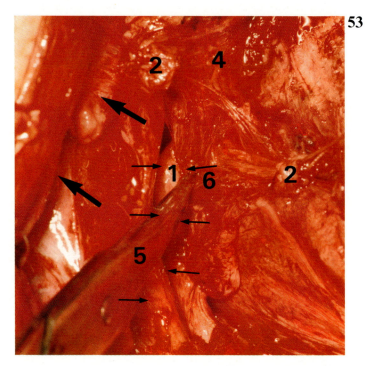

52 and 53 Exposure and lateral displacement of left ureter

The roof of the ureteric tunnel with the uterine vessels on its upper surface is divided between the ligatures in Figure 52 and the exposed ureter and its intact mesentery are displaced laterally by the scissors in the direction of the large arrows in Figure 53. The procedure is exactly as on the right side and the same numbers apply.

Stage 8: Mobilisation of uterus from rectum and bladder

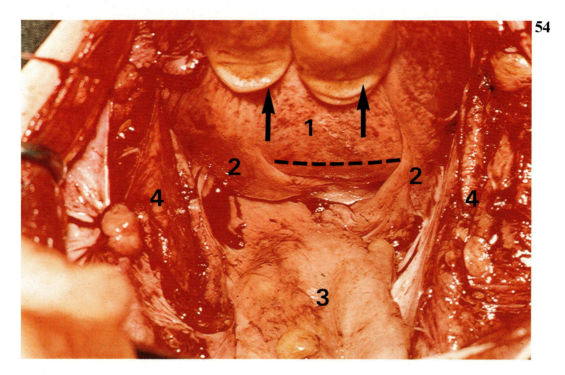

54 Preparing to open recto-vaginal space

The uterus (1) is held upwards by the fingers in the direction of the arrows to expose the utero-sacral ligaments (2) and (2) and the rectum (3) lying posteriorly. The ureters are seen laterally (4) and (4). The dotted line indicates the incision to be made into the peritoneum to gain access to the recto-vaginal space.

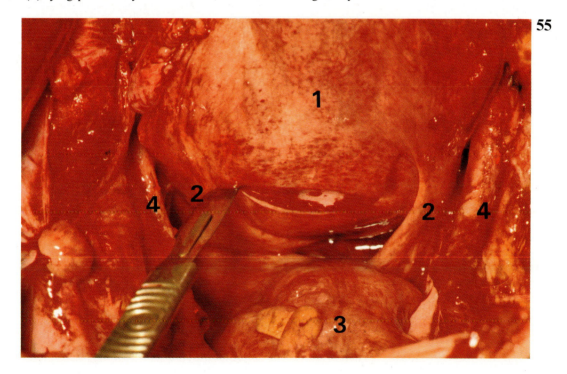

55 Opening recto-vaginal space

The scalpel incises the peritoneum between, and deep to, the attachments of the utero-sacral ligaments in the line previously indicated. The level is carefully chosen as that where the firmly attached uterine peritoneum becomes more loosely applied and is just mobile on the posterior cervical surface.

167

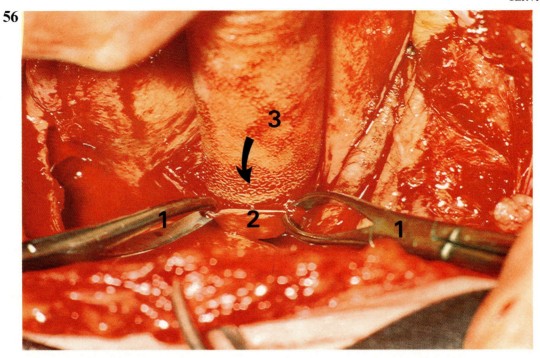

56 Establishing a recto-vaginal opening

The recto-vaginal space is a potential one and has to be opened up by the surgeon. The tissue forceps (1) and (1) hold the lower, loosely attached edge of the peritoneal incision (2) while the surgeon's forefinger (3) is introduced into the opening and inserted downwards in the direction of the arrow to establish a space as far as the pelvic floor. The finger tip is kept close to the vagina which contains the gauze pack and the space opens up quite easily.

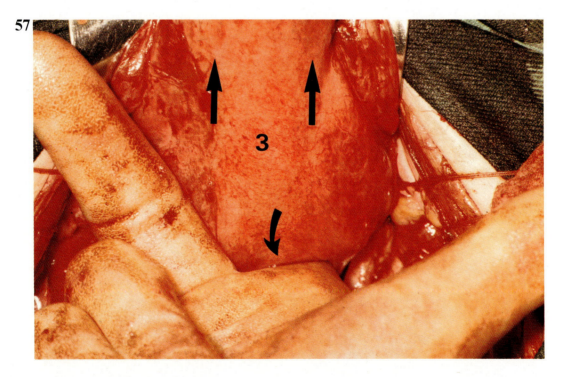

57 Separating the upper vagina from the rectum

The firm gauze pack in the vagina forms a column which the finger follows downwards and it is a simple matter to free the vagina posteriorly and separate the rectum from it. This separation is carried well laterally so that there is no question of the rectum being caught up and damaged when the parametrium is divided during hysterectomy. The uterus is held upwards in the direction of the arrows and the right forefinger acts as a blunt dissector.

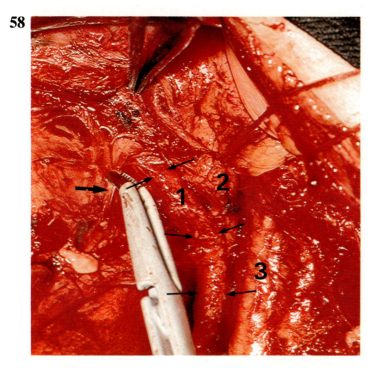

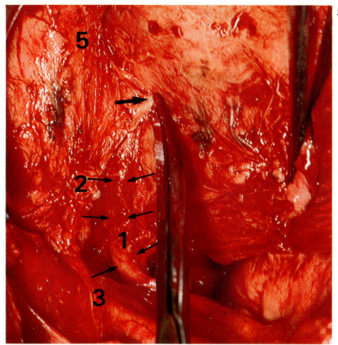

58 to 60 Further separation of the bladder from uterus

When the rectum has been freed posteriorly it is possible to elevate the uterus further into the wound allowing separation of the bladder to a deeper level anteriorly, and this is now done. In Figure 58 a vascular attachment (arrowed) just medial to the right ureter (1) is touched with the diathermy before division. The uterine pedicle is at (2) and the external iliac artery (3). In Figure 59 the bladder is further separated in the midline by dividing adhesions with the scissors where arrowed. The left ureter is at (1) and the bladder (5). In Figure 60 the finger displaces the area of the right uretero-vesical junction (4) downwards to expose the vagina (6) which is distended by the gauze pack. The ureter is outlined in each photograph.

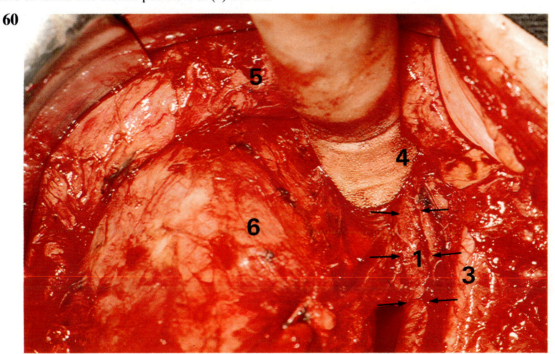

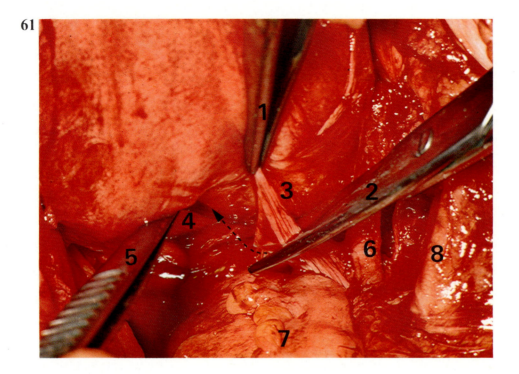

61 and 62 Dividing pelvic peritoneum postero-laterally to expose utero-sacral ligaments

Although the broad ligament has been opened up and the recto-vaginal space defined and enlarged, the uterus still has a peritoneal attachment between these areas and this covers the upper surface of the utero-sacral ligaments besides

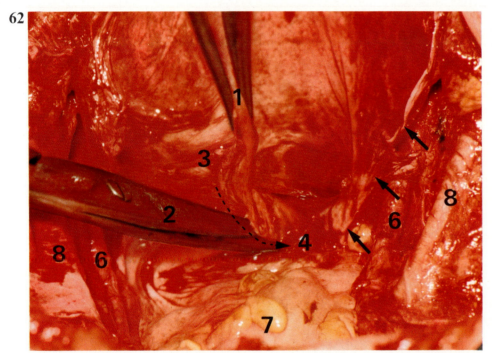

extending laterally for about 2 cm. This must be divided to give access when clamping the utero-sacral ligaments, and also to ensure that the rectum can be retracted well out of the way when doing so. This is a very important step in the operation. In Figure 61 the dissecting forceps (1) holds the outer border of this sheet of peritoneum while the scissors (2) divide it from the base of the right broad ligament (3) towards the recto-vaginal space (4) which is indicated by forceps (5). The right ureter is at (6), the rectum (7) and the right external iliac artery (8). In Figure 62 division of the peritoneum is seen to be complete on the right side and the peritoneal edge is arrowed. The same procedure is being carried out on the left side and the same numbers are used as on the right.

**Stage 9: Securing lower uterine attachments
(Isolating cervix and parametrium)**

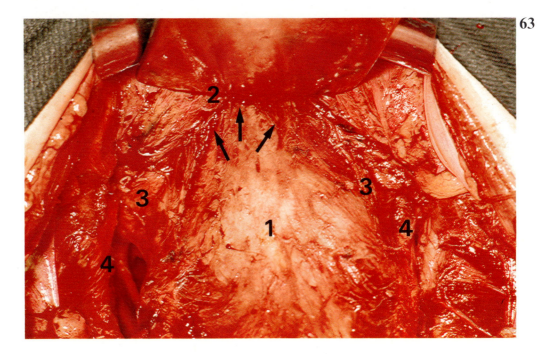

63 Removal of the vaginal pack

The gauze pack is withdrawn from the vagina at this stage and it is seen that the uterus and upper vagina are deeply separated from the bladder anteriorly (arrowed). The uterus is now attached solely by the fan-shaped parametrium on each side and this is largely formed by the utero-sacral ligament posteriorly and the cardinal ligament more anteriorly and distally. The cervix is at (1), bladder (2), parametrium (3) and ureters (4).

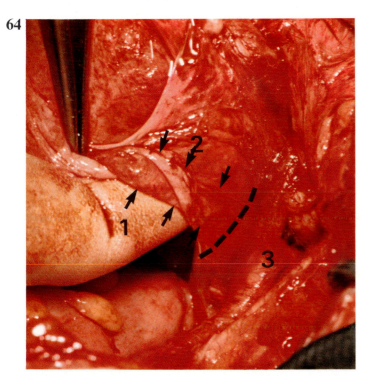

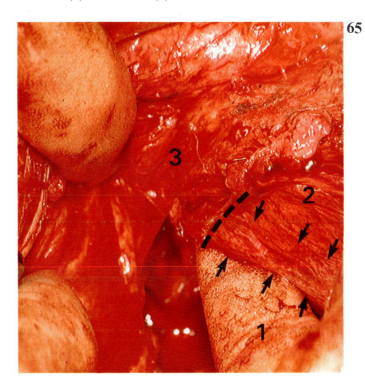

64 and 65 Displaying utero-sacral ligaments and parametrium

In Figure 64 the forefinger (1) lifts the right parametrium (2) upwards to display its utero-sacral constituent (arrowed) and which forms its posterior edge. The line of excision will be where indicated by the dotted line. In Figure 65 the same structures are shown on the left side and the numbers are similar. The ureter is at (3) in each photograph.

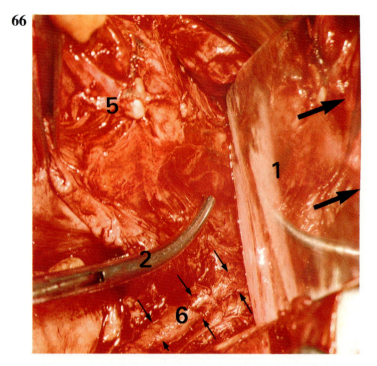

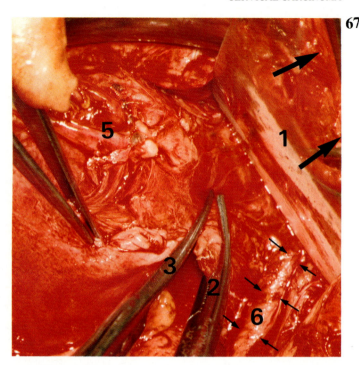

66 and 67 Dividing utero-sacral ligament portion of right parametrium

In Figure 66 a Kelly retractor (1) acting in the direction of the arrows safeguards the ureter and bladder while a curved Oschner forceps (2) is applied at the site of the dotted line (Figure 64). In Figure 67 the ligament is divided by the scissors (3) to leave a cuff of tissue distal to the forceps and the ureter is still shielded by the retractor. The cervix is at (5) and the pelvic portion of the ureter is visible at (6) in each photograph, and is outlined.

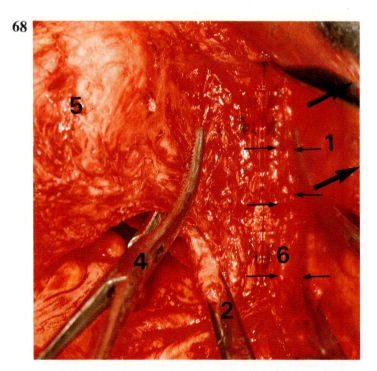

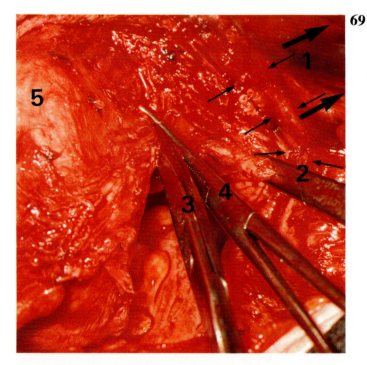

68 and 69 Dividing cardinal ligament portion of right parametrium

In Figure 68 the retractor is still in position while a second forceps (4) clamps the deeper cardinal ligament portion of the parametrium, and in Figure 69 this is being detached with the scissors. The numbers are as in Figures 66 and 67, and the ureters are again outlined.

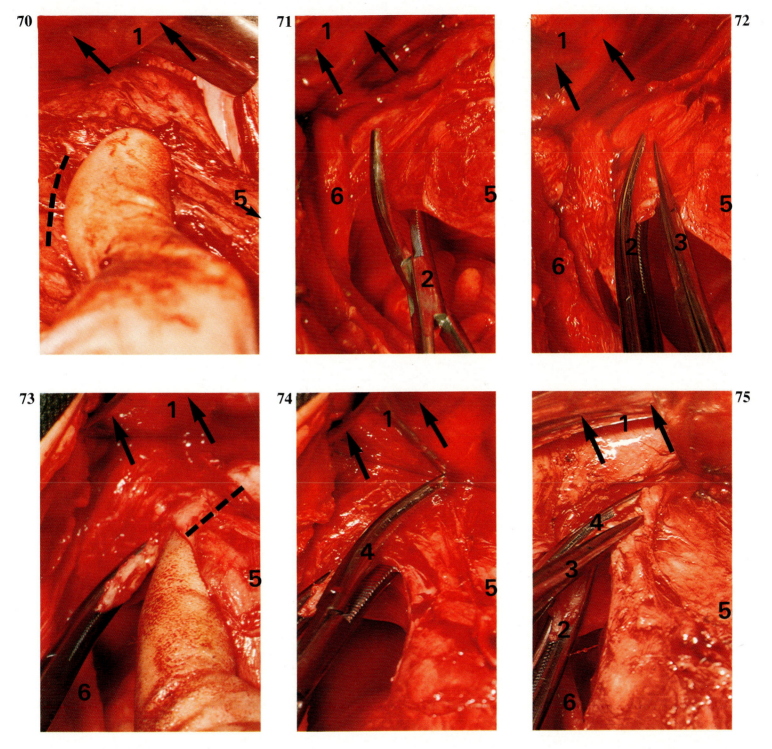

70 to 75 Steps in division of left parametrium

The same procedure is carried out as on the right side in Figures 64 to 69 and the steps are in the same progression. The structures are: Kelly retractor (1), forceps on utero-sacral ligament portion of parametrium (2) and on cardinal ligament portion (4), scissors (3), cervix (5). The two ligamentous parts of the parametrium are displayed on the fingers in turn (Figures 70 and 73) and the incision is made along the dotted line in each case. Where visible, the ureter is at (6).

76

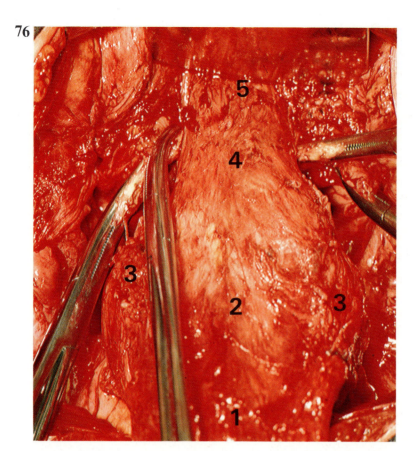

76 Uterus, cervix, parametrium and upper vagina freed from lower uterine attachments (anterior view)

The uterus (1), cervix (2), parametrium (3) and upper vagina (4) have been divided from their lateral attachments and it only remains to separate them from the vagina (5). The two forceps on each side were those applied in Figures 65 to 75 and they secure the two portions of the parametrium.

77

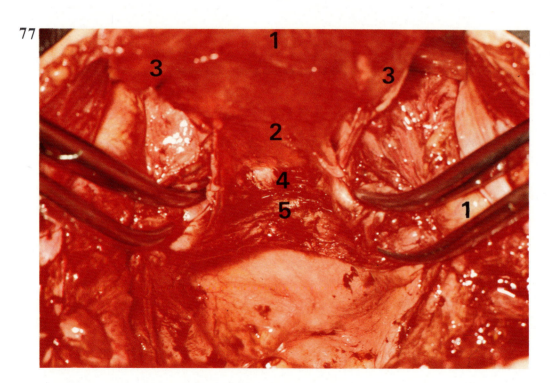

77 Uterus, cervix, parametrium and upper vagina freed from lower uterine attachments (posterior view)

The stage of the operation is shown in a posterior view and the same numbers are used. The same two forceps are on the parametrium of each side.

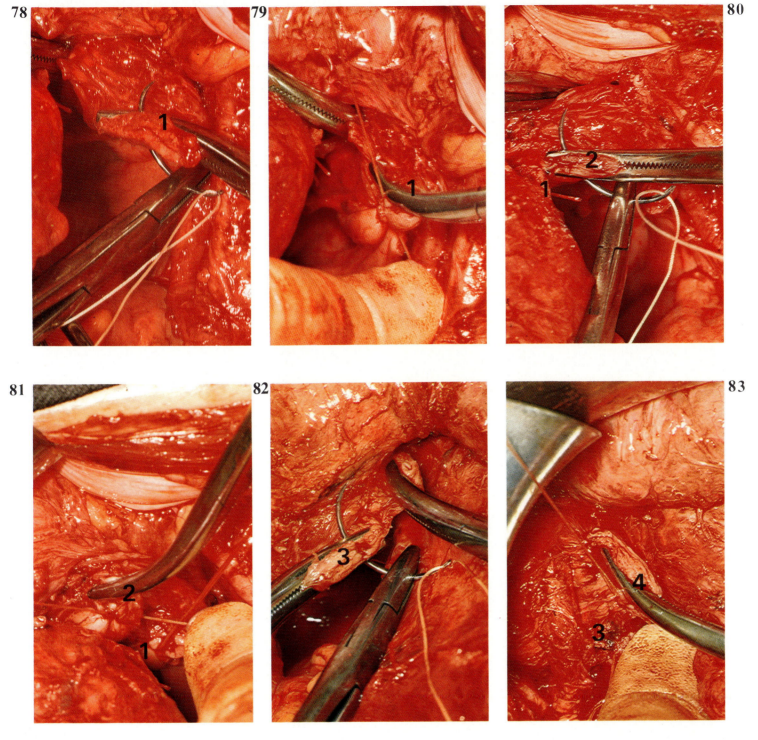

78 to 83 Ligation of utero-sacral and cardinal ligament pedicles of the parametrium

Commencing on the right, the utero-sacral ligament (1) is transfixed in Figure 78 and tied first round the point and then round the heel of the forceps in Figure 79. The right cardinal ligament (2) is transfixed in Figure 80 and tied in Figure 81. The left utero-sacral ligament (3) is transfixed in Figure 82 and the left cardinal ligament (4) is ligated in Figure 83.

Stage 10: Removal of uterus, cervix, parametrium and upper vagina

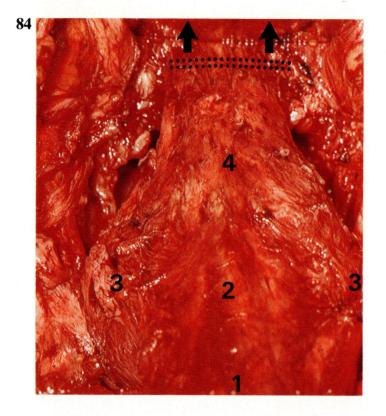

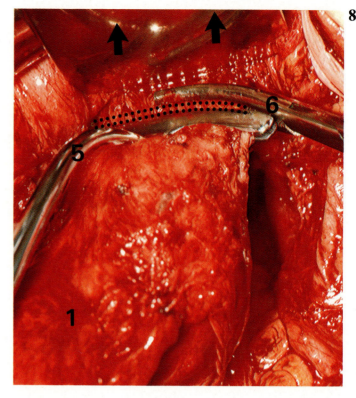

84 to 86 Defining and clamping upper vagina prior to transection

In Figure 84 the retractor held in the direction of the arrows displaces the bladder to show the considerable length of upper vagina available for removal (4). The uterus (1), cervix (2) and parametrium (3) are numbered as previously and the vaginal transection will be made at the dotted line. In Figure 85 a Berkeley-Bonney clamp (5) is seen applied just above the level of the dotted line to act partly as a tractor or handle on the specimen and partly to prevent escape of malignant cells when the vagina is opened. Distal to it an Oschner forceps is applied to the vaginal angle on the right side (6). A similar forceps (7) is being placed on the left side in Figure 86. The Berkeley-Bonney clamp is in no way essential and two long curved clamps, such as Oschner or Kocher's forceps applied on either side serve equally well.

87 Transection of vagina

The scalpel (8) cuts across the anterior and posterior walls of the vagina between the Berkeley-Bonney clamp (5) and the Oschner forceps (6) and (7) as shown. At this considerable depth in the pelvis, care is taken to retain a cuff of tissue beyond the blades of the forceps to minimise the risk of the ligatures slipping.

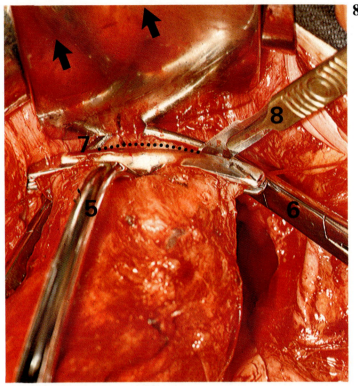

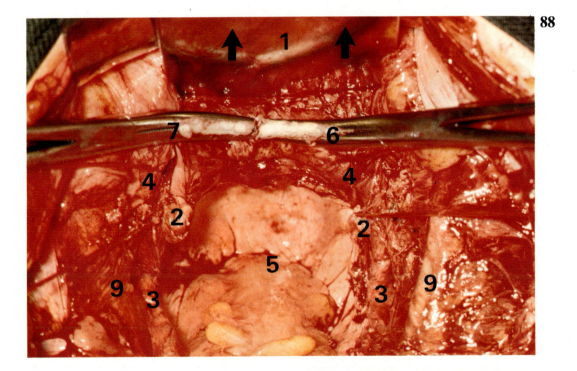

88 View of pelvic floor following removal of uterus

The forceps (6) and (7) are still on the vaginal angles. The other structures are: retractor guarding bladder (1), utero-sacral ligament pedicles (part of parametrium) (2), cardinal ligament pedicles (part of parametrium) (4), ureters (3), rectum (5), external iliac arteries (9).

Stage 11: Closure of vaginal vault

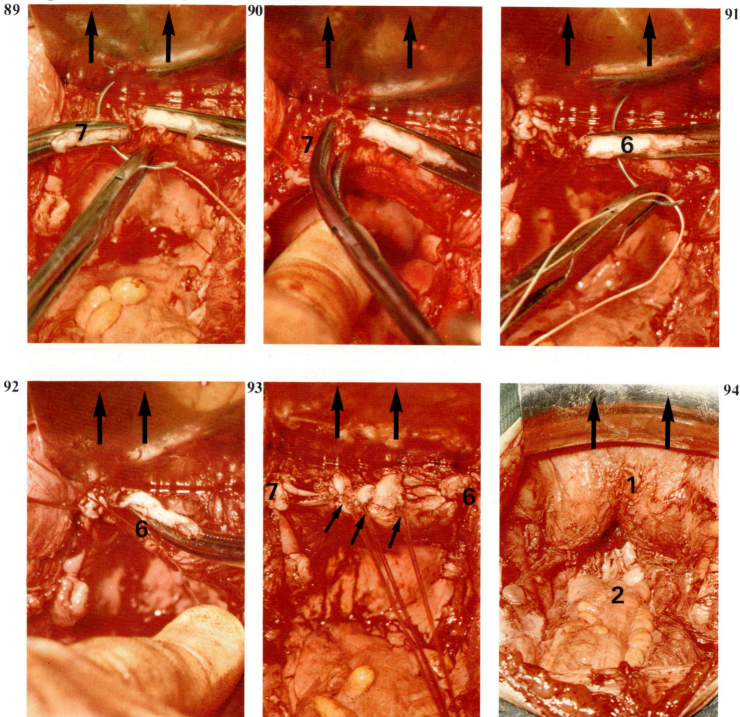

89 to 94 Steps in transverse closure of vaginal vault

The left vaginal angle pedicle (7) is transfixed in Figure 89 and ligated in Figure 90. The same is done on the right side in Figures 91 and 92. In Figure 93 the vaginal angles (6) and (7) are held laterally by their uncut sutures and 3 mattress stitches (arrowed) have been used to close the vaginal vault transversely between them. In Figure 94 the bladder (1) has been released from behind the speculum and falls posteriorly and caudally to lie in apposition with the rectum (2) so that the vault of the vagina is no longer visible from the abdomen.

Stage 12: Pelvic lymphadenectomy (left side)

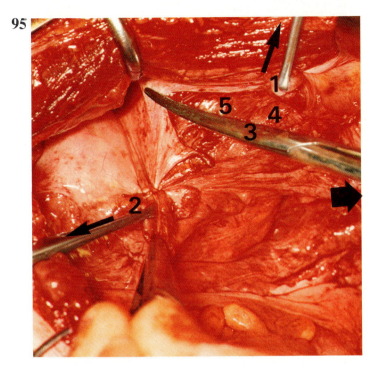

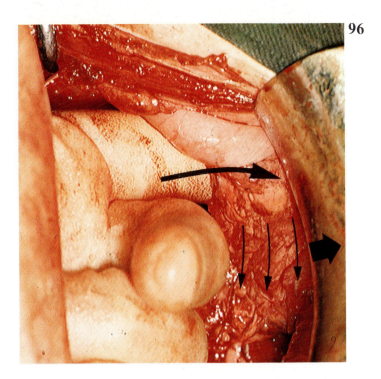

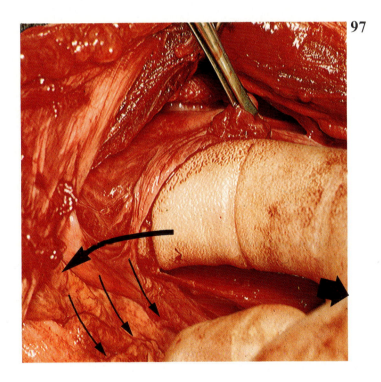

95 Lateral extension of opening into broad ligament

To gain access to the large vessels and the pelvic side wall, the round ligament and ovarian pedicles are held in tissue forceps (1) and (2) respectively in the direction of the arrows, while the scissors (3) divide the peritoneum to expose the external iliac artery (4) and the psoas muscle (5). The genito-femoral nerve is usually seen lying on the muscle.

96 and 97 Digital clearance of glands from external and common iliac arteries

In Figure 96 the forefinger is hooked under the anterior leaf of the lateral incision and tunnels forward along the line of the external iliac artery in the direction of the arrow, as far as the obturator fossa. The finger then literally sweeps the peritoneum, extraperitoneal fat and the glands medially and posteriorly from the surface of the great vessels and pelvic side wall to open up the para-vesical space. In Figure 97 the finger hooks under the posterior leaf of the lateral peritoneal incision and tunnels upwards along the external and common iliac arteries in the direction of the arrow, before sweeping the tissues medially from the pelvic side wall in a similar fashion. The ureter is always immediately apparent on the extraperitoneal surface during this latter manoeuvre.

The left forefinger is used in Figure 96 and the right in Figure 97. The direction in which the peritoneum is swept is indicated by the fine arrows. The very broad arrow points in the general direction of the symphysis pubis in these and in the previous photograph.

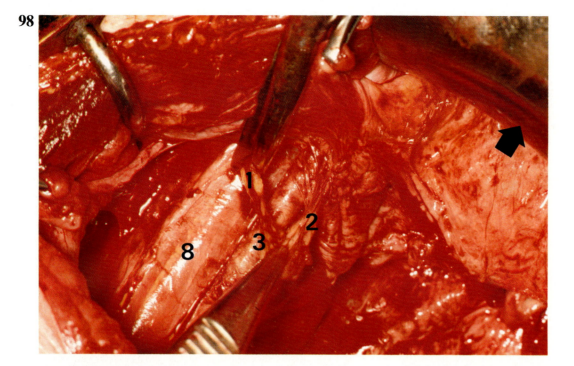

98 Clearing glands from surface of psoas muscle

Glands of the lateral external iliac chain (1) sometimes adhere to the psoas muscle sheath and are separated by scissors snips and drawn medially by the dissecting forceps to join the main mass of glands (2). The external iliac artery is at (3) and the psoas muscle (8). The angle at which the structures are shown is explained by the Trendelenberg position of the patient. The symphysis pubis is indicated by the very broad arrow in this and in the following photograph.

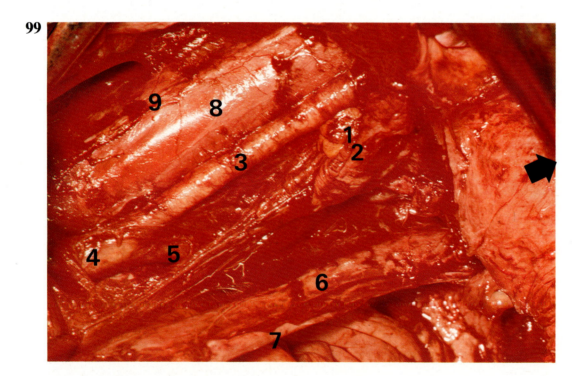

99 Large vessels and pelvic side wall exposed

The lateral and middle chains of external iliac glands (1) have been displaced medially with the main mass of fat and glands (2); the common iliac (4), the external iliac (3) and the internal iliac artery (5) are now displayed. The ureter (6) is well medial near the peritoneal edge (7). The psoas muscle is at (8) and the genito-femoral nerve (9).

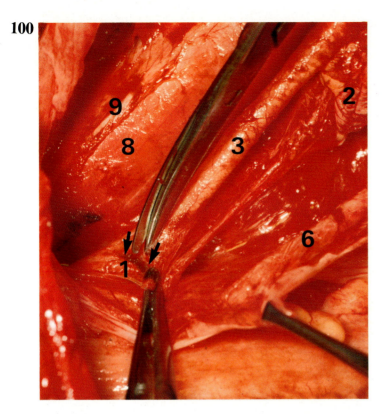

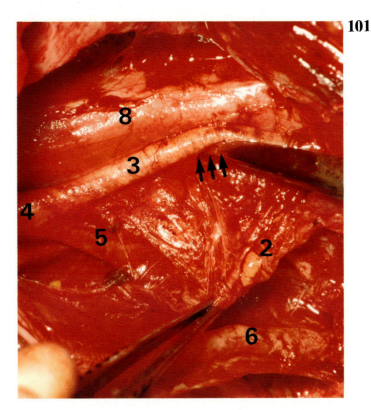

101

100 to 103 Dissection of glands from external and common iliac arteries

In Figure 100 the scissors have cleared the external iliac artery of glands and continue proximally to separate common iliac glands (1) from the artery in the plane of separation arrowed. In Figure 101 the most medial chain of glands is being separated in a plane (arrowed) between the external iliac artery and vein. In Figure 102 dissection continues in the direction of the arrows between the external iliac artery and its accompanying vein (7) which is now

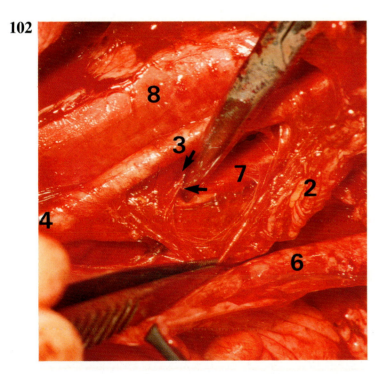

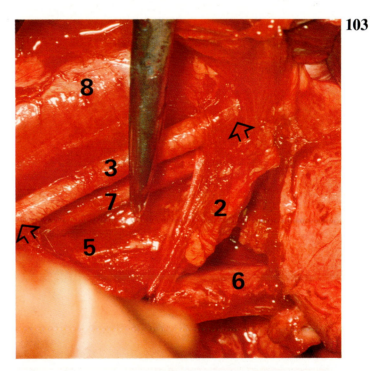

visible. In Figure 103 the vessels are dissected clear of glands from the bifurcation of the common iliac artery to the region of the inguinal ligament (between broad arrows). The internal iliac artery is just visible (5). In all four photographs main structures are: external iliac artery (3), psoas muscle (8), common iliac artery (4), ureter (6).

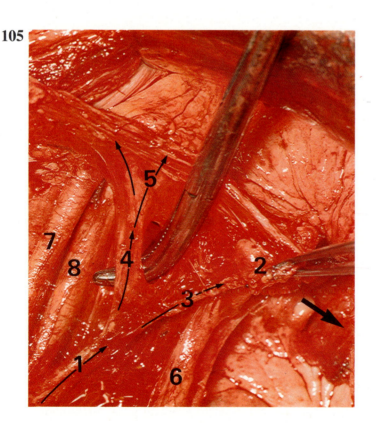

104 Definition of internal iliac artery

The scissors release the fibrous attachments of the internal iliac artery (1) as it runs distally and before dividing into its main branches. The uterine branch (3) is distal to the points of the scissors and runs into the uterine pedicle (2) which is pulled medially by tissue forceps in the direction of the arrow and across the line of the ureter (6) although it is in fact a lateral relation of the ureter. The course of the uterine artery as it runs from the internal iliac artery to the ligated pedicle is indicated by fine arrows. To aid orientation the external iliac artery and vein are at (7) and (8) respectively.

105 Dissecting anterior branches of internal iliac artery

The outline of the uterine branch (3) is seen running into the uterine pedicle (2) and the Phillips' forceps displays the obliterated umbilical artery (4) as it runs distally and gives off a superior vesical branch to the bladder (5). The direction of blood flow in the various branches is indicated by fine arrows. The other structures in the photograph are numbered as in Figure 104.

It was Bonney's practice to detach the obliterated umbilical artery at its origin from its internal iliac artery and remove a segment of the vessel *en bloc* with the internal iliac glands as far as the angle of the bladder. The step is unnecessary and may be dangerous in depriving the bladder of its superior vesical artery blood supply. The glands are not closely applied to the vessel and it can easily be displaced while the glands are enucleated.

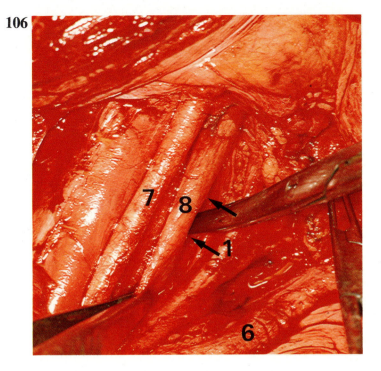

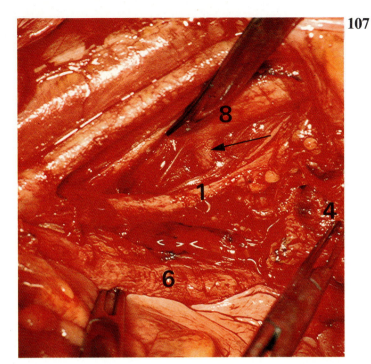

106 to 109 Dissection of internal iliac (hypogastric) and obturator glands (i)

The internal iliac glands lie in an angle between the external iliac vein (8) and the anterior branch of the internal iliac artery (1), against the side wall of the pelvis and partially surrounding the obturator nerve in that position. In Figure 106 the external iliac vein (8) is steadied with the dissecting forceps while the scissors open up a plane of separation beneath it towards the pelvic side wall (as arrowed). In Figure 107 the process continues at a deeper level and a large tributary of the vein is indicated by an arrow. In Figure 108 the finger is introduced to find a plane of separation against

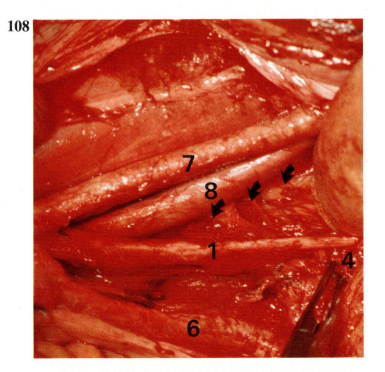

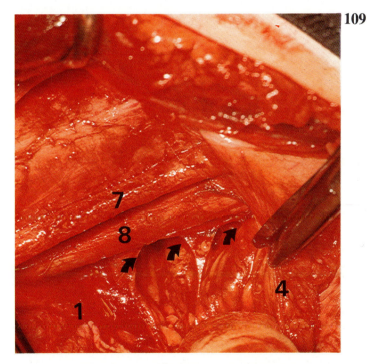

the pelvic side wall and to separate the fat and glands medially from it in the line of the arrows. In Figure 109 the space is largely opened up and the scissors are being used to dissect out the mass of fat and glands which has been displaced by the finger from the pelvic side wall and is at (4) in Figures 107–109.

110

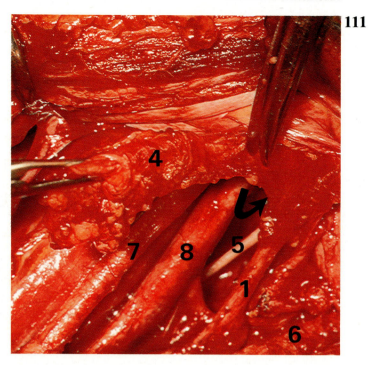

111

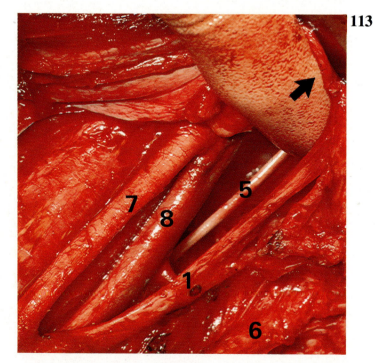

110 to 113 Dissection of internal iliac (hypogastric) and obturator glands (ii)

Sharp dissection of the gland groups continues except where they have to be separated from the obturator nerve digitally. The nerve is shown already stripped (5) in Figure 110 and the

gland mass (4) is being elevated. In Figure 111 the glands are held in the forceps while separation towards the obturator foramen (3) continues with the scissors. In Figure 112 the

112

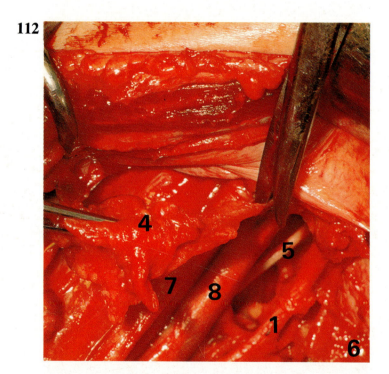

113

gland mass has been freed from the side wall. It is still *en bloc* with the external iliac glands and has some light attachments to the bladder angle. In Figure 113 the angle between the external iliac vein (8) and the internal iliac artery (1) is held

open with the forefinger and is seen to be quite clear of glands and fat. The external iliac artery is at (7) and the ureter (6) in these photographs.

114

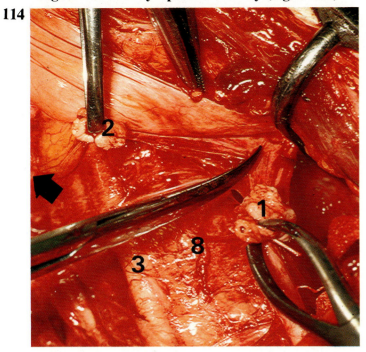

115

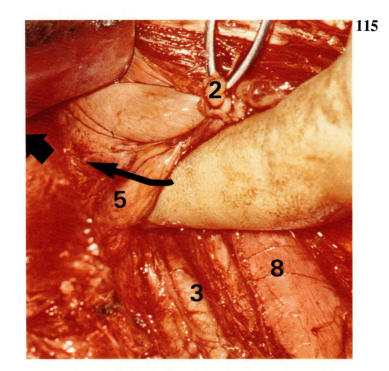

116

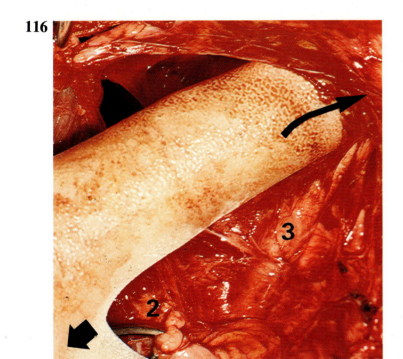

117

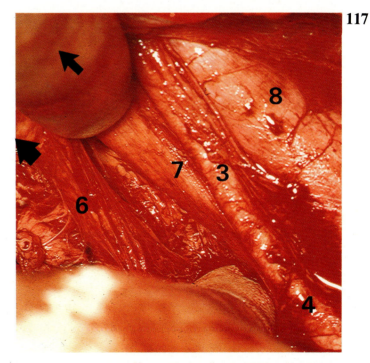

114 to 117 Extension of broad ligament opening and digital clearance of glands from large vessels on pelvic side wall

The procedure described for Figures 95, 96, and 97 is repeated. In Figure 114 division of the peritoneum between the ovarian (1) and round ligament (2) pedicles exposes the external iliac artery (3) and the psoas muscle (8). In Figure 115 the forefinger opens up the para-vesical space anteriorly by separating the fat and glands (5) medially off the side wall; in Figure 116 posteriorly a similar medial sweep of the peritoneum, fat, glands and ureter exposes the common and external iliac vessels. In Figure 117 the finger holds the separated structures medially. The ureter is at (6), the common iliac artery (4) and the external iliac vein (7). The double manoeuvre of stripping the pelvic side wall has rotated the plane of the photograph in Figure 116. Orientation is aided by a very broad arrow pointing in the general direction of the symphysis pubis in each case.

118

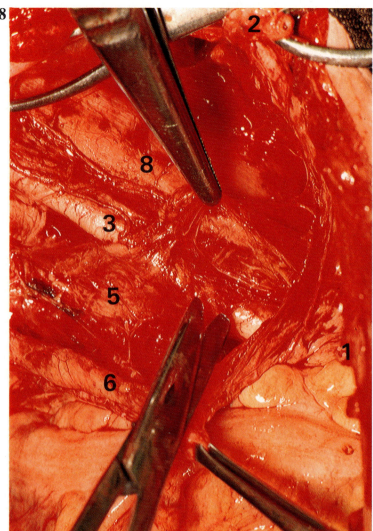

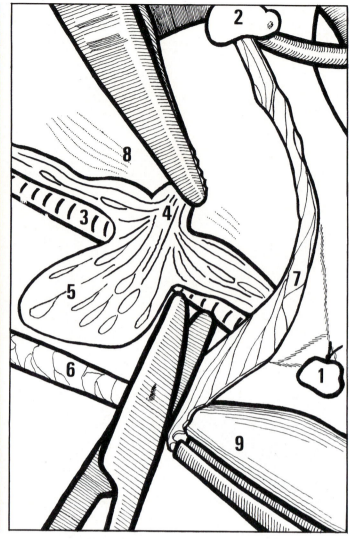

118 Commencing gland dissection on right side

The photograph serves as a revision when commencing
gland dissection and once the fat and glands have been
digitally swept from the pelvic side wall. Ovarian and round
ligament pedicles are at (1) and (2), the external iliac artery
(3), the psoas muscle (8), the fat and glands (5) and the
ureter (6). Digital separation does not remove glands and
lymphatics cleanly and the scissors are freeing lymphatic
glands and vessels from the psoas muscle sheath and the
lateral aspect of the external iliac artery. The lymphatic
tissue is held up in the dissecting forceps and represents the
lateral chain of external iliac glands. In Figures 119 to 121
the external iliac vessels are stripped of all lymphatic tissue
anteriorly, medially and between artery and vein; all this can
be done relatively easily and safely. A procedure whereby
the external iliac artery and vein are both separated from the
side wall of the pelvis and lifted from their bed in a search
for lymph glands is sometimes described. We believe that
this is not only unnecessary but unsafe and could lead to
severe venous bleeding. There are no recognisable glands to
be found between the vessels and the side wall in this area
and lymphography repeatedly shows the glands entirely
anterior and medial to the external iliac vessels.

Diagram 10
1 Ovarian pedicle
2 Round ligament pedicle
3 External iliac artery
4 External iliac glands – lateral chain in forceps
5 Fat and glands of pelvic side wall
6 Ureter
7 Peritoneal edge
8 Psoas muscle
9 Rectum

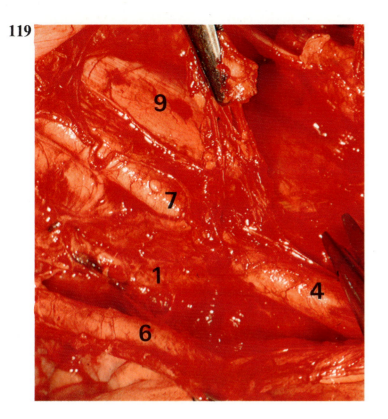

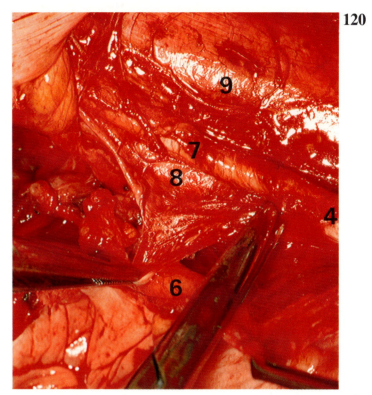

119 to 121 Dissection of external and common iliac glands

The procedure is exactly as on the left side. In Figure 119 the glands are stripped distally from the common and external iliac arteries and they represent the median chain of lymphatics. In Figure 120 the medial chain is sought between the external iliac artery and vein and in Figure 121 the whole chain is separated medially off the common and external iliac vessels. The structures are: common iliac artery (4), external iliac artery (7), external iliac vein (8), internal iliac artery (1), psoas muscle (9), ureter (6).

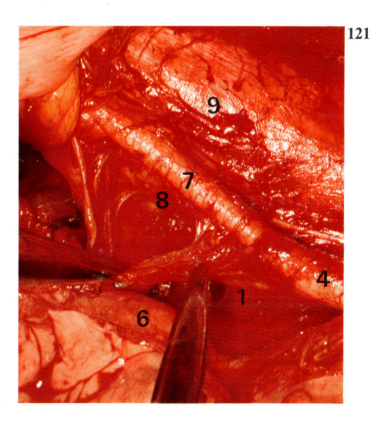

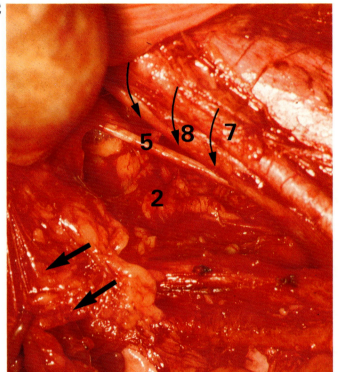

122

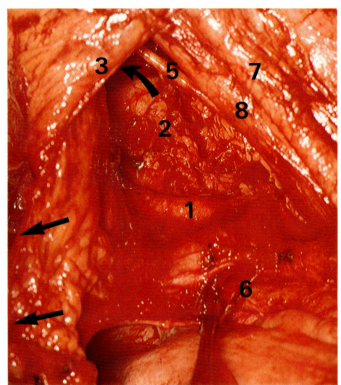

123

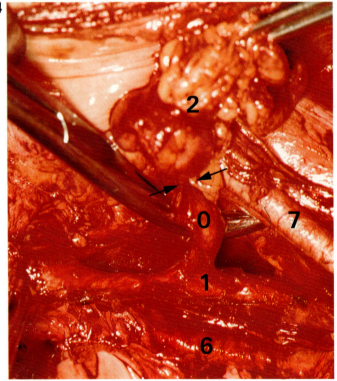

124

122 to 124 Dissection of internal iliac (hypogastric) and obturator glands

The procedure is as described on the left side in Figures 106 to 113 and only those points requiring emphasis are repeated here. In Figure 122 a plane of separation is found immediately under the external iliac vein (arrowed) and the fat and glands (2) are partially separated from the side wall with the finger to expose the obturator nerve (5). The external iliac mass of glands has been swept medially as arrowed. In Figure 123 the internal iliac glands have been separated well anteriorly from the obturator fossa (3 and arrowed) and are ready to be removed from the angle between the external iliac vein and the internal iliac artery. The obturator fossa is now quite empty except for the obturator nerve. In Figure 124 the glands have been removed from the angle on the pelvic side wall and are shown to be lightly adherent to the obliterated umbilical artery (0) which is displayed on the Phillips' forceps as it comes off the anterior branch of the internal iliac (hypogastric) artery (1). There is no difficulty in separating the glands from the artery in the region of the fine arrows, and no need to remove a segment of this artery which gives an important blood supply to the bladder through its superior vesical branch. The ureter is at (6) and the external iliac artery (7).

125 Detachment of glands at vesical angle

The detached external (2) and internal iliac (2) groups of glands merge distally and are adherent to the lateral aspect of the bladder in the area of the dotted line. It is important to separate them without injury to the bladder yet removing the gland tissue completely and it can be difficult to distinguish collections of fat from lymph glands in obese patients. The separation is best done by blunt dissection and sealing off small vessels with the diathermy. The external iliac artery and vein are at (7) and (8) respectively.

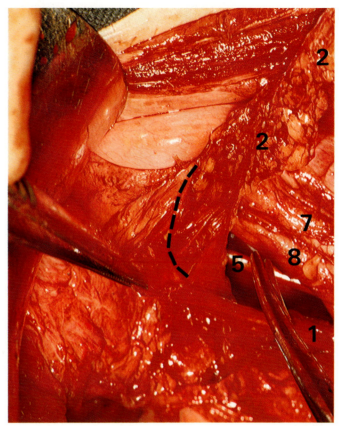

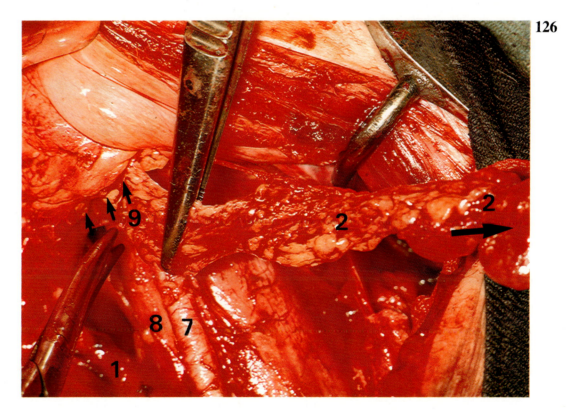

126 Complete detachment of gland mass

The photograph shows the external (2) and internal (2) gland groups held laterally in the direction of the large arrow while the scissors finally detach lymphatic tissue from the larger vessels in the region of the inguinal ring (9). The small arrows indicate where the gland tissue was separated from the bladder angle. The external iliac artery and vein are at (7) and (8) respectively.

Stage 14: Reperitonisation, pelvic drainage and wound closure

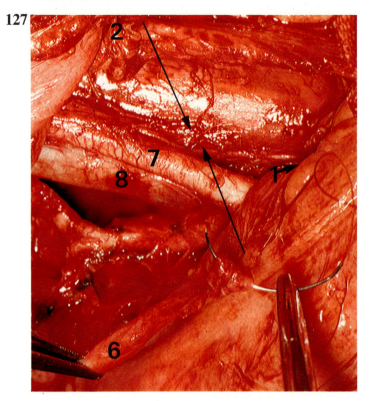

127

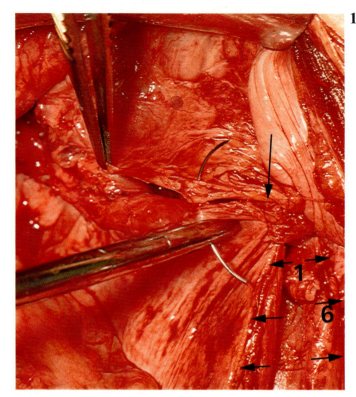

128

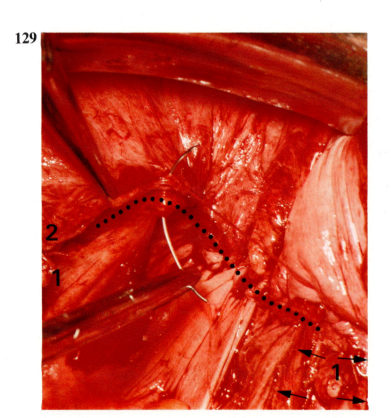

129

127 to 129 Closure of peritoneum across vaginal vault

The pelvic peritoneum is open transversely above the vault of the vagina and is also open towards the pelvic brim on each side along the general line of the ureter. Only the central part is closed in the first instance, leaving the upward extensions for insertion of drains and closure at a later stage. In Figure 127 the round-bodied needle carrying a PGA No. 00 suture picks up the posterior layer of peritoneum medial to the right ovarian pedicle (1), avoiding the ureter. The anterior leaf of the peritoneum is then picked up adjacent to the ligated right round ligament (2); the two leaves of peritoneum are approximated as the stitch is tied. The anchor stitch is arrowed in Figure 128 and the ovarian pedicle (1) is still visible laterally, with the peritoneum open along the line of the ureter; the edges indicated by fine arrows. A purse string anchoring stitch to bury the ovarian pedicle should not be attempted in this situation, as it is liable to kink the ureter when it is tied. The stitch continues across the pelvis towards the ovarian and round ligament pedicles on the left side in Figure 129, and when tied off will leave the ovarian pedicle uncovered with a similar open peritoneal space extending proximally along the general line of the ureter. The dotted line shows the transverse peritoneal closure.

The two long arrows in Figure 127 show the line of approximation of the two layers of peritoneum when tying the anchor stitch.

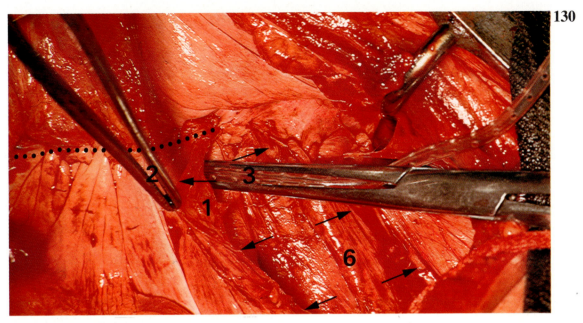

130 Insertion of Redivac drain from right side

The line of transverse closure of the peritoneum is 'broken'
and the edges of the still-open right side are indicated by
fine arrows. The dissecting forceps (2) steadies the medial
peritoneal edge while the sinus forceps inserts the distal end
of a Redivac drain (3) under the closed central area of
peritoneum to overlie the vaginal vault. The drain will be
brought out to the right side of the abdominal wound.

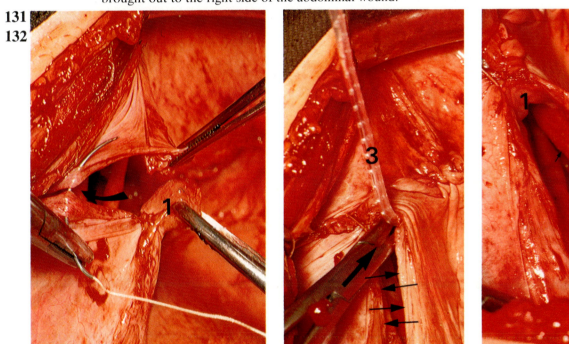

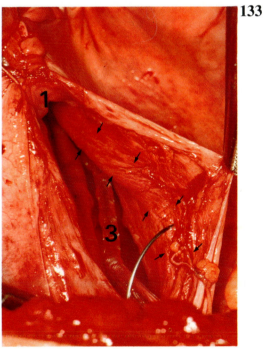

131 to 133 Further steps in placing Redivac drains

Figure 131 shows the closure of the right-sided peritoneal
opening commencing lateral to the transverse closure. The
ovarian pedicle (1) is still uncovered and will have to be
everted extraperitoneally. This is effected as shown in the
direction of the arrow. In Figure 132 the left-sided Redivac
drain is being inserted in the direction of the arrow with sinus
forceps, and in Figure 133 the peritoneal opening on the
left side is being closed over the drain. The ovarian pedicle
(1) is also uncovered but will be everted as the gap is
closed from above downwards. The ureter is clearly seen on
the medial leaf of peritoneum and is outlined. It is not
kinked or stretched and it is very important that this be so. If
the ovarian pedicle were drawn towards the round ligament
pedicle when closing the peritoneum transversely, there
would be danger of kinking the ureter.

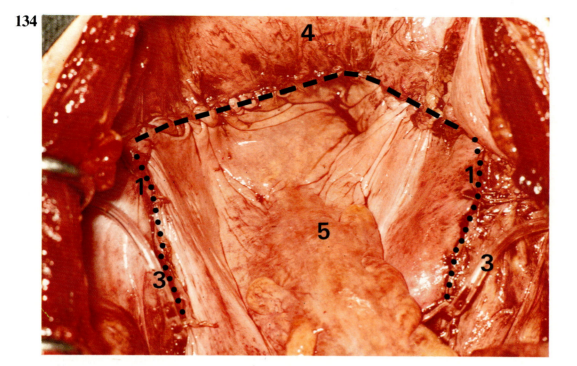

134 Peritonisation completed

The transverse peritoneal closure is indicated by the broken line and the two upward extensions by the dotted lines. The ovarian pedicles are in the areas (1) and (1). The Redivac drains (3) and (3) are seen emerging from the upper ends of the lateral peritoneal closures. The bladder is at (4) and the rectum (5).

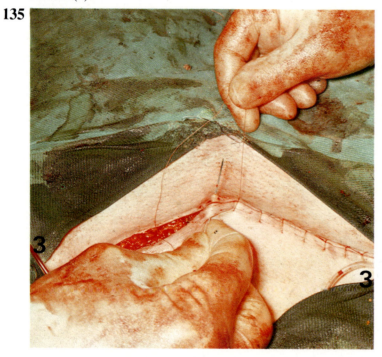

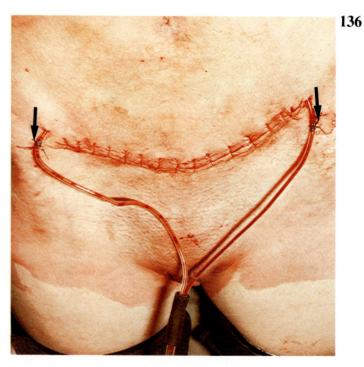

135 and 136 Skin closure and appearance of wound at end of operation

The skin is being closed by a continuous locking stitch of PGA No. 1 material in Figure 135 and the drains are seen emerging lateral to the wound. In Figure 136 skin closure is complete with the drains attached to the skin where arrowed, and suction drainage is already established.

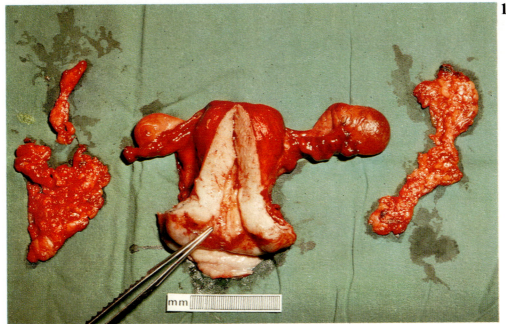

137 Specimen

The uterus has been opened anteriorly and the dissecting forceps indicates the central area of the cervical growth. The upper third of the vaginal skin has been removed and the internal and external iliac gland groups have been removed *en bloc* from each side.

Results of treatment of cervical carcinoma by surgery and other methods

The Annual Report (1976) gives the figures from 23 Institutions each treating a minimum of 200 cases of Stage 1 and Stage 2 carcinoma of the cervix. Peel (1978) has recently reviewed this report and points out that three of the four centres which achieved a five-year survival rate of more than 90 per cent for Stage 1 carcinoma of the cervix made use of radical surgery in more than 80 per cent of cases. In Table 1, Peel sets out five-year survival figures from some of these centres which compare the results of surgery with those of radiotherapy in recent years. These figures show that early cancer of the cervix can be treated effectively by surgery alone, by radiotherapy alone or by a combination of the two.

Table 1
Results of Treatment of Carcinoma of the Cervix

Author	Number of Cases	Percentage Five-Year Survival								Notes
		Stage 1		Stage 2 (all cases)		Stage 2A		Stage 2B		
		Overall	Positive Nodes	Overall	Positive Nodes	Overall	Positive Nodes	Overall	Positive Nodes	
RADIOTHERAPY										
Joslin (1976)	249	94.0		57.0						Combined intracavitary and external beam therapy (actuarial survival)
SURGERY COMPARED WITH RADIOTHERAPY										
Newton (1975)	58	81.0								Radical surgery only
	119									
	61	74.0								Radiotherapy only
Masabuchi et al (1969)	562	90.5	57.1	74.4	50.8					Radical surgery ±DXR (66% stage 1; 37% stage 2)
	602	88.2		68.7						Radiotherapy only (34% stage 1; 63% stage 2)
SURGERY WITH RADIOTHERAPY										
Meigs (1962)	486	83.0	44.0	55.0	27.0					
Stallworthy & Wiernik (1975)	292	82.0	62.0	77.0	42.0					All use preoperative intracavitary irradiation and postoperative external irradiation if nodes involved
Kolstad (1973a and b)	537	88.3	62.9							
Currie (1971)	434	86.3	44.0			75.0	61.7	58.9	40.0	
Christiensen & Fogleman (1976)	320	81.5				71.4		49.0		Meigs-Taussig operation
	350	88.5				68.7		58.2		Okaybayashi operation Postoperative irradiation if nodes positive
Hoskins et al (1976)	224	87.0				92.0				Performed by oncology trainees under supervision

From Peel (1978)

Suggested reading

Annual report on the results of treatment in carcinoma of the uterus, vagina and ovary (Vol. 16, 1976), edited by H. L. Kottmeier. Radiumhemmet, Stockholm.

Buchsbaum, H. J. & Schmidt, J. D. (1978). The urinary tract in radical hysterectomy. *Gynecologic and Obstetric Urology*, 113–127. W. B. Saunders, Philadelphia.

Burch, J. C., Chalfant, R. L. & Johnson, J. W. (1965). Technique for prevention of ureterovaginal fistula following radical hysterectomy. *Annals of Surgery*, 161, 832–837.

Coppleson, M. (1976). Management of preclinical carcinoma of the cervix. *The Cervix*, 453–473, edited by J. Jordan & A. Singer. W. B. Saunders, London, Philadelphia.

Green, T. H. (1966). Ureteral suspension for prevention of ureteral complications following radical Wertheim's hysterectomy. *American Journal of Obstetrics and Gynecology*, 28, 1–10.

Jordan, J. (1978). Personal communication.

Mattingley, R. F. & Borkowf, H. I. (1978). Acute operative injury to the lower urinary tract. *Clinics in Obstetrics and Gynaecology*, 5, 1, 138–147.

Novak, F. (1956). Procedure for the reduction of the number of uretero-vaginal fistula following Wertheim's hysterectomy. *American Journal of Obstetrics and Gynecology*, 72, 506–510.

Ohkawa, K. (1978), as quoted by H. J. Buchsbaum. The urinary tract in radical hysterectomy. *Gynecologic and Obstetric Urology*, 113–127. W. B. Saunders, Philadelphia.

Peel, K. R. (1978). The surgery of cervical carcinoma. *Clinics in Obstetrics and Gynaecology*, 5, 3, 659–673.

Symmonds, R. E. (1966). Morbidity and complication of radical hysterectomy with pelvic node dissection. *American Journal of Obstetrics and Gynecology*, 94, 663–667.

Suggested reading (colposcopy)

Bourke, L. & Matthews, B. (1978). *Atlas of Colposcopy*. F. A. Davis, Philadelphia.

Cartier, R. (1977). *Practical Colposcopy*. Karger, Basel.

Coppleson, M., Pixley, E. & Reid, B. (1978). *Colposcopy*. Second edition. Thomas, Springfield.

Dexeus, S., Carrera, J. & Coupez, F. (1977). *Colposcopy*. W. B. Saunders, Philadelphia.

Kolstad, P. & Stafl, A. (1976). *Atlas of Colposcopy*. Second edition. University Press, Baltimore.

4: Uterine carcinoma

Surgery is accepted as the correct primary treatment for endometrial carcinoma but there are varying opinions on the extent of the operation and on the place and timing of adjuvant radiotherapy. The authors propose to define the various groups of patients requiring treatment and subsequently suggest the most appropriate surgical management for each. The extent and technique of each operation is subsequently described and illustrated.

The following classification of clinical groups includes practically all patients with endometrial carcinoma.

Group 1 Preclinical and early clinical lesions

This group is usually made up of peri-menopausal women who suffer from irregular bleeding, who have had curettage and are known to have hyperplastic endometrium. These patients may have repeated dilatation and curettage operations and the histological findings are often difficult to interpret. The pathologist is not certain that there is malignant change but is unhappy with the cell changes and general hyperplasia. A certain number of patients eventually have hysterectomy and, when the uterus is examined in detail, a proportion is found to have early malignancy. The group of patients described is liable to develop malignancy; Gusberg and Kaplan (1963) showed that between 12 and 23 per cent of women with atypical endometrial hyperplasia eventually develop a malignant tumour. These women are nearly all in good general health.

Group 2 Established endometrial carcinoma

These are cases of adenocarcinoma of the endometrium already diagnosed by curettage and awaiting treatment. Within this group, the general condition of the patient and the accompanying medical conditions often dictate the extent of surgical treatment, whatever may be the ideal. Patients with endometrial cancer are predominantly elderly and may suffer from hypertension, obesity, cardiovascular or pulmonary conditions. Approximately 80 per cent of them are fit for extensive surgery, usually in the form of an extended hysterectomy without pelvic lymphadenectomy. Of the remaining 20 per cent, some are fit for limited surgery such as a simple and expeditious hysterectomy after careful preparation in hospital. The percentage so treated depends on the inclination and the skill of the surgeon.

Group 3 Advanced and inoperable disease

There is a residue of patients in whom advanced disease, severe medical complications and obesity make extensive surgery completely inappropriate.

Selection of appropriate operations for clinical groups

With this particular disease there is the opportunity of using individualized management, i.e. tailoring surgery and adjuvant methods to meet the particular circumstances of the individual case. This approach has been described by the author elsewhere (Lees and Bar Am, 1978).

Group 1

High risk patients in **Group 1** should certainly have hysterectomy, and a total abdominal hysterectomy with bilateral salpingo-oophorectomy with the removal of a cuff of vagina is adequate. In these cases found to have frank invasive carcinoma and hyperplastic endometrial change, the results are excellent. Adjuvant radiotherapy is not required and it is probably safe to conserve ovarian function if particularly requested, although that is not so important in this particular age group. The operation is essentially the same as that described for pre-clinical carcinoma of the cervix (page 127) and is not described again.

Group 2

Established cases in **Group 2** should have radical hysterectomy if the general condition allows. This takes the form of an extended hysterectomy with an emphasis on wide local removal of the growth to obviate vault recurrence. The necessity or wisdom of doing a pelvic block dissection of glands in these medically unfit patients has been the subject of discussion in relevant literature for some time and is now doubted in most quarters: the authors agree with this viewpoint.

A Wertheim pan-hysterectomy was often used but it is now generally accepted that the bulk of cases of endometrial carcinoma can be suitably treated by an extended or radical hysterectomy without pelvic lymphadenectomy. It should be remembered that effective radiotherapy can now be given in high dosage to the lateral pelvic and para-aortic fields, if indicated. An operation of this type is described in the text.

The senior author, on the basis of a large personal experience, has developed a type of extended hysterectomy with partial vaginectomy which is thought to have some advantages. The operation is described on page 221.

Group 3

Patients from **Groups 2** and **3** who are either medically unfit or in whom the growth is too advanced for the type of surgery described, can derive great benefit from hysterectomy, even if it is incomplete in the sense that no great amount of parametrium or vagina is removed. Abdominal or, sometimes, vaginal hysterectomy can relieve the patient of a discharging and debilitating growth, and give a five-year salvage rate of approximately 40 per cent. Undoubtedly, if it is possible to perform, this kind of surgery is worthwhile. The operation does not differ in any way from the standard procedures already described.

Results of treatment

The Annual Report (1976) gives the five-year survival rates for each of the four stages of endometrial carcinoma for the period 1962–1968 (Table 1). These are compiled from 14,506 cases from 47 different centres and there is considerable variation in treatment methods.

Table 1

Five-year Survival Rate Calculated for Each of the Four Stages for the Period 1962–1968

Stage	No. of Patients Treated	No. of Patients Alive	Survival Rate
1 (carcinoma confined to the corpus)	10,699	7,695	71.9
2 (carcinoma involving corpus and cervix)	1,980	984	49.7
3 (carcinoma extending outside uterus but not outside true pelvis)	1,355	416	30.7
4 (carcinoma extending outside true pelvis or involving mucosa of bladder or rectum)	472	44	9.3
	14,506	9,139	63.0

The overall five-year survival rate obtained in 4,197 cases treated in 1962–1963 and presented in the previous Annual Report (Vol. 15, 1973) was 60.2 per cent. In this present report (Vol. 16, 1976) the corresponding figure for the period 1962–1968 was 63.0 per cent.

It can also be seen that about sixty per cent of cases reported to the Stockholm registry for the Annual Report were treated by surgery with or without pre- or postoperative irradiation (Table 2). Forty per cent of cases were treated by irradiation alone.

Table 2

Summary of the Therapy Applied in Carcinoma of the Corpus in the Years 1962–1968 at 47 Institutions

Stage	No. of Cases in which the Planned Treatment was				Total No. Treated
	Hyst. (with or without postop. rad.)	Preop. Rad. + Hyst. (with or without postop. rad.)	Primary Radiation Alone	Other	
1	4,409	2,752	3,534	4	10,699
2	449	399	1,128	4	1,980
3	382	125	836	12	1,355
4	92	28	307	45	472
1–4	5,332	3,304	5,805	65	14,506

Diagnostic dilatation and curettage

When investigating cases of possible endometrial carcinoma, only a minority of patients are found to have the disease. The one outstanding suspicious symptom is uterine bleeding or bloodstained serous discharge; it is generally post- but sometimes peri-menopausal in onset.

Possible non-malignant causes of this symptom include atrophic vaginitis, endometrial and cervical polypi and particularly 'withdrawal bleeding' due to fluctuation of oestrogen levels following irregular or poorly controlled administration of exogenous oestrogens. As far as other growths are concerned one would expect to recognise a clinical cervical lesion on speculum examination. Ovarian tumours, particularly feminizing ones, and many of the solid ovarian carcinomata may produce symptoms in the form of post-menopausal bleeding.

It is axiomatic that a diagnostic curettage be done in all cases but there is a temptation to adopt different standards in differing circumstances and this merits comment. For example, a slightly bloodstained yellow discharge in the presence of obvious senile vaginitis, or a small non-recurring

bleed a few days after discontinuing hormone tablets taken, perhaps irregularly and inadequately, for menopausal symptoms might seem to be adequately covered by an out-patient Vabra-type curettage. As the reader is aware the chances of cure are greatly diminished by missing the diagnosis at an early stage and, in this as in any other cancer, there is no place for dilution of standards in investigation. A full-scale curettage is mandatory. Surgeons of experience can all remember cases where established routine procedure saved them from making a mistake and, although we regret referring back to the possibility of medical litigation, the surgeon who disregards the basic rules in such matters is left with little defence. Certainly one will do very many tedious examinations with negative findings but there is no alternative.

It should be noted that certain recognised additional symptoms greatly increase the likelihood of finding carcinoma and these include pain during the bleeding, friable debris in the blood or discharge and general symptoms if the disease is advanced.

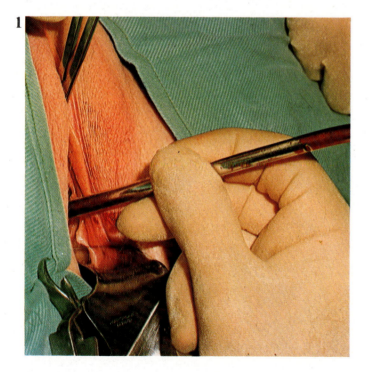

1 Dilatation of the cervix
Dilatation of the cervix in suspected endometrial carcinoma should be done very cautiously. The uterine cavity may be quite short and the fundus largely replaced by growth so that even a blunt dilator can penetrate it with surprising ease. The inexperienced reader should refer to the technical precautions described in Volume 1 (pages 14–15). There may be venous bleeding from the uterus between the insertion of succeeding dilators and this nearly always indicates the presence of malignancy. Friable debris in the blood provides even stronger evidence.

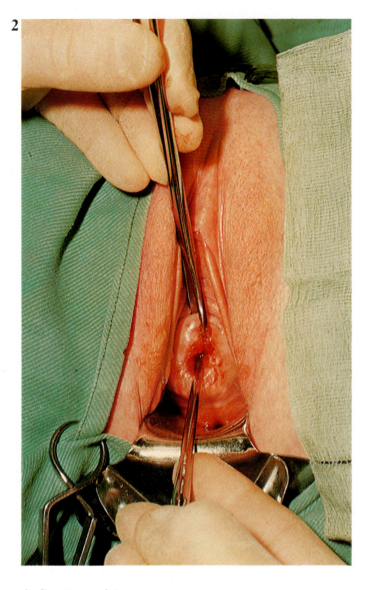

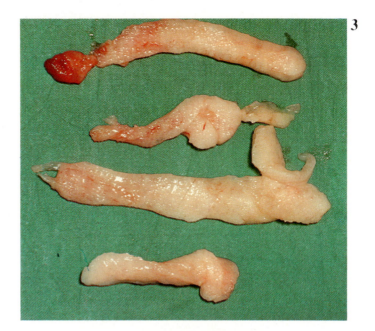

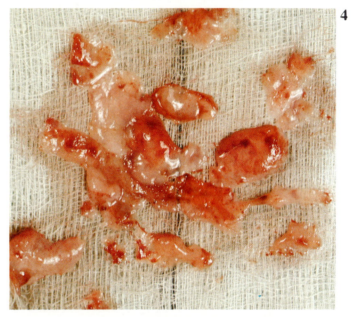

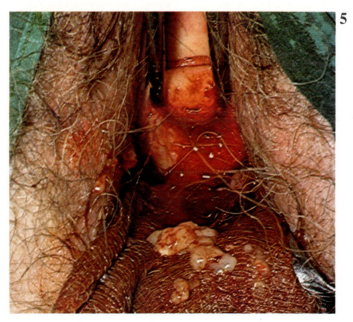

2 Curettage of the uterus

Curettage is performed with a moderately blunt-ended curette; extreme gentleness is paramount so as to avoid perforation of a malignant uterus. The curettings are transferred to a gauze swab placed lateral to the vulva either as they are obtained or on retrieval from the posterior vaginal fornix.

Figures 3, 4 and 5 show the types of benign and malignant endometrium which may be obtained.

3 Hyperplastic endometrium – benign

Smooth, pale glistening appearance with no surface breakdown suggests either cystic hyperplasia or excess administration of oestrogens as the aetiology in the post-menopausal state.

4 Endometrial polyp

Typical endometrial polypi with smooth glistening surface from a patient with predominantly intermenstrual bleeding.

5 Endometrial adenocarcinoma

Profuse curettings with marked necrotic change are typical. The appearance is cheesy with loss of glistening surface.

Histological confirmation is required, of course, in all the specimens.

199

Extended abdominal hysterectomy

The term extended hysterectomy is variously interpreted and the operation is sometimes no more than a total abdominal hysterectomy and bilateral salpingo-oophorectomy with removal of a cuff of vagina. Something much more extensive is required if vault recurrence is to be avoided and the aim of the operation must be to remove not only the uterus and its appendages entire, but also a wide area of vaginal vault skin and parametrial tissue. This should be done without spill or dissemination of malignant cells. The concept of tumour spread by malignant cells advancing along distinct lymphatic pathways to more distant parts of the body has been replaced, to some extent, by the more realistic idea of a local neoplastic explosion with direct tumour cell invasion of the surrounding tissues. If the surgeon keeps this picture in mind the requisite type of operation is better appreciated.

From the technical point of view, the first point to be remembered is that extensive local removal cannot be effected without dissection and lateral displacement of the ureters; such a step is essential if the operation is to be adequate. As far as the pelvic lymph glands are concerned, there was a period during which complete gland removal was recommended and attempted but authoritative opinion now questions the need and, indeed, the wisdom of doing so (De Muelenare (1973), Boronow (1976)). The trend is towards the use of the newer forms of radiotherapy for demonstrable lateral pelvic extension; this aspect has recently been reviewed by Maier (1978).

Statistics from the Royal Prince Alfred Hospital, Sydney, Australia, and contributed by Dr M. Coppleson, are taken from the Annual Report (1976) as an appropriate parameter in estimating what can be expected from radical surgical management of the disease (Table 3). A modified Wertheim hysterectomy was the treatment of choice in the majority of cases considered good surgical risks and management generally corresponds with our own. Radiation was given postoperatively in cases in which the growth was anaplastic, had invaded deeply into the myometrium, or/and had involved the adnexa, the cervix or vagina.

Recent personal experience in Sheffield has encouraged a move away from ultra-radical surgery to something more moderate. In a first series of 102 cases, where 76 patients were treated by radical hysterectomy, partial vaginectomy following preoperative internal radiotherapy, the five-year survival rate was 64 per cent. There were no vault recurrences but two patients died of pulmonary embolism. In a second series of 92 cases, 61 patients were similarly treated with radical hysterectomy and partial vaginectomy, but lymphadenectomy was omitted and replaced by biopsy of the three lymph gland groups on each side of the pelvis. Radiotherapy was given by linear accelerator to the pelvic side walls as required. The five-year survival rate in this series was 80 per cent. The elimination of vault recurrence was maintained and there were no fatal cases of pulmonary embolism (Lees 1978).

Table 3

Number of Cases Treated by	
Hysterectomy or radical hysterectomy	193
Preoperative radiation plus hysterectomy	2
Radiation	7
Other therapy	1

Stage	Patients Treated No.	Patients Treated %	Patients Alive at 5 Years No	Patients Alive at 5 Years %
1	177	87.2	139	78.5
2	13	6.4	4	30.7
3	11	5.4	3	27.3
4	2	1.0	1	50.0

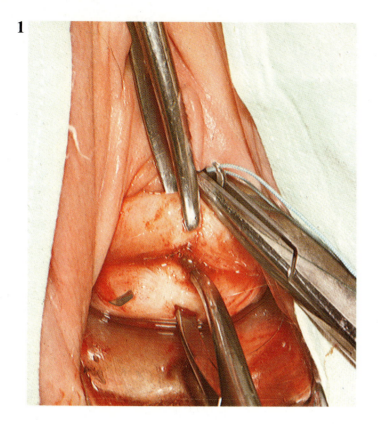

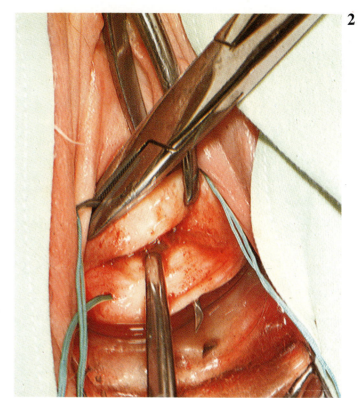

1 to 3 Closure of cervix at commencement of operation

The cervix is closed by a deep X stitch of PGA No. 2 or other strong suture to prevent the escape of malignant cells during operation. An Auvard speculum exposes the cervix and in Figure 1 the cutting needle carrying the stitch deeply transfixes both lips of the cervix obliquely from left anterior to right posterior. In Figure 2 the stitch continues in the same way but from right anterior to left posterior. In Figure 3 the ends have been tied and cut short to show the cervix sealed by the completed stitch.

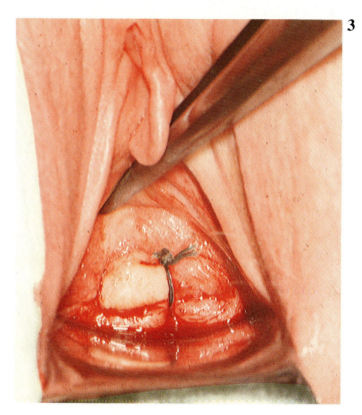

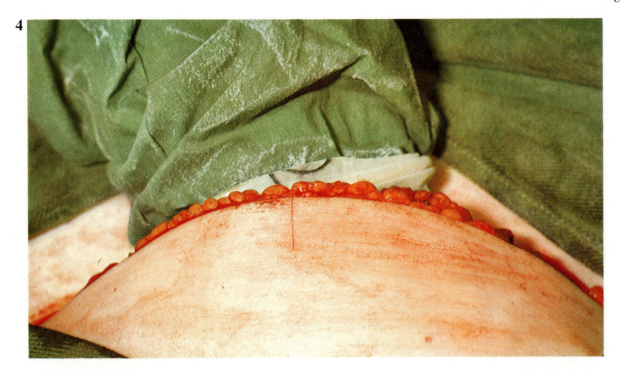

4 Exploration of abdomen

This step is very important and should never be omitted. The condition of the uterus and the appendages is of first importance but a routine examination of the whole abdomen is also carried out. The main purpose is to detect any extra-uterine spread of the growth but examination of the principal abdominal structures sometimes reveals findings that have an important bearing on immediate and subsequent management.

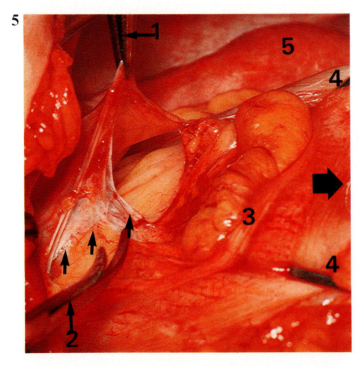

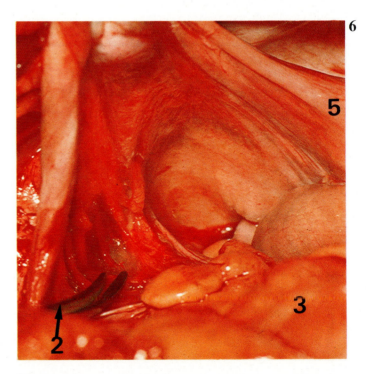

5 and 6 Release of descending colon from left appendages

The sigmoid colon is often adherent to the infundibulo-pelvic fold on the left side. It interferes with access and should be detached. In Figure 5 the dissecting forceps (1) holds the peritoneum of the posterior layer of the broad ligament on the left while the scissors (2) detach the colon (3), where arrowed. The tissue forceps (4) pull the colon postero-medially in the direction of the broad arrow. The uterus is at (5). In Figure 6 the colon is now well clear while the uterus is lifted upwards and forwards and the site of the adhesion of the colon is now seen on the left side. The same numerals apply.

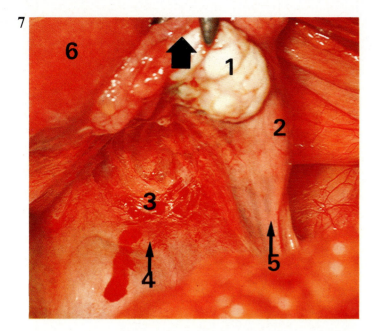

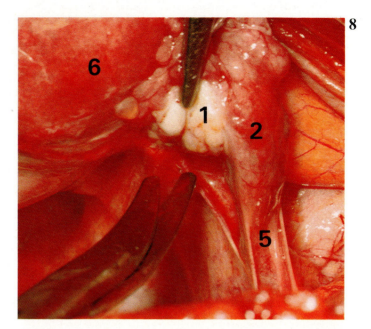

7 to 9 Freeing and elevating right appendages

The type of adhesions seen around the right appendages in the illustrations may result from a large amount of preoperative irradiation but could equally well be the result of previous pelvic infection. In either case, the first requirement is to divide the adhesions and elevate the appendages so that hysterectomy can proceed and, at the same time, so that the line of the right ureter is kept accessible. The reason for this will soon be apparent. In Figure 7 the right ovary (1) and right tube (2) are lifted upwards by the tissue forceps in the direction of the arrow and the parietal peritoneum is left ragged (3) by separation of the structures. The ureter is seen (4) and the ovarian pedicle (5). The uterus is at (6). The scissors continue the upward separation of the appendages in Figures 8 and 9 with the separation practically completed in Figure 9. The same numerals apply in each photograph.

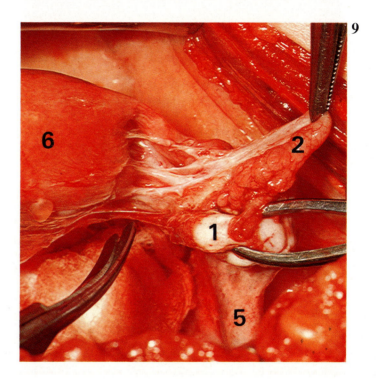

Stage 1: Exposure of the ureters

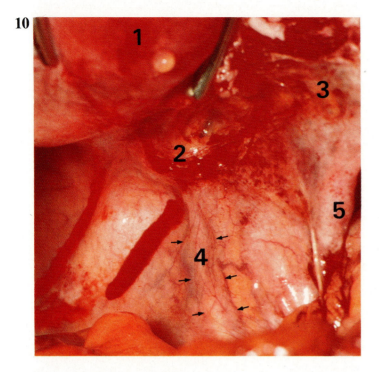

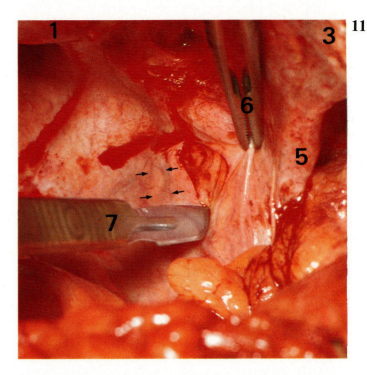

10 and 11 Definition of right ureter

In Figure 10 the uterus (1) is lifted upwards and forwards to disrupt its adhesion to the pelvic floor (2) and the right appendages are seen laterally (3). The right ureter is easily recognised extraperitoneally at (4) and the right ovarian pedicle is at (5). In Figure 11 a fold of the posterior layer of the broad ligament, where it overlies the right ureter, is held by dissecting forceps (6) while an incision is made with the scalpel (7) through the peritoneum only, on the lateral side of, and quite clear of the ureter (outlined). A scalpel incision is neat and definitive but could endanger the ureter and scissors should be preferred as safer.

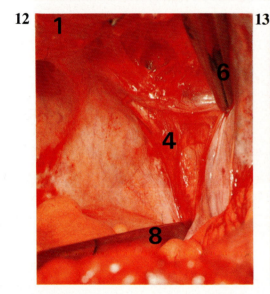

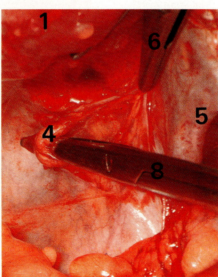

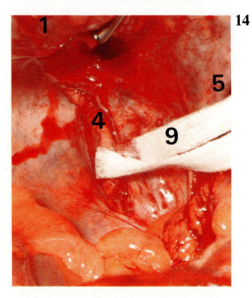

12 to 14 Exposure of right ureter

In Figure 12 the scissors (8) commence dissection of the right ureter extraperitoneally and in Figure 13 it is seen raised on the points of the scissors. A broad tape (9) for subsequent identification is placed under the ureter in Figure 14.

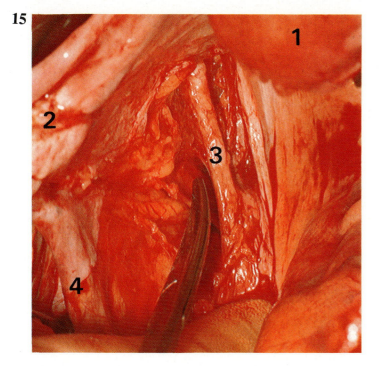

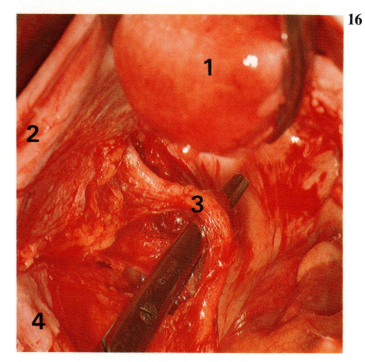

15 to 17 Exposure of left ureter
Three stages in the exposure of the left ureter are shown.
The posterior aspect and the base of the left broad ligament
were opened up exactly as on the right side once the ureter
had been visualised. The uterus is at (1), the left appendages
(2), the ureter (3), and the ovarian pedicle (4).

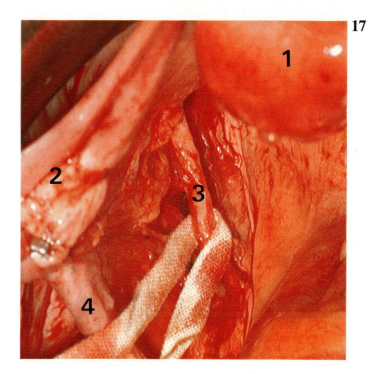

Stage 2: Division of upper uterine attachments

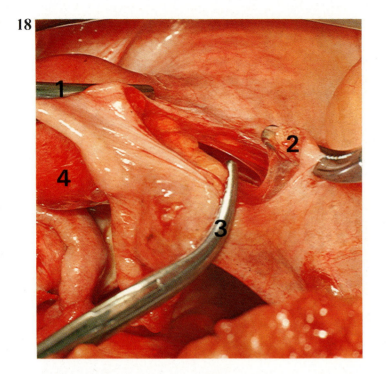

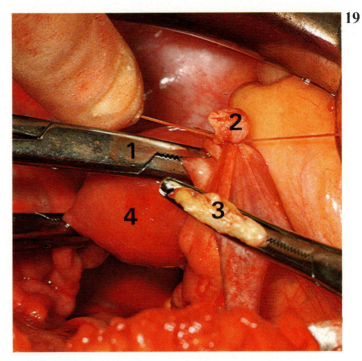

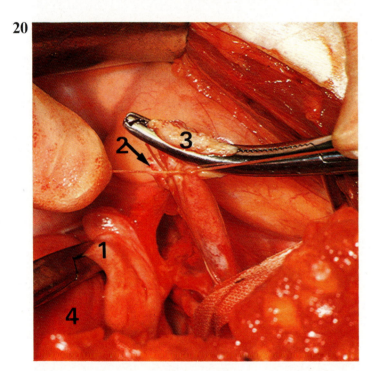

18 to 20 Securing right upper uterine attachments

In Figure 18 the right broad ligament is held by forceps (1) and the cut end of the right round ligament is held in forceps (2). A further pair of forceps (3) has been applied to the ovarian pedicle. In Figure 19 the round ligament pedicle is being ligated following transfixion and the ovarian pedicle is being similarly dealt with in Figure 20. The fundus of the uterus is at (4) in each photograph.

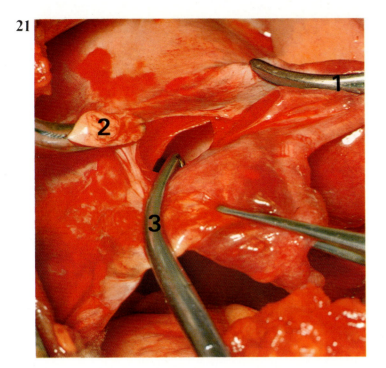
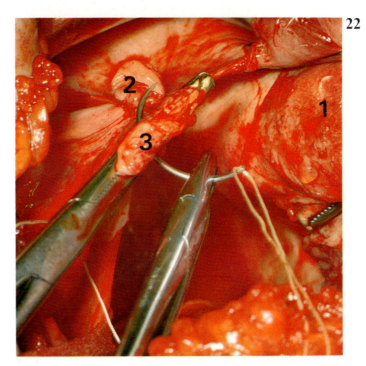
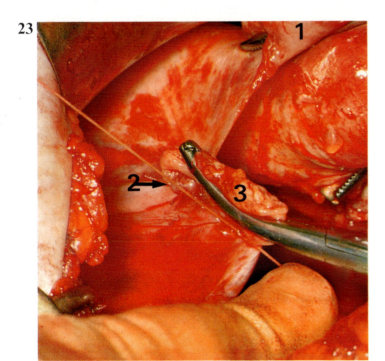
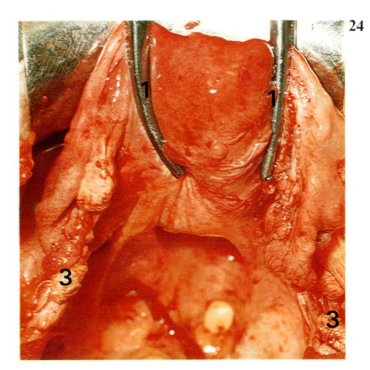

21 to 24 Securing left upper uterine attachments

The same procedure is carried out on the left side; the numbering is similar. In Figure 21 the left ovarian pedicle is clamped ready for division, in Figure 22 it is being transfixed with the ligature carrying needle and in Figure 23 it is being tied off. Figure 24 shows the uterus held up by the broad ligament forceps with the detached appendages laterally. The ligated ovarian pedicles are at (3).

Stage 3: Opening up broad ligaments

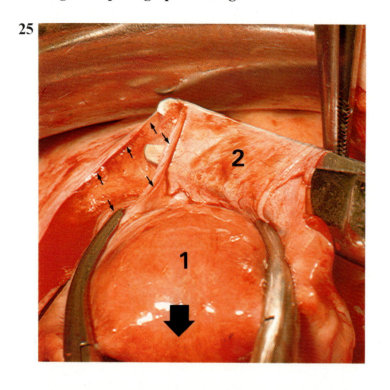

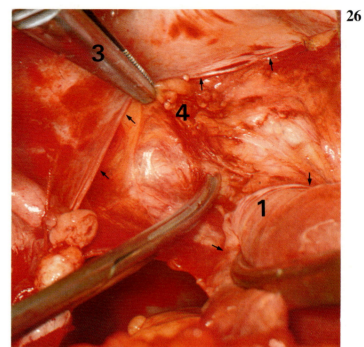

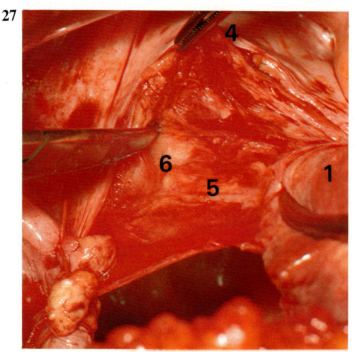

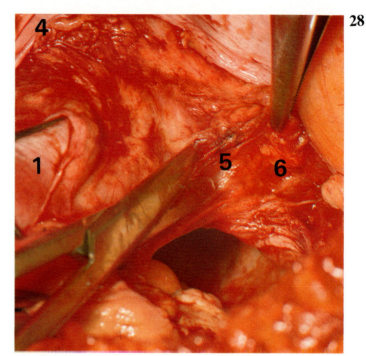

25 to 28 Division of anterior layer of broad ligament to define bladder and uterine vessels

The upper part of the posterior layer of the broad ligament has already been opened when exposing the ureters. In Figure 25 the uterus (1) is held back in the direction of the broad arrow and the utero-vesical fold of peritoneum has already been divided (fine arrows) on the left side. The peritoneum is seen raised on the scissors prior to division on the right side (2). In Figure 26 the divided edge of peri- toneum is held in dissecting forceps (3) and is now arrowed on both sides. The points of the scissors dissect the bladder (4) from the anterior aspect of the uterus (1) and the cervix. In Figure 27 the uterine vessels (5) are defined and stripped of areolar tissue as far as the parametrium. In this position they overlie the ureteric tunnel (6). A similar procedure is carried out on the right side in Figure 28; the numbers refer to the structures as in Figures 25–27.

29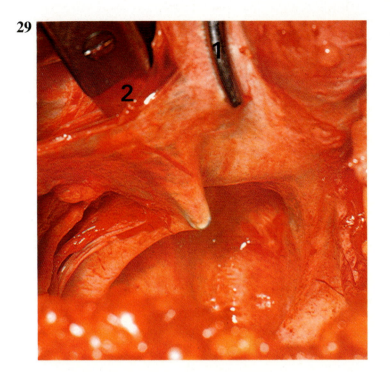

30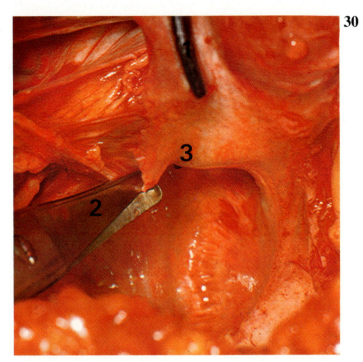

31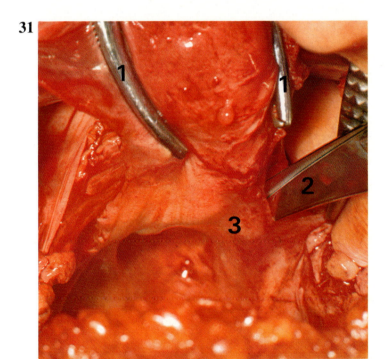

32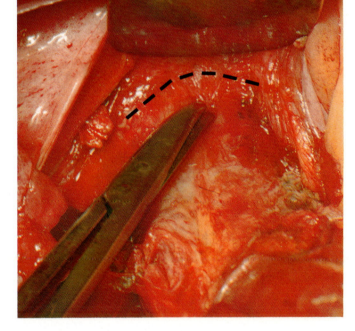

29 to 31 Completing division of posterior layer of broad ligament to further free uterus

In Figure 29 the heavy curved forceps (1) hold the left broad ligament and the scissors (2) tunnel the posterior layer of the broad ligament prior to dividing it. In Figure 30 the scissors have divided the peritoneum as far down as the left utero-sacral ligament (3). In Figure 31 a similar division is made of the right side as far as the utero-sacral ligament (3).

32 Completing separation of bladder anteriorly

In Figure 32 attention is again turned to the anterior aspect of the uterus where a deep retractor supports the bladder while the scissors free the base of the bladder from the anterior aspect of the cervix and upper vagina along the dotted line.

Stage 4: Exposure of ureters

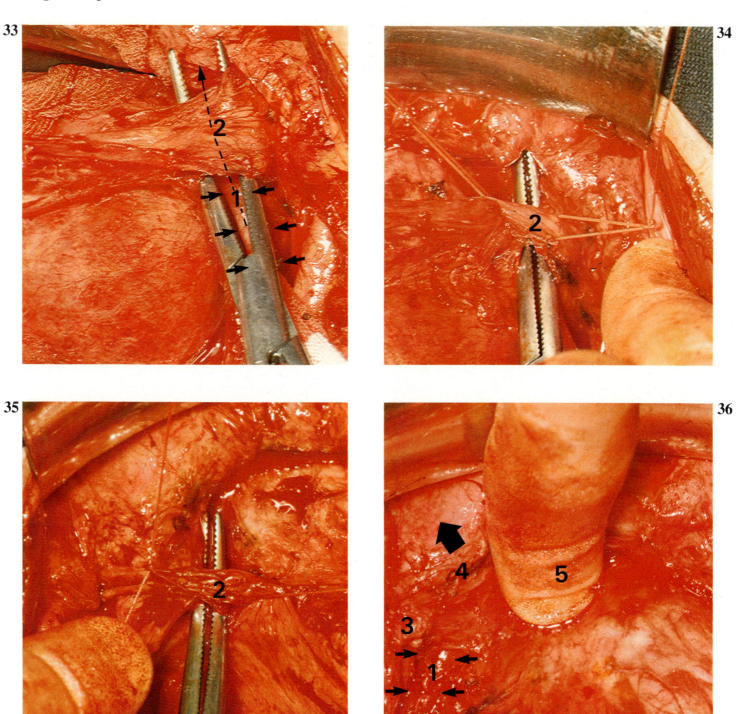

33 to 36 Exposure of ureters in the ureteric tunnel

The line of the right ureter (arrowed and (1)) is followed into the ureteric tunnel by large Spencer-Wells forceps in Figure 33. The roof of the tunnel with its uterine vessels (2) is then defined, doubly ligated and is ready to be divided in Figure 34. The same stage has been reached on the left side in Figure 35. The exposed ureters can then be displaced laterally so as to allow access to a substantial portion of vaginal vault. Figure 36 shows the left ureter (1) lying medial to the ligated left uterine pedicle (3) and being displaced along with the angle of the bladder (4) from the upper vaginal angle with the finger (5) (in the direction of the arrow).

Stage 5: Securing lower uterine attachments

The uterus is still attached by the utero-sacral ligaments. Part of each cardinal ligament forming the roof of the parametrial (ureteric) tunnel was divided when exposing the ureters; any remaining fibres will be clamped and divided with the vaginal angle pedicle when the uterus is removed. The utero-sacral ligaments, however, are tethering the uterus infero-posteriorly and must be detached from the uterus to increase its mobility and accessibility to the vaginal angles.

37 Detaching utero-sacral ligaments

The left utero-sacral ligament is detached from the uterus with scissors cutting distal to the holding forceps; the same is then done on the other side. The ligaments are at (1) and (1).

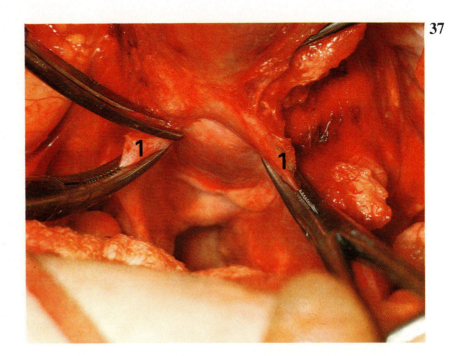

37

38

38 Freeing the uterus posteriorly

Both utero-sacral ligaments have been separated off the uterus and are held in forceps (1) and (1). The scalpel (2) has completed a stroke across the posterior aspect of the cervix at the level of its inferior border to divide the peritoneum (arrowed) where it is attached to the posterior aspect of the cervix, and also to divide any superficial fibrous tissue which is still anchoring the uterus. Immediately this is done, the uterus can be lifted up from the pelvic floor and the utero-sacral ligaments and the peritoneal edge between them fall back to expose the posterior fornix of the vagina. By blunt dissection and leverage on the forceps, it is simple to strip the peritoneal covering from the upper third of the posterior vaginal wall.

211

39

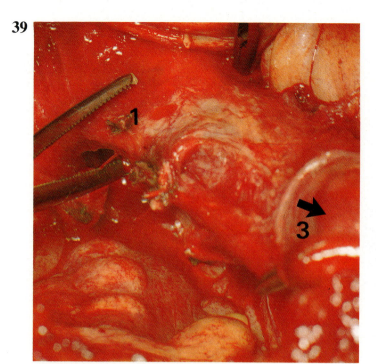

40

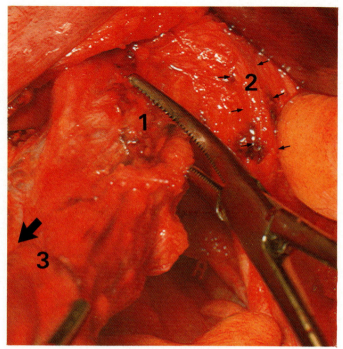

41

39 to 41 Wide excision of vaginal vault

In Figure 39 the uterus is pulled in a medial and cephalad direction, as arrowed, and the upper vagina is being clamped on its left lateral edge about the junction of the upper and middle thirds (1). In Figure 40 the same procedure is carried out on the right side and, in this instance, the right ureter is plainly visible (2). These two clamps include in their grasp any remaining fibres of the cardinal ligaments. In Figure 41 a large Kelly retractor pulls back the bladder to show the considerable depth anteriorly at which the vagina will be divided. The lower uterine wall is at (3) in each photograph.

42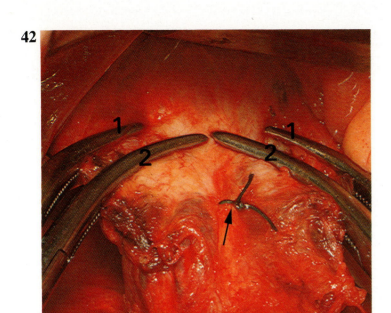

43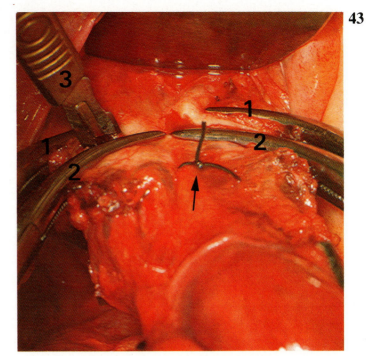

42 to 44 Removal of uterus and wide cuff of vagina

In Figure 42 the level of the external cervical os is indicated by the stitch (arrowed) and shows that the cuff is fully adequate in length. Above the two clamps already in place (1) and (1), two further occluding forceps are applied across the vagina (2) and (2). In Figure 43 the scalpel (3) divides the vagina between the two sets of forceps and in Figure 44 the uterus and vaginal cuff have been removed, leaving the original clamps (1) and (1) and the open vaginal vault (4).

44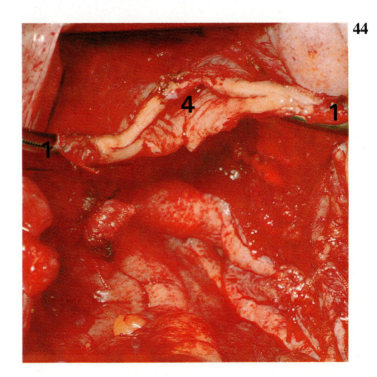

Stage 6: Closure of vaginal vault

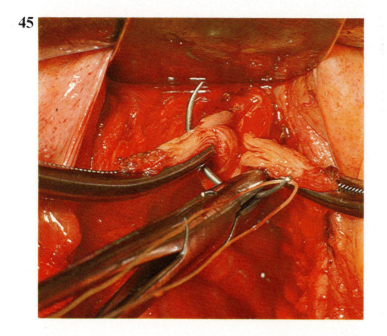

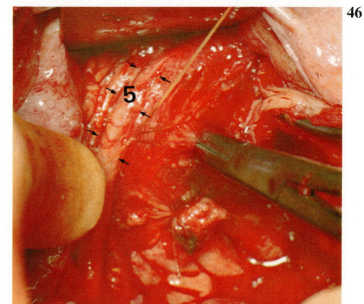

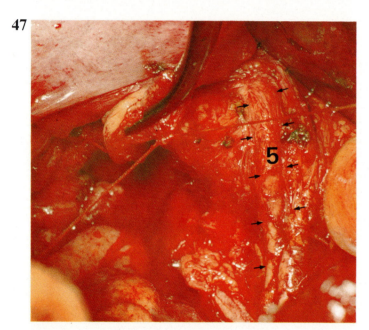

45 to 47 Securing vaginal angles

The left vaginal angle is transfixed by the needle carrying the ligature in Figure 45 and the angle pedicle is being ligated in Figure 46. In Figure 47 the right vaginal angle is being similarly ligated. The remaining fibres of the cardinal ligaments are included in these pedicles. In both Figures 46 and 47, the ureter (5) is clearly seen and is arrowed.

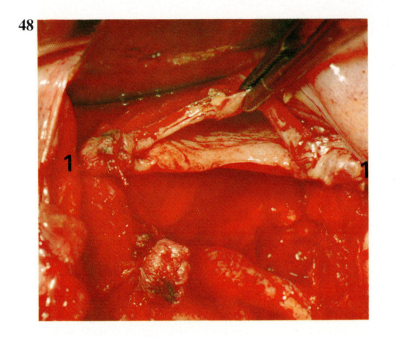

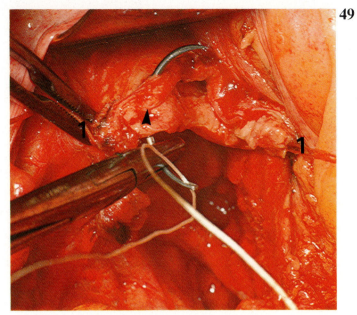

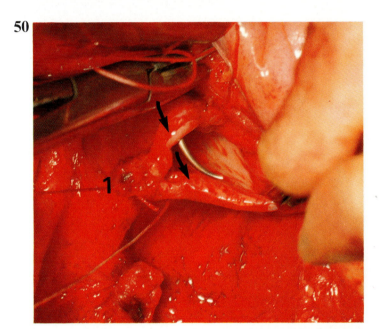

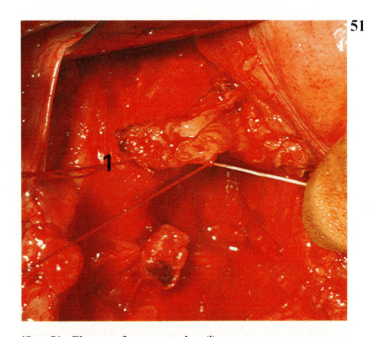

48 to 51 Closure of upper vagina (i)

In Figure 48 the vaginal angles are held apart by the uncut
sutures (1) and (1) and the dissecting forceps on the anterior
edge hold the vaginal cavity open. The left-sided mattress
suture is inserted postero-anteriorly (arrowed) in Figure 49
and returned antero-posteriorly (arrowed) in Figure 50.
The stitch is tied off in Figure 51.

52

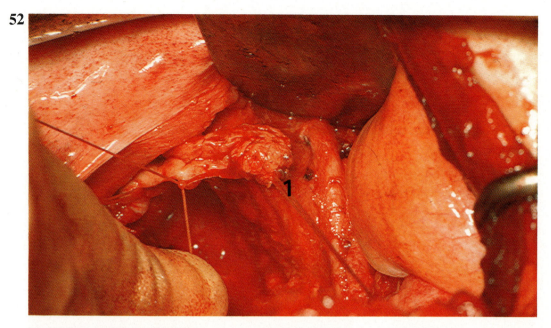

52 Closure of upper vagina (ii)
The same procedure is repeated on the right side with the
mattress suture shown being tied.

53

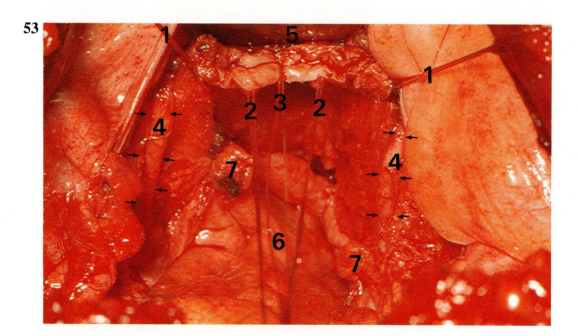

53 Transverse closure of upper vagina completed
The uncut vaginal angle sutures (1) and (1) are still used
as tractors and the two mattress sutures (2) and (2) with a
single stitch medially (3) complete the closure. The ureters
are clearly seen and are numbered (4). The bladder is protected by the Kelly retractor (5) and the rectum is at (6).
The ligated utero-sacral pedicles which will now be incorporated in the vault are numbered (7) and (7).

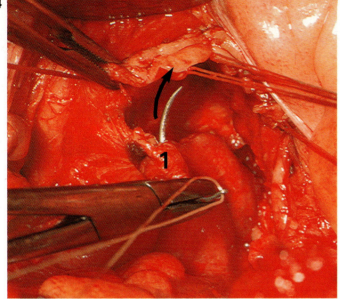

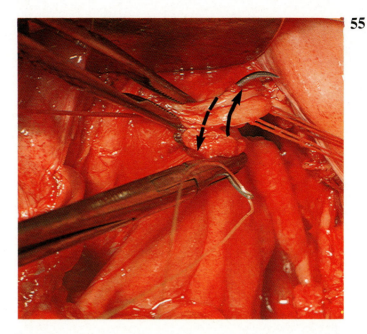

55

54 to 56 Attachment of left utero-sacral ligament to vaginal vault

The pedicle of the utero-sacral ligament is attached to the posterior aspect of the vaginal vault by a mattress suture as shown. In Figure 54 the ligament (1) has been picked up on the needle which is about to transfix the closed vaginal vault close to where it is held by dissecting forceps (arrowed).

In Figure 55 the procedure continues in the direction of the solid arrow and the needle will then return through the same structures in the reverse direction as indicated by the broken arrow. This has been completed in Figure 56 and the mattress suture is tied, fixing the utero-sacral pedicle firmly to the vaginal vault.

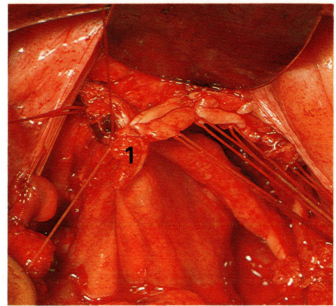

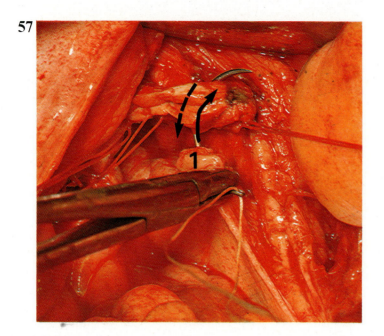

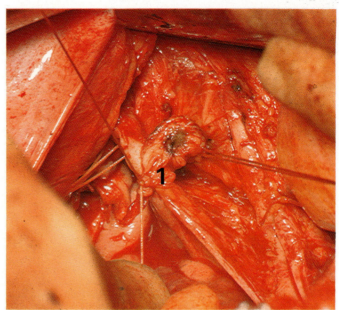

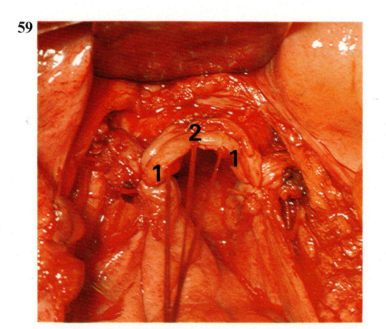

56

57 to 59 Attachment of right utero-sacral ligament to vaginal vault

A similar mattress suture is placed on the right side. The ligament is numbered (1) and the outward and return course of the needle through the closed vault of the vagina is indicated by solid and broken arrows respectively in Figure 57. The stitch is tied in Figure 58 and in Figure 59 the completely supported vault is shown with the centre stay suture at (2) and the ligaments attached to the vault at (1) and (1).

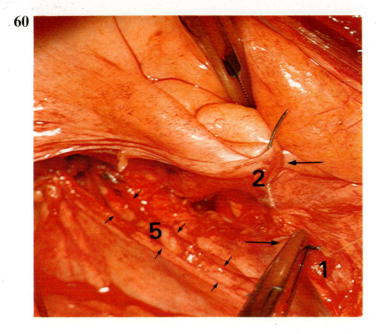

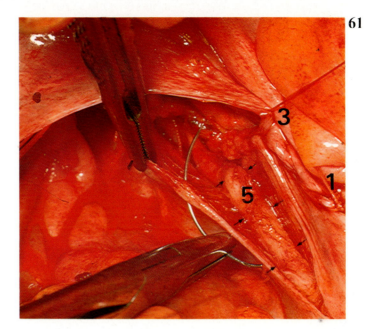

Since the ureters have been exposed in practically their entire pelvic length, it is not very convenient to close the peritoneum by a single continuous stitch curving across the pelvic floor. The best method is to close the central peritoneum in the usual way by a continuous suture from the round and ovarian ligaments on one side to the other, and leaving the gaps along the line of the upper ureter on each side to be closed later. These openings are in fact ideal for laying the Redivac type drains across the vaginal vault and extraperitoneal space and can be lightly sutured together **subsequently**. This two-stage method of closing the peritoneum, and the reasons for doing so, was described for the Wertheim operation in Figures 127 to 129 (page 190).

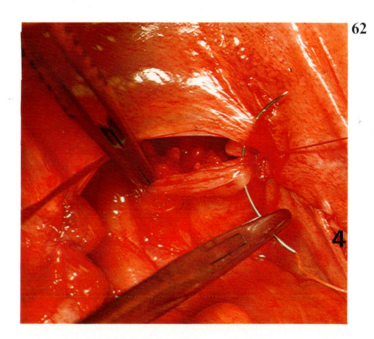

60 to 62 Closure of peritoneum across centre of pelvis

In Figure 60 a fine needle carrying a continuous PGA No. 00 suture picks up the posterior leaf of pelvic peritoneum medial to the ovarian pedicle (1) and the anterior leaf lateral to the round ligament pedicle (2) and as arrowed. When tied, the anchor stitch everts the round ligament pedicle but the ovarian pedicle is purposely left uncovered since there is often a relative shortage of pelvic peritoneum and a purse

string type stitch would be under tension and could kink or distort the ureter. In Figure 61 the anchor stitch (3) is tied and the round ligament pedicle is beneath it. The ovarian pedicle (1) is uncovered and is seen laterally. The needle meantime picks up a second bite of the posterior peritoneal edge and in Figure 62 proceeds across the pelvis. The open gap in the peritoneum on the right side is numbered (4). The ureter (5) is outlined in Figures 60 and 61.

63

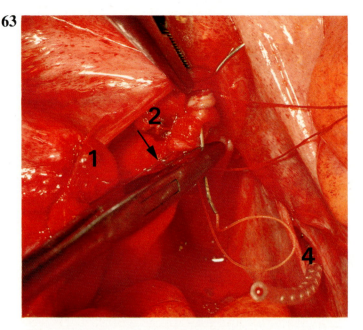

64

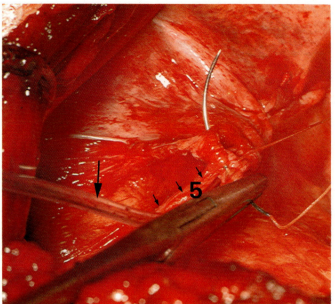

63 and 64 Extra-peritoneal drainage

In Figure 63 the transverse peritoneal closure nears completion on the left and will cover the round ligament pedicle (2) but again avoids the ovarian pedicle (1). A Redivac drain has already been inserted from the left side (arrowed) but is largely hidden by the needle-holder proximally although it can be seen emerging distally through the open peritoneal gap on the right side (4). In Figure 64 the drain is clearly seen as the left-sided peritoneal gap is closed by a fine continuous suture. The left ureter (5) lies immediately underneath and emphasises the ease with which it could be distorted.

65

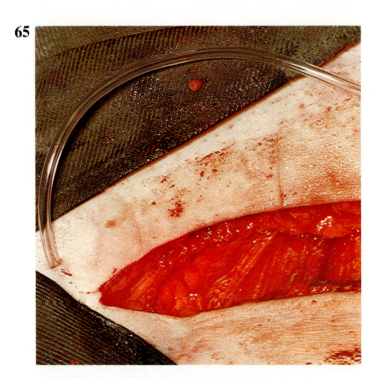

66

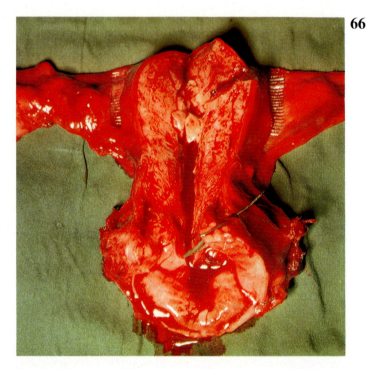

65 Redivac drain brought through abdominal wall

The needle attached to the proximal end of the Redivac drain is brought from the left iliac fossa intra-peritoneally and then through the abdominal parietes lateral to the transverse incision, so the drain lies as shown. The drain may be kept retro-peritoneal. As there is no angulation or possibility of kinking, drainage is not interfered with and the wound is not involved or weakened by the presence of the drain.

66 Specimen

The uterine cavity and cervical canal have been opened anteriorly and the naked eye appearance shows that the preoperative radiotherapy has induced macroscopic regression of the endometrial growth. The size of the vaginal cuff is seen to be adequate; this is of great importance in the management of this disease since subsequent local vault recurrence indicates complete failure of treatment.

Radical hysterectomy and partial vaginectomy with pelvic node biopsy
(Lees' modification)

This operation was developed to overcome the difficulty in obtaining an adequate amount of vagina and parametrial tissue by a purely abdominal approach. The problem of access in the usually obese, elderly and medically unfit women with endometrial carcinoma is well recognised. This two stage procedure involves an initial vaginal approach with partial vaginectomy and division of lower uterine supports, followed by an abdominal entry for hysterectomy which has been facilitated by the detachment of the lower pelvic supports. Some surgeons may feel that the orthodox extended hysterectomy meets their needs. However, in certain cases others will find this modification helpful. Results obtained by the senior author in 137 cases treated by this technique, and referred to on page 200 have been extremely satisfactory.

The operation commences by closing the cervix with stitches and then raising the vaginal skin from the underlying tissues over the upper half of the vagina. The vagina is circumscribed about its mid-point and the whole of the vault skin is raised from its underlying tissues as a pouch. The mouth of this pouch is closed with a purse string suture to form a second watertight barrier to the escape of intra-uterine debris and cells. The utero-vesical pouch is opened as in a vaginal hysterectomy. The pouch of Douglas is then opened, giving access to the utero-sacral ligaments. These latter structures are secured well back from the uterus, detached, transfixed and ligated. The uterus is thus freed posteriorly in the depth of the pelvis and subsequent hysterectomy is easy and atraumatic. The whole uterus and cervix are pushed up into the pelvic peritoneal cavity and the vaginal vault closed transversely by a series of interrupted vertical mattress sutures.

The abdominal hysterectomy is performed through a transverse incision, which gives better access than a vertical one in obese patients and is immeasurably stronger post-operatively. The uterus is gently removed by first securing the round and ovarian ligaments and completing the separation of the bladder from the uterine cervix. The ureters are identified and followed forward to expose them in the ureteric tunnels and the uterine vessels on each side are secured in the process of dividing the roof of the tunnel. The ureters are then displaced laterally to allow access to the cardinal ligaments. Since the utero-sacral ligaments are already detached, the pedicles of the cardinal ligaments are only about 1.5 cm in diameter. These ligaments are clamped and cut well laterally, and the uterus is lifted out of the pelvis. The closed vault of the vagina can scarcely be seen or reached at this stage because it is so deep in the pelvis; this emphasises the enormous advantage gained from the initial vaginal approach. The amount of tissue removed from the vagina and paracolpos is fully adequate and classes the operation as a very radical one. Before closing the peritoneum across the pelvic floor and vaginal vault, gland biopsies are taken from each of the three groups – common iliac, external iliac and hypogastric – on each side. The histological appearance of the glands together with the degree of differentiation of the original tumour indicates the need, or otherwise, for postoperative irradiation.

If biopsy shows that the growth has already spread to the glands of the pelvic side wall, the prognosis is necessarily poor but radiotherapy may still be effective and modern methods are obtaining improved results. We have satisfied ourselves that, in the circumstances described, the results of such treatment are superior to what could be obtained by radical surgical procedures of the Wertheim type.

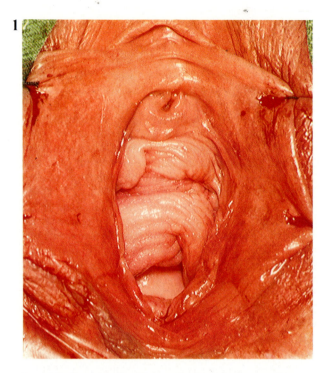

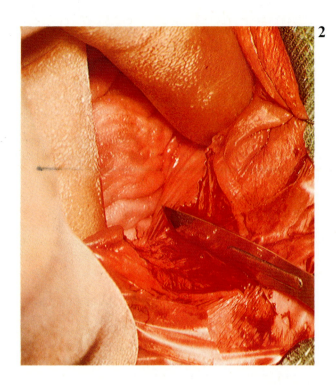

1 and 2 Preparation for vaginal part of operation

Figure 1 shows the patient in lithotomy position with the labia stitched back to give good access to the upper vagina.

In Figure 2 an episiotomy-type relief incision is made postero-medially on the left side to improve access still further.

Stage 1: Closing cervix with X-stitch

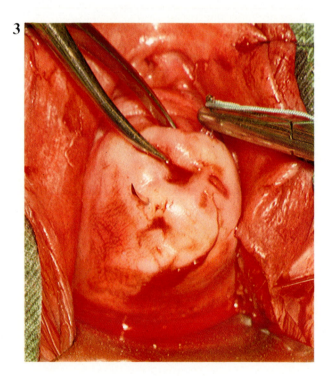

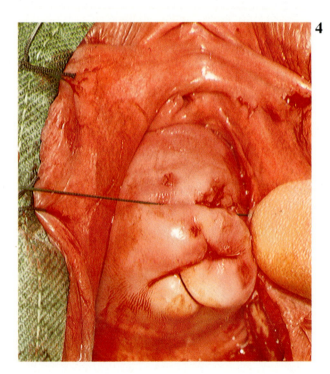

3 and 4 Inserting X-stitch in cervix

The anterior lip of the cervix is held in a tissue forceps and the stitch of PGA No. 1 suture is carried on a cutting needle. In Figure 3 the needle transfixes the cervix deeply from the left side of the anterior lip to the right side of

the posterior lip, as shown, and then returns from left posterior to right anterior to complete the X-stitch. In Figure 4 the ends of the stitch are being firmly tied to close off and seal the cervical canal.

Stage 2: Circumcision of vaginal skin at mid-point

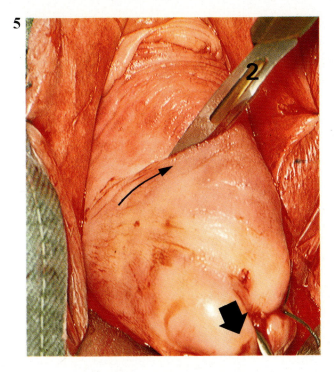

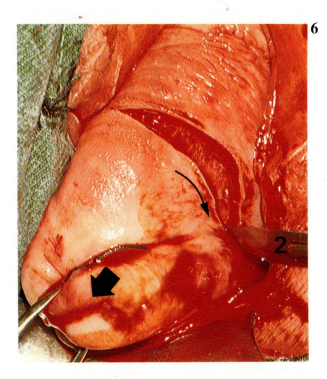

5 and 6   Circumcision of vaginal skin (i)
The anterior lip of the cervix is held in Littlewood's forceps (1) and the large arrows indicate the direction in which it is being held. In Figure 5 the scalpel (2) cuts through the full thickness of the skin of the anterior vaginal wall about its mid-point and beginning on the right side (in the direction of the fine arrow). The incision continues in the same plane across the left side in Figure 6 (arrowed).

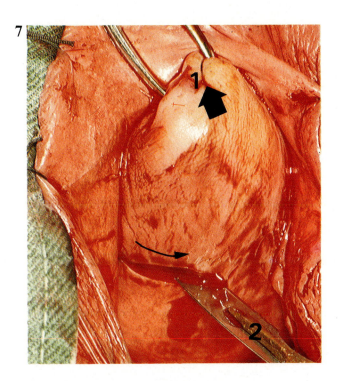

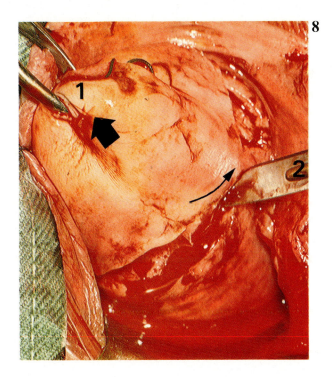

7 and 8   Circumcision of vaginal skin (ii)
The cervix (1) is now held up by the Littlewood's forceps and the incision continues across the right and the left posterior walls as arrowed in Figures 7 and 8 respectively. The circular incision is now completed.

Stage 3: Formation and closure of upper vaginal sac

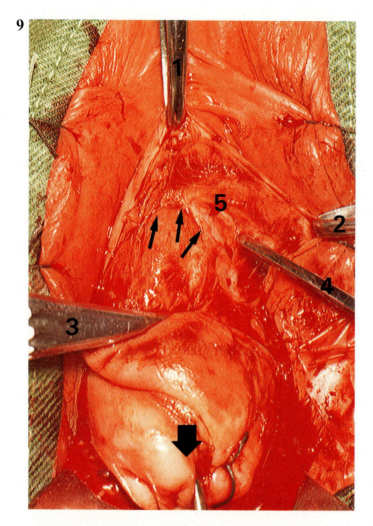

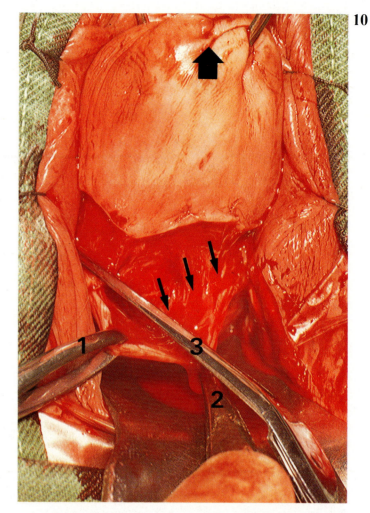

9 Undercutting upper edge of lower vagina (anterior)

It is important to release the remaining vaginal skin from the underlying bladder and pubo-cervical fascia and, in addition, one has to anticipate closing the top of the shortened vagina when the present stage of the operation is completed. For both these reasons the vaginal edge must be undercut and freed. In the photograph the edge is held by tissue forceps at (1) and (2) while dissecting forceps (3) retract the upper vaginal skin to allow the scissors (4) to establish a plane of separation (arrowed) between the skin and the pubo-cervical fascia covering the bladder (5).

10 Undercutting upper edge of lower vagina (posterior)

The posterior vaginal edge is held in tissue forceps (1) and (2) while the angled scissors (3) are used partly as a blunt dissector and partly to snip the tissues in freeing the upper edge of what will be the shortened vagina. A good plane of separation between the skin and the underlying recto-vaginal fascia and rectum is arrowed.

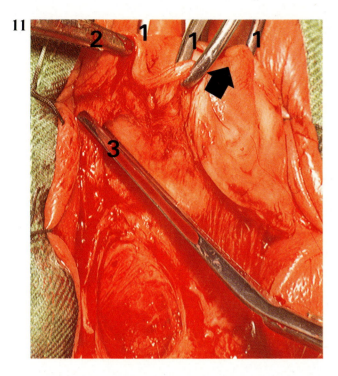

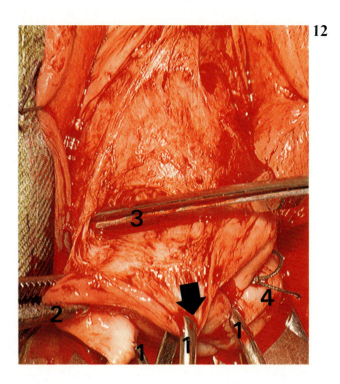

11 and 12 Freeing pouch or sac of upper vaginal skin (i)

With the edges of the upper vaginal skin held in tissue forceps (1), (1), (1) and steadied by the dissecting forceps (2) the posterior aspect is freed with the angled scissors (3) as shown in Figure 11. In Figure 12 the same procedure is followed anteriorly and the same numbers apply. The stitch inserted to close the cervix is seen (4).

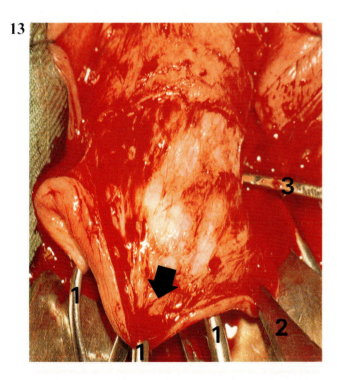

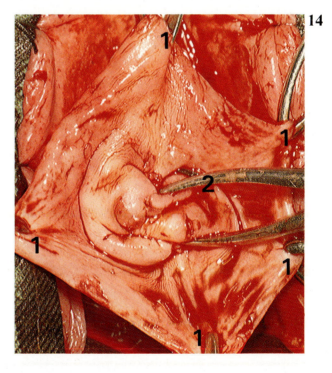

13 and 14 Freeing pouch or sac of upper vaginal skin (ii)

The process continues anteriorly at a somewhat higher level in Figure 13 and the whole area of upper vaginal skin has been raised from the underlying tissues and is ready to be formed into a pouch which will enclose the cervix. The area of skin is clearly seen on Figure 14 where the five pairs of tissue forceps on the skin edges are at (1) and the forceps on the anterior lip of the cervix at (2).

15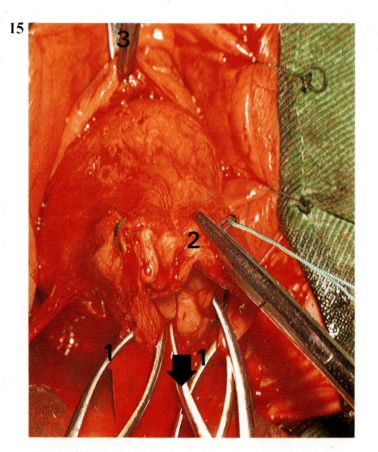

16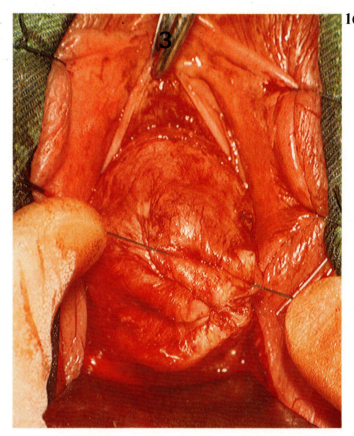

15 and 16 Closing upper vaginal pouch with purse string suture

The skin edges are held in the Littlewood's forceps (1) while the needle (2) carrying a strong suture takes a series of bites of tissue round the skin edge to form a watertight purse string closure of the mouth of the sac. The tissue forceps (3) is holding the upper edge of the vagina. In Figure 16 the purse string suture is being tied off firmly as shown.

Stage 4: Opening peritoneal sac

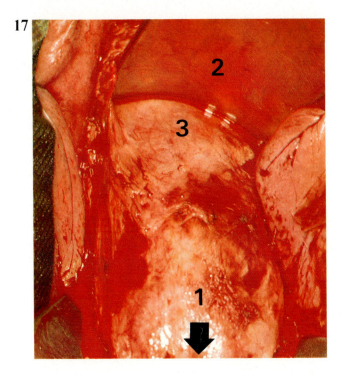

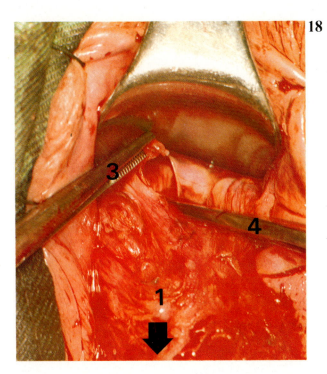

17 and 18 Opening anterior uterine pouch

The cervix enclosed in the upper vaginal sac (1) is held downwards in the direction of the arrow while the retractor (2) holds back the bladder to expose the utero-vesical pouch

(3) in Figure 17. In Figure 18 the pouch is seen held by dissecting forceps (3) and has just been opened by the scissors. This opening between the bladder and the uterus is then enlarged.

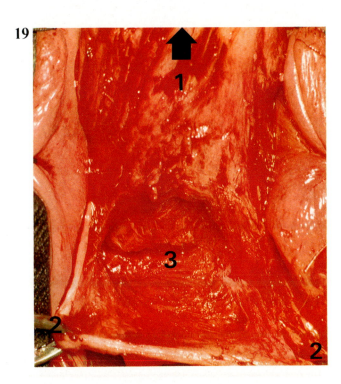

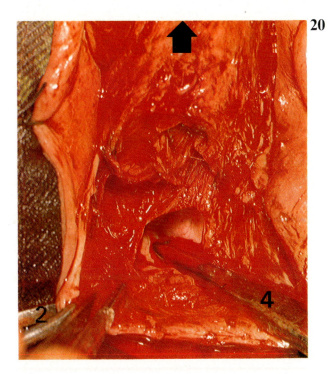

19 and 20 Opening posterior uterine pouch

The cervix in the vaginal sac (1) is held upwards in this instance (arrowed) and the tissue forceps (2) and (2) retract

the upper vaginal edge to expose the area behind the cervix (3) in Figure 19. In Figure 20 the scissors (4) have just opened the posterior pouch or pouch of Douglas.

Stage 5: Securing utero-sacral ligaments

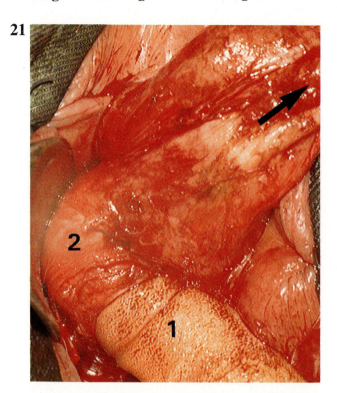

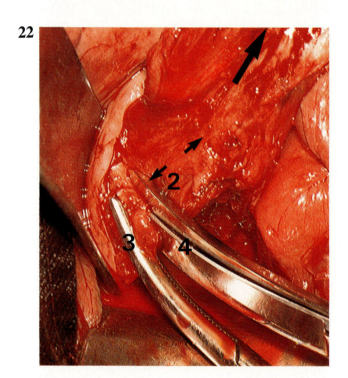

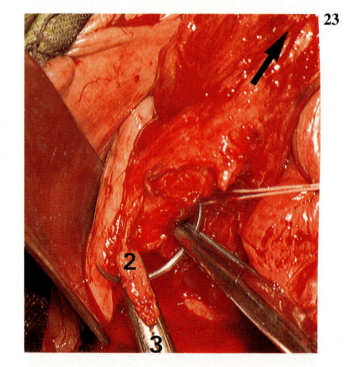

21 to 23 Detaching utero-sacral ligament (right)

The forefinger (1) is introduced into the open pouch of Douglas and easily identifies the right utero-sacral ligament (2) by hooking it laterally as shown in Figure 21. The ligament (2) is then clamped and divided as far from the uterus as possible, as in Figure 22. The forceps is at (3) and the scissors (4) and the considerable distance from the uterus is indicated by the arrows. In Figure 23 the utero-sacral pedicle is transfixed with PGA No. 1 suture prior to ligation. The large arrow indicates the longitudinal axis of the uterus as it is held anteriorly and medially in each photograph.

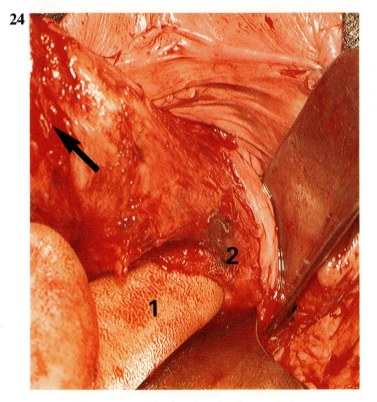

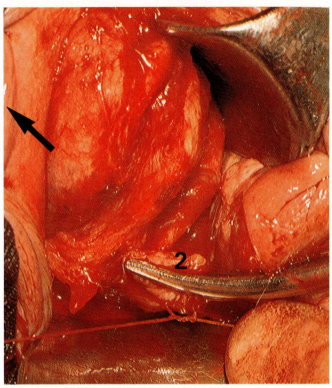

24 and 25 Detaching utero-sacral ligament (left)

The same procedure is followed on the left side with the finger (1) introduced into the pouch of Douglas in Figure 24 and hooked laterally to identify the utero-sacral ligament (2) which is followed as far postero-laterally from its uterine attachments as possible before being clamped and detached. In Figure 25 the pedicle is being ligated.

Stage 6: Closure of vaginal vault

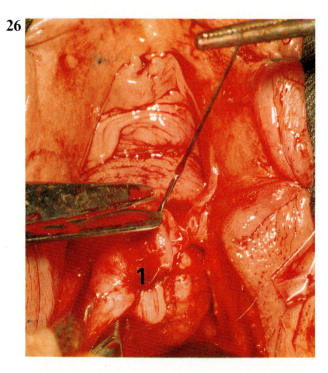

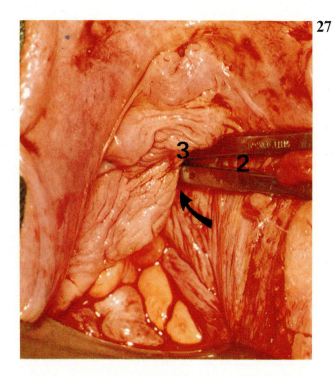

26 and 27 Cervix and closed upper vaginal sac elevated into pelvis

In Figure 26 the purse string suture on the closed vaginal sac (1) is cut and in Figure 27 the forceps (2) elevates the whole uterus, cervix and vaginal sac into the pelvis in the direction of the arrow. The anterior lower vaginal skin edge is at (3).

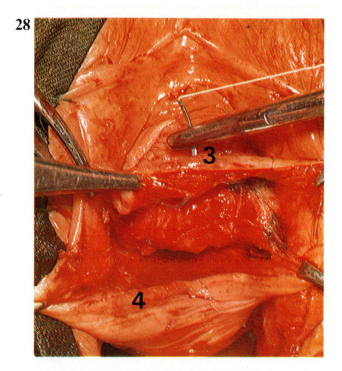

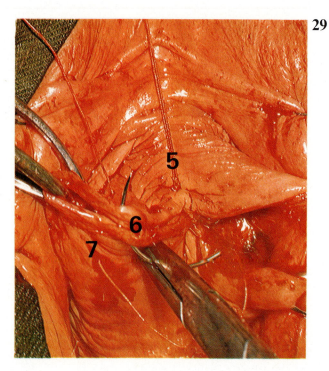

28 and 29 Suturing vaginal vault

In Figure 28 a needle carrying PGA No. 1 suture transfixes the anterior vaginal skin edge at its mid-point (3) and will pick up the posterior edge at the corresponding point (4).

The stitch is completed and held uncut (5) in Figure 29 while further vertical mattress stitches (6 and 7) close the right side of the vault.

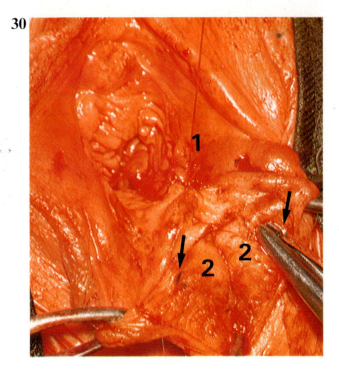

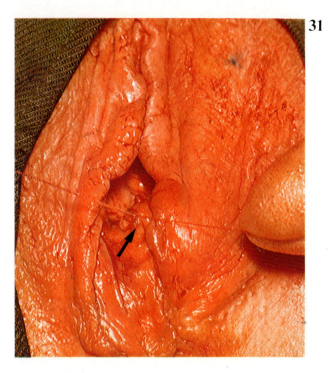

30 and 31 Repair of relief incision

The upper skin edge of the episiotomy-type incision is held up by the uncut anchor suture (1) while the needle (arrowed) traverses the two muscle edges (2) and (2) in Figure 30. Two such stitches are required. In Figure 31 the continuous skin stitch has been completed and is being tied off (arrowed).

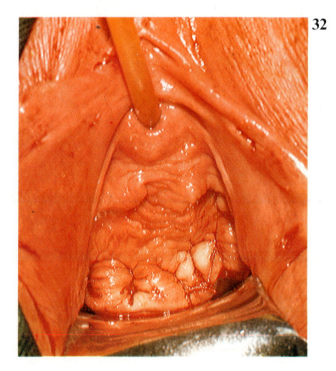

32 Vaginal vault closed

The speculum displays the vaginal vault closed transversely. The vagina is seen to be shortened but it is functionally adequate and will subsequently lengthen if the patient is sexually active. A Foley catheter is *in situ* for three days postoperatively.

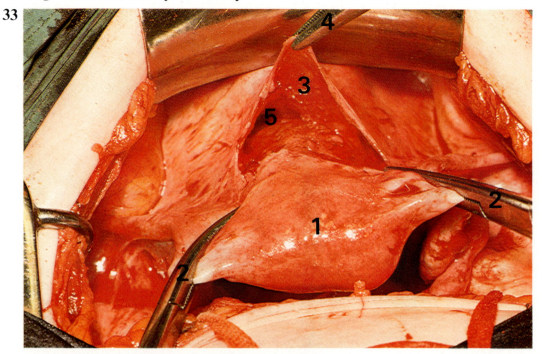

33 Appearance abdominally – anterior uterine pouch open
The uterus (1) is held by forceps (2) and (2) on the broad
ligaments and the bladder (3) elevated by the dissecting
forceps on its visceral peritoneum (4) to display the open
utero-vesical pouch (5).

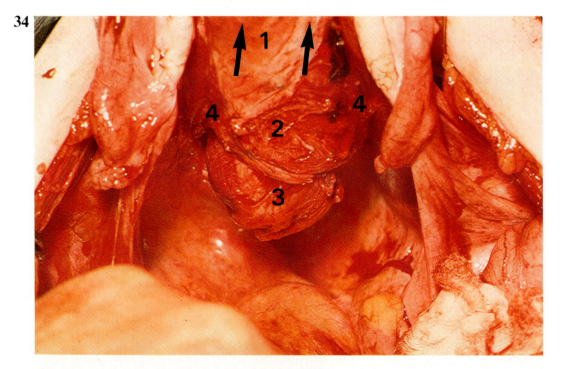

34 Appearance abdominally – pouch of Douglas open
The uterus (1) is held upwards in the direction of the arrows
to show the cervix (2) and closed upper vaginal pouch (3)
protruding through the open pouch of Douglas and lying
free in the posterior pelvis. The cut uterine ends of the utero-
sacral ligaments are at (4) and (4).

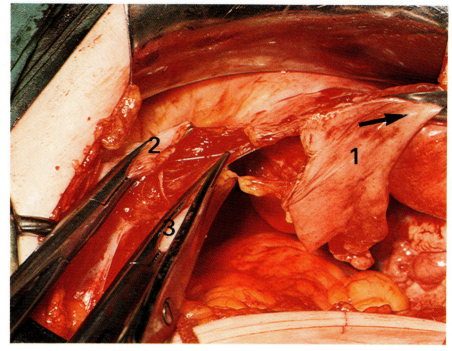

35 Securing upper uterine attachments (left)
The appendages (1) are held medially by the curved forceps on the broad ligament. The round ligament has already been detached (2) and the scissors are cutting through the ovarian pedicle (3).

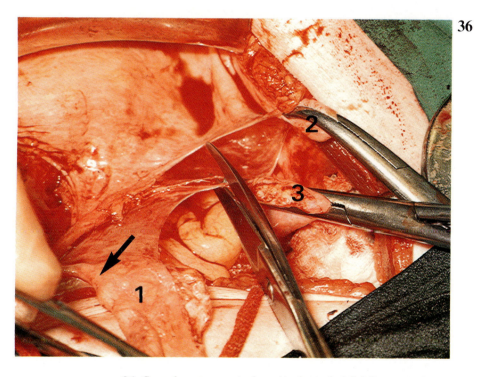

36 Securing upper uterine attachments (right)
The same procedure is being re-enacted on the right side and the same numerals apply.

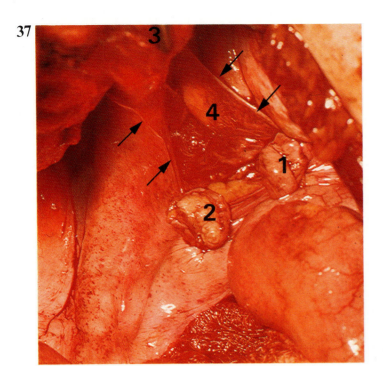

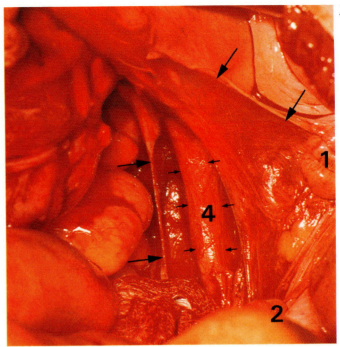

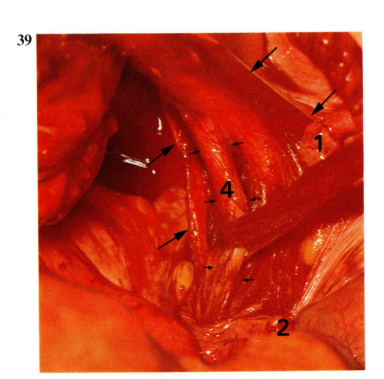

37 to 39 Definition of right ureter

In Figure 37 the round ligament pedicle is numbered (1) and the ovarian pedicle (2). A curved forceps holds the uterine end of the broad ligament (3) and the anterior and posterior layers of the right broad ligament are indicated by fine arrows. The outline of the right ureter is seen at (4). In Figure 38 the broad ligament has been opened up to display the ureter (4) and in Figure 39 the ureter has been underrun with a broad tape. The widely separated anterior and posterior layers of the broad ligament are still arrowed in Figures 38 and 39 and the ureter is outlined by very fine arrows.

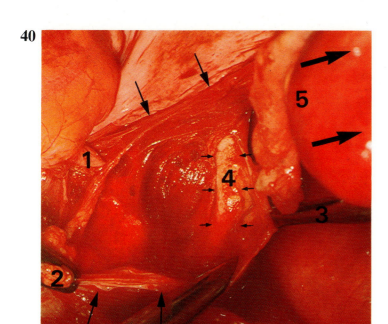

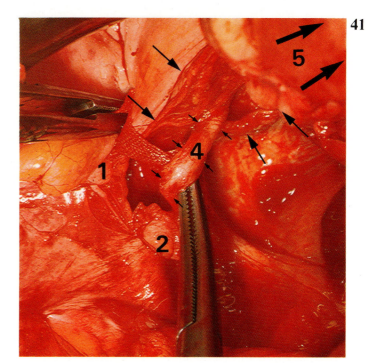

40 and 41 Definition of left ureter

The same procedure is followed as on the right side. The round ligament pedicle is at (1) and the ovarian pedicle (2). The anterior and posterior layers of the left ligament are indicated by fine arrows. In Figure 40 the tissue forceps (3) stretch the posterior layer of the broad ligament to show the ureter lying extra-peritoneally (4). The uretus and left appendages (5) are held medially by the broad ligament forceps in the direction of the large arrows. In Figure 41 the ureter has been freed sufficiently to allow it to be underrun by a marker tape. The same numerals apply in each photograph.

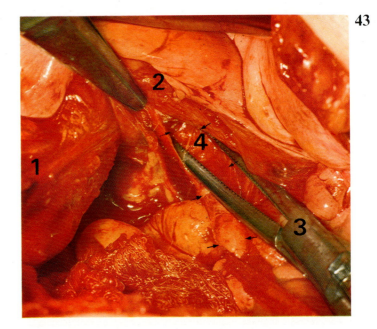

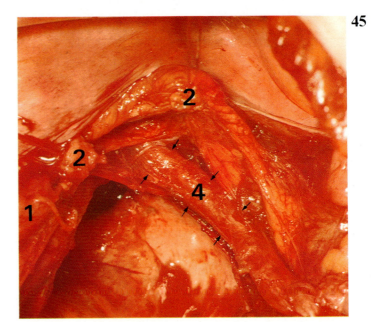

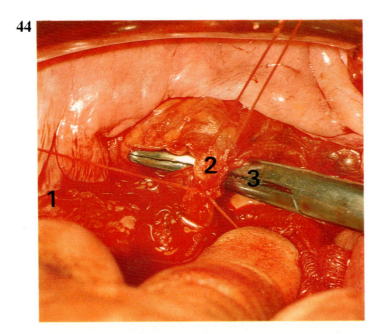

42 and 43 Definition of right ureteric tunnel
With the uterus lying medially at (1), the dissecting forceps
grasps the uterine vessels (2) as they cross the roof of the
ureteric tunnel while the long Spencer-Wells forceps (3)
follow the line of the ureter (4) into the tunnel and ensure
that the roof is quite clear of the ureter itself. Two stages
of the manoeuvre are shown in the successive figures.

44 and 45 Dividing uterine pedicle as it crosses right ureter
The closed Spencer-Wells forceps (3) lies in the line of the
ureter within the tunnel and hides it from view in Figure 44.
The uterine pedicle is meantime doubly ligated and in Figure
45 has been cut between the ligatures (2) and (2) to expose
the ureter (4).

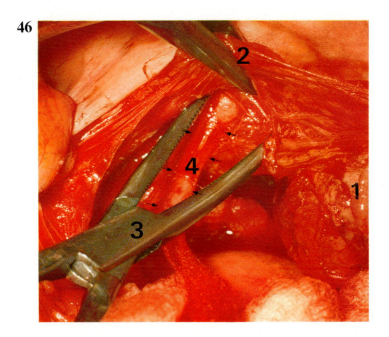

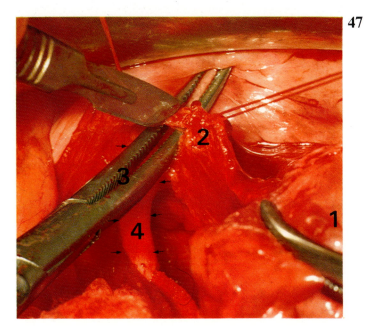

47

46 to 48 Dividing uterine pedicle as it crosses the left ureter
Exactly the same procedure is carried out on the left side.
The same numerals apply.

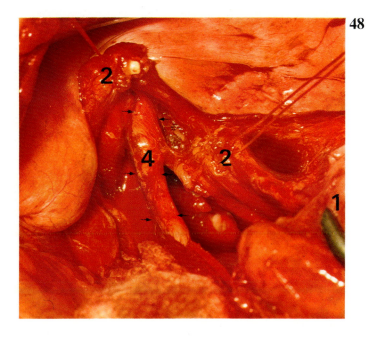

49

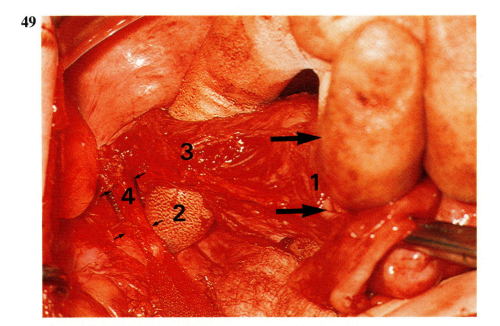

49 Defining left cardinal ligament

The anterior and posterior uterine pouches were opened and the uterosacral ligaments divided in the vaginal part of the operation. The uterine pedicles were detached abdominally when exposing the ureters and the cardinal ligaments are the only remaining lower uterine attachments. In the photograph the uterus (1) is pulled medially, as arrowed, and the surgeon's forefinger (2) displays the left cardinal ligament (3).

50

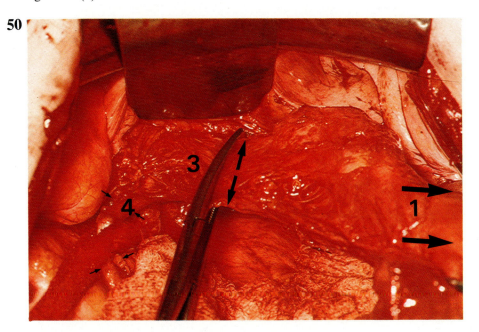

50 Clamping left cardinal ligament

The cardinal ligament (3) is of manageable thickness, which is obviously important at this depth in the pelvis. A curved Oschner forceps clamps the complete pedicle in one bite (arrowed) well clear of the uterus (1) and at a safe distance from the left ureter (4).

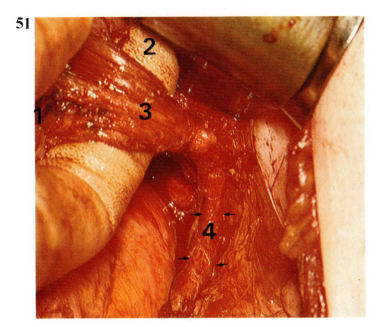

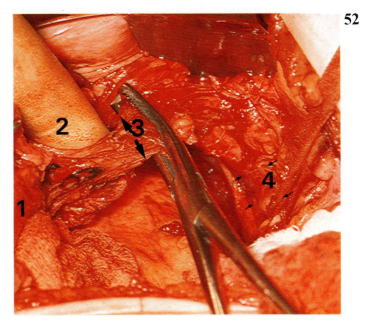

51 and 52 Defining and clamping right cardinal ligament
The same procedure is carried out on the right side and the
same numerals apply.

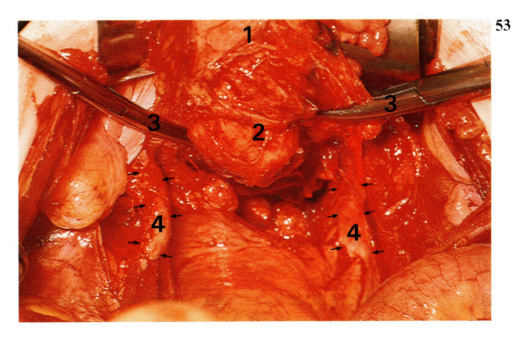

53 Cardinal ligaments secured
The cardinal ligaments are held well clear of the cervix by
curved forceps (3) and (3). The uterus is at (1) and the
upper vaginal sac and cervix at (2). The ureters are clearly
visible (4) and (4).

54

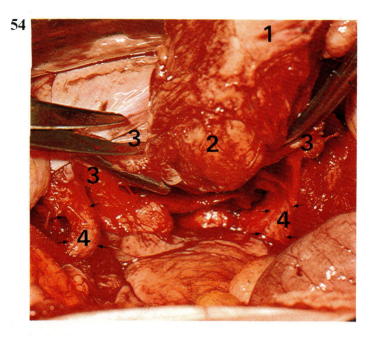

55

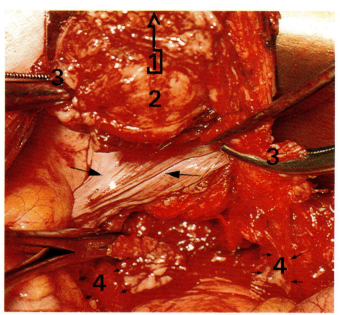

54 to 56 Removal of uterus

In Figure 54 the left cardinal ligament is being cut with the scissors. In Figure 55 division is repeated on the right side and shows more clearly that 0.5 cm of tissue is left as a cuff distal to the forceps to obviate any slipping. The uterus, cervix and vaginal sac are almost completely de-tached and the left cardinal ligament is free. The glistening vaginal skin is arrowed. In Figure 56 the ligature on the left cardinal ligament is tied but uncut, and the right cardinal ligament is in process of being ligated. The same numerals apply: uterus (1), cervix within vaginal sac (2), cardinal ligaments (3), ureters (4).

56

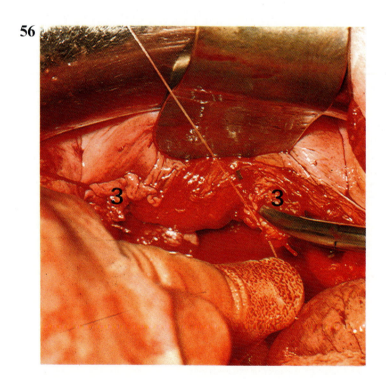

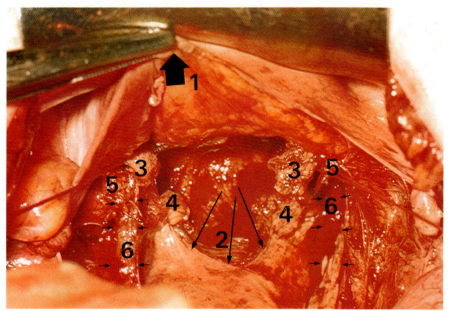

57 Deep pelvic view following hysterectomy

The uterus has been removed and the bladder (1) is elevated by the dissecting forceps in the direction of the arrow. The anterior surface of the rectum (2) is devoid of peritoneum, the line of reflection being shown by fine arrows. The ligated cardinal ligaments (3) and (3) are held on uncut sutures and posterior to these are the utero-sacral ligaments previously ligated (4) and (4). The uterine vascular pedicles are at (5) and (5) and the ureters are seen (6) and (6).

This photograph illustrates the depth at which the vagina has been divided; even with the bladder retracted it is not possible to see the closed vaginal vault. It would not be possible to achieve removal of this amount of vaginal tissue by an entirely abdominal approach. Note the distance of the detached utero-sacral pedicles from the vaginal vault.

58 specimen

The preoperative radiotherapy has localised the growth in the isthmal region (arrowed) and an adequate amount of vaginal skin is seen to have been removed.

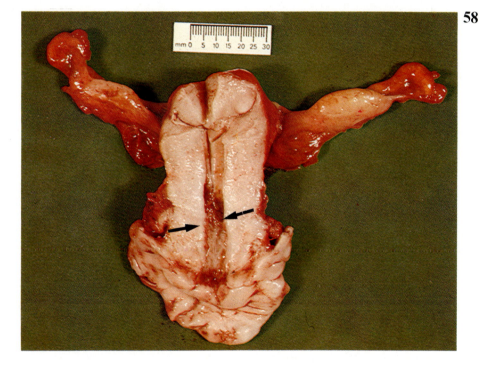

Suggested reading

Annual report on the results of treatment in carcinoma of the uterus, vagina and ovary (Vol. 16, 1976), edited by H. L. Kottmeier, Radium-hemmet, Stockholm.

Boronow, R. C. (1976) Endometrial cancer: not a benign disease. *Obstetrics and Gynaecology*, 47 (5), 630.

De Muelenare, G. F. G. O. (1973). The case against Wertheim's hysterectomy in endometrial carcinoma. *Journal of Obstetrics and Gynaecology of the British Commonwealth*, 80, 728.

Gusberg, S. B. & Kaplan, A. L. (1963). Precursors of corpus cancer. *American Journal of Obstetrics and Gynecology*, 87, 659.

Lees, D. H. (1978). The surgery of endometrial carcinoma. *Clinics in Obstetrics and Gynaecology*, 5, 3, 675.

Lees, D. H. & Bar-Am, A. (1978). A rational approach to the surgical treatment of endometrial carcinoma. *Endometrial Cancer*, 139–148, edited by M. G. Brush, R. J. King & R. W. Taylor. Ballière-Tindall, London.

Maier, J. G. (1978). Radiotherapy treatment of endometrial cancer. *Gynecologic Oncology*, 258, edited by L. McGowan. Appleton-Century-Crofts, New York.

5: Ovarian carcinoma

The treatment of ovarian carcinoma is predominantly by surgery but results are generally recognised as unsatisfactory and compare badly with those of cancer of the cervix and endometrium. If the growth has spread beyond the ovary when first seen, the pelvic and sometimes the abdominal peritoneum will be involved so that there is little hope of complete surgical removal. The reasons for this are worth recounting because they indicate the areas where special care should be exercised in management of the disease.

Ovarian cancers are treacherous in that their development is 'silent'. They are often diagnosed only because they become obvious from their size or because of some complication which demands treatment. Although young women are known to develop ovarian malignancy, there is a general reluctance by clinicians to believe that seemingly benign ovarian tumours and cysts are, in fact, cancer. Ovarian growths may derive from germ cells, stromal cells or germinal epithelium so that there is a bewildering number of neoplastic possibilities and some are wildly anaplastic. Spread is direct within the peritoneal cavity and by the blood stream so that dissemination is both early and widespread. In treating them it must be remembered that if surgery fails radiotherapy has very little to offer; chemotherapy has an important place in treatment but its full potential has not yet been realised.

In view of what has been said, special consideration must be given to the surgery of ovarian malignancy and the following points deserve particular attention:

1 Laparotomy for adnexal tumours should be done with the possibility of ovarian malignancy in mind. It is always a possibility in young women, while in the middle-aged and elderly an ovarian tumour should be regarded as probably malignant until proved otherwise.

2 Because of these risks the patient should be made aware of the dangers and the surgeon must always have a mandate to do what is found to be necessary at operation.

3 Since an extensive and difficult surgical procedure may be necessary, the decision on whether or not to attempt removal of the tumour can be an agonising one as it may affect the life of the patient. Therefore much depends on the training and surgical skill of the operator.

The choice and the extent of the original operation are very important and the reader must have guidance on these matters. The question cannot be considered fully in an Atlas on surgical technique and, at the same time, reference to the text-books reveals conflicting views. (Barber (1974), Mattingley (1977), Hudson (1978), Munnell (1978).) The authors have cut across theoretical considerations and put forward an orthodox practical scheme of management based on the extent of the disease as seen at laparotomy and an estimate of what is surgically possible. If the growth can be removed completely, the only remaining question is whether omentectomy should be added to the total hysterectomy and bilateral salpingo-oophorectomy. In the special circumstances of a very young woman desiring children and where the type of growth is known, there might be a question of more conservative surgery and that is discussed below. If the growth is not completely removable the aim must still be to excise the primary tumour and the maximum amount of tumour tissue. No two cases are similar but the operations described in the Atlas were specifically chosen to cover the great majority of cases seen. The first and most important decision has been made when the growth is classified as completely removable or not. As regards terminology, the adjective 'radical' does not necessarily or even usually mean an extended major operation and in many instances it means no more than a total hysterectomy and bilateral salpingo-oophorectomy. It is used to denote an operation in which the relevant structures are either completely removed or as much of them as possible is removed and it may of course include additional procedures such as omentectomy or appendicectomy. In contradistinction 'conservative' denotes a partial procedure such as oophorectomy or simply biopsy. We believe it important to preserve these simple and recognised subdivisions where all is so complex and we note that others also use them (Munnell, 1974).

Peritoneal cytology ought to have a worthwhile application in making decisions at operations but necessary delays and difficulties of interpretation seem inseparable from the procedure and we do not consider that it is suitable for routine use. Keegel, Pixley and Bauchsbaum (1974) have reported their experience with the method.

Selection for surgical treatment and choice of operation

In dealing with a case of obvious malignancy the first consideration is whether or not the growth can be completely removed. The two possibilities are dealt with separately:

I When complete surgical removal is possible

1 Radical Surgery: total abdominal hysterectomy and bilateral salpingo-oophorectomy

This is the traditional operation. It is applicable where clinical diagnosis has been made and whether the staging be 1a, 1b, or 2a, i.e. confined to one or both ovaries and at most involving uterus or fallopian tubes but not peritoneum/omentum. It has not been our custom routinely to remove the omentum; there are recent reports which suggest that it may be wise to do so and that is considered in the text.

2 Conservative Surgery: oophorectomy

In a special group of young women a less radical operation with conservation of the uterus and the other ovary is admissible. The question is discussed and a representative case described on page 256.

II When complete surgical removal is not possible

1 Radical Surgery: removal of the ovarian primary growth with the maximum amount of tumour tissue

The operation is applicable in Stage 2b cases (i.e. carcinoma extending to other pelvic tissues), and some Stage 3 cases (i.e. with widespread intraperitoneal metastases) and its use is based on evidence that subsequent chemotherapy is effective in direct proportion to the reduction in the malignant cell population. The operation always includes removal of the omentum. A case is described on page 266.

2 Conservative Surgery: laparotomy and biopsy of tumour

The surgeon's decision on whether to attempt the above operation depends on several factors including the general condition of the patient and his own experience. If surgical removal, even partial, seems impossible without jeopardy to the patient's life, then the correct procedure is to make a full assessment of the condition as it affects the whole abdomen and to take adequate biopsies. It is possible that chemotherapy and radiotherapy will so improve matters as to give the opportunity of a 'second look' operation, when removal may be possible. Although such operations are much discussed, the opportunities to do them are few and they can be tedious and difficult. Cases vary so greatly that there is no set procedure and a description is not therefore attempted in the Atlas.

Results of treatment

The Annual Report (1976) finds enormous variation in the material and histology reported by the participating institutions. In view of the lack of uniformity in the statistics it has not been possible to compare the therapeutic results in the various centres. It appears that the majority of patients have been treated by surgery alone or by surgery combined with radiotherapy and/or chemotherapy. Table 1 sets out the available figures for the numerous types of ovarian cancer and these merit study by all engaged in treatment.

It is assumed that at all stages of management and review the surgeon will observe and be guided by 'Clinical Staging for Primary Cancer of the Ovary' as recommended by F.I.G.O. The relevant information has been extracted from the Annual Report and is reproduced on pages 337–339 of the Atlas.

Table 1

Carcinoma of the Ovary

Obviously malignant cases and cases of low potential malignancy (examined between 1963–1968, at 33 centres)*

Clinical Stage and 5-Year Survival Rate (F.I.G.O. staging)	Histological Groups					Cases of Low Potential Malignancy (all histological types) 385***
	1 (Serous cystomas) 2128	2 (Mucinous cystomas) 609	3 (Endometrioid and (4) Mesonephric tumours) 706	5 (Concomitant or undifferentiated carcinoma) and (6) No histology 1145	Total 4588**	
Stage 1a (growth limited to one ovary, no ascites)						
Number of patients examined	348	209	143	89	789	133
Number alive at 5 years (%)	216 (62%)	166 (79%)	96 (67%)	48 (54%)	526 (67%)	124 (93%)
Stage 1b/c (growth in both ovaries, no ascites. c=1a or 1b with ascites)						
Number patients examined	205	88	50	46	389	86
Number alive at 5 years (%)	100 (49%)	53 (60%)	30 (60%)	19 (41%)	202 (52%)	77 (89%)
Stage 2a (extension &/or metastases to uterus &/or tubes)						
Number patients examined	86	27	51	21	185	24
Number alive at 5 years (%)	42 (49%)	15 (56%)	28 (55%)	7 (33%)	92 (50%)	23 (96%)
Stage 2b/c (extension other pelvic organs, including peritoneum. c=2a or 2b with ascites)						
Number patients examined	331	83	147	124	685	55
Number alive at 5 years (%)	124 (37%)	38 (46%)	64 (43%)	34 (27%)	260 (38%)	40 (73%)
Stage 3 (involving one/both ovaries with intra-peritoneal metastases or growth limited to true pelvis with histologically proven spread to small bowel or omentum)						
Number patients examined	736	138	194	450	1518	47
Number alive at 5 years (%)	88 (12%)	17 (12%)	10 (5%)	15 (3%)	130 (9%)	18 (38%)
Stage 4 (involving one/both ovaries with distant metastases)						
Number patients examined	401	57	118	252	828	12
Number alive at 5 years (%)	24 (6%)	3 (5%)	5 (4%)	9 (4%)	41 (5%)	2 (17%)
Special Group (probable ovarian cancer but impossible to determine origin)						
Number patients examined	—	—	—	144	144	—
Number alive at 5 years (%)	—	—	—	3 (2%)	3 (2%)	—

*modified from the Annual Report (1976) Vol. 16   **50 patients have not been staged   ***28 patients have not been staged

I Surgical removal is possible
1. Radical operation: total abdominal hysterectomy and bilateral salpingo-oophorectomy

The case to be described represents the group of ovarian malignancy in which the tumour can be removed completely.

It is not possible to estimate the stage of an ovarian growth on a clinical or pathological basis and since practically all patients come to laparotomy, the staging is made on the operative findings. The growth in this instance was judged to be 1a on the F.I.G.O. classification. This means that it involved one ovary only with no evidence of other pelvic spread and no accompanying ascites. The patient was over 40 years of age and the universally accepted management of such a case is total hysterectomy and bilateral salpingo-oophorectomy. Majority opinion would agree with the authors that removal of the omentum is not indicated; this will be referred to again later.

The surgical approach is through a transverse lower abdominal incision and the growth is mobilised and delivered into the wound. There is usually a manageable pedicle in such cases and salpingo-oophorectomy is carried out. Thereafter hysterectomy and removal of the other appendages is completed. The difficulty of obtaining information on the results of surgical treatment has been referred to but in cases such as this, and where there is no attachment of growth to the parietal peritoneum, the prognosis is generally very good.

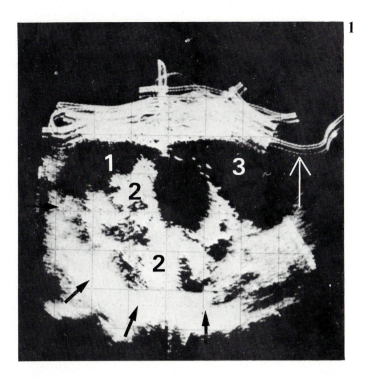

1 Negative of ultrasonic scan

The longitudinal cut of a B Scan (ultrasonic) from a Diasono-graph 4102 shows the outline of the cyst (1) containing solid areas (2). The appearance is characteristic of ovarian malignancy and the extent of the tumour is indicated by arrows. The bladder is at (3) and the perpendicular arrow marks the symphysis pubis.

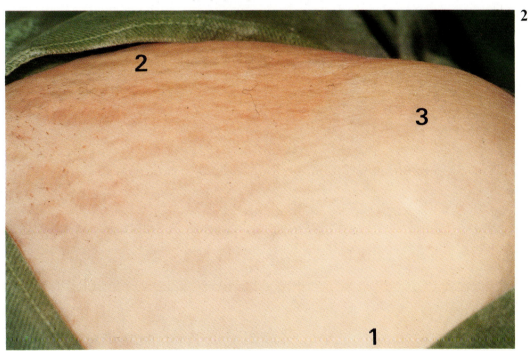

2 Lower abdomen prior to operation

The symphysis pubis is in the area (1) and the umbilicus at (2). The abdomen is generally distended and there is a cystic swelling on the left side (3). The striae are the result of the cystic enlargement and closely resemble those of pregnancy.

Stage 1: Opening abdomen

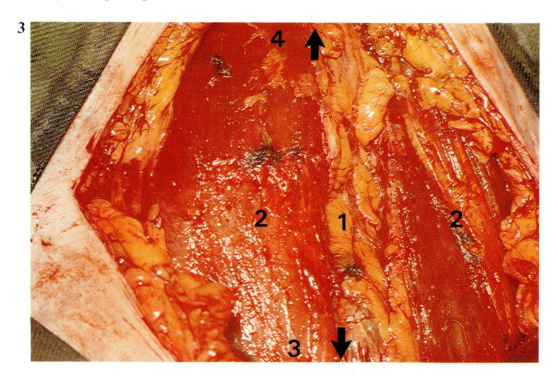

3 Transverse incision

The incision is placed slightly higher than the corresponding transverse incision used in routine gynaecological surgery so that it can be extended laterally above the iliac spines if necessary. The rectus sheath has been incised and retracted in the direction of the arrows to expose the peritoneum (1) between the recti muscles (2) and (2). The umbilicus is in the direction of (3): the symphysis of (4), in each photograph.

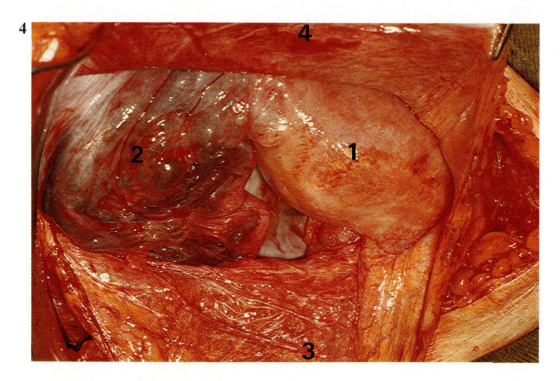

4 Appearance on opening abdomen

The uterus (1) is displaced to the right and anteriorly by a large left-sided ovarian swelling (2) with large vessels running over its upper pole.

5

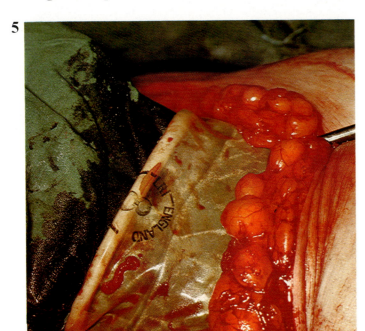

6

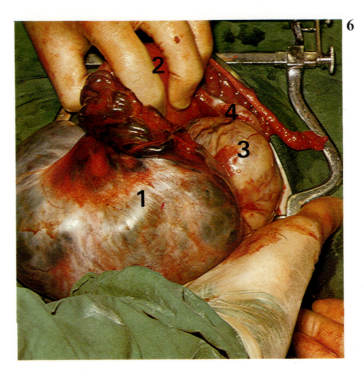

5 Exploration of the abdomen

The size, consistency and fixity of the cyst are established by manual exploration of the pelvis and abdomen at this stage. Tumours of this size preclude examination of the upper abdomen. That is postponed until the mass has been removed but must not be forgotten subsequently.

6 Delivery of tumour into wound

There were only a few adhesions and it was possible to deliver the cystic swelling into the wound in the manner shown. It is generally possible and preferable to maintain the upper pole of the cyst (1) in the centre of the wound while sliding the hand under and posterior to the growth towards the pouch of Douglas and then using the open hand as a spoon with which to slowly deliver the tumour through the wound opening. The left hand is using the uterus (2) as a handle to aid the delivery in this case. The area (3) is a solid part of the left ovarian tumour. The right ovary (4) is small and of normal appearance.

Stage 3: Left salpingo-oophorectomy

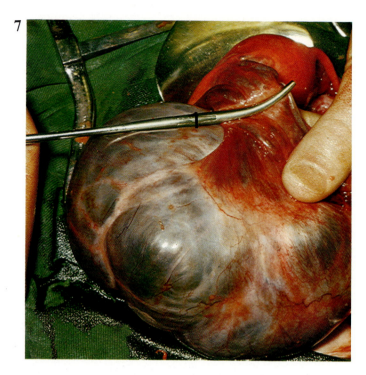

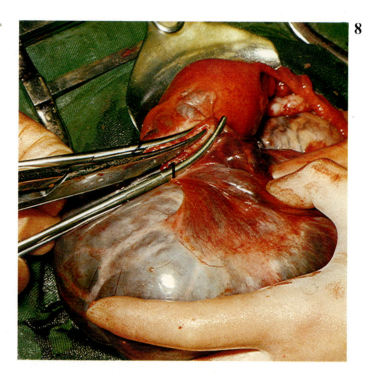

7 to 10 Removal of growth (left salpingo-oophorectomy)

The partly cystic and partly solid tumour is now free and has a narrow pedicle so that the correct procedure is to remove it forthwith and allow hysterectomy and pelvic clearance to proceed without hindrance from the large mass. In Figure 7 a first clamp (1) is applied to the pedicle which contains ovarian vessels and the left fallopian tube. In Figure 8 a second clamp (2) has been applied and the scissors are cutting between them. In Figure 9 the growth has been detached from the uterus and each part of the pedicle is held in strong forceps. The uterus is at (3) in the photograph. The specimen is shown in Figure 10.

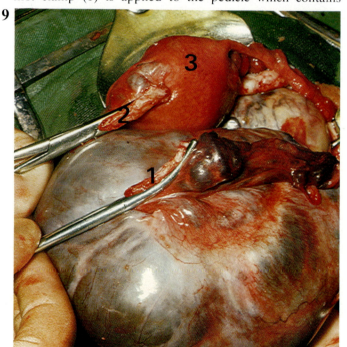

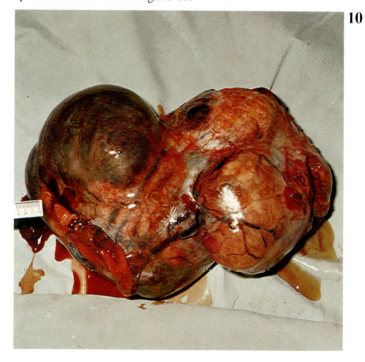

Stage 4: Proceeding to hysterectomy

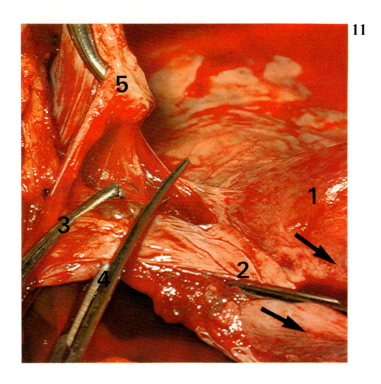

11 to 13 Dividing upper uterine attachments

In Figure 11 the uterus (1) and the uterine pedicle of the tumour (2) are held medially in the direction of the arrows while the ovarian pedicle or infundibulo-pelvic ligament is clamped by forceps (3) and is being divided by scissors (4). The left round ligament (5) has already been clamped and detached from the uterus. In Figure 12 the ovarian and round ligament pedicle are at (3) and (5) respectively and the anterior layer of the left broad ligament is held up by forceps (6) while the scissors raise the peritoneum of the utero-vesical pouch prior to dividing it. The same procedure is being followed on the right side in Figure 13 and the same numbers are used.

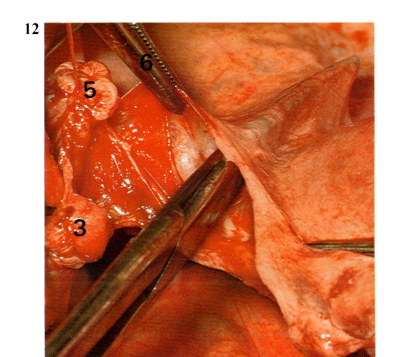

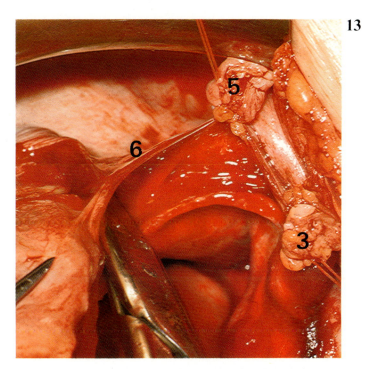

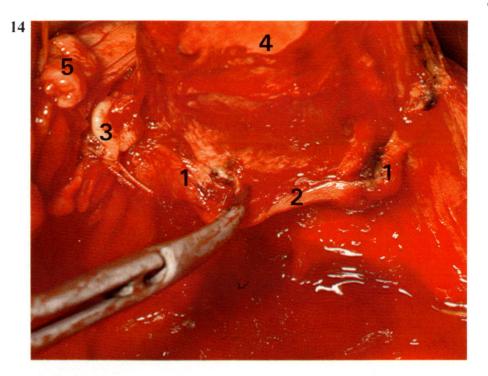

14 Freeing posterior uterine attachments

The uterus was very firmly held by the utero-sacral ligaments in this case and both ligaments (1) and (1) with the intervening fold of peritoneum (2) have been detached from the uterus and stripped downwards to make the uterus more mobile. The diathermy is sealing off a bleeding vessel. The uterus is at (4) and the left ovarian and round ligament pedicles are at (3) and (5).

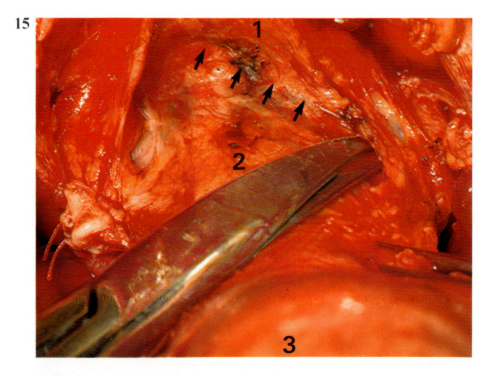

15 Freeing anterior uterine attachments

The scissors are used partly as a blunt dissector and partly to snip attachments in separating the bladder (1) from the cervix (2) as shown and the plane of cleavage is arrowed. The fundus of the uterus is at (3).

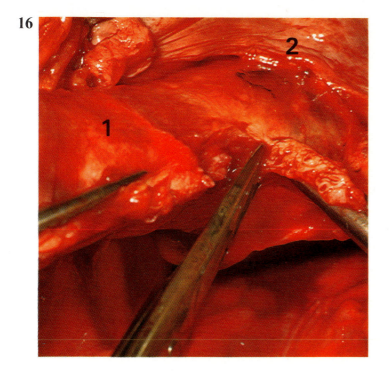

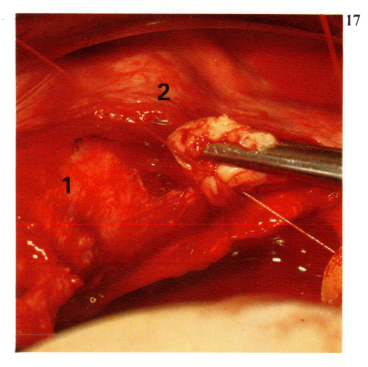

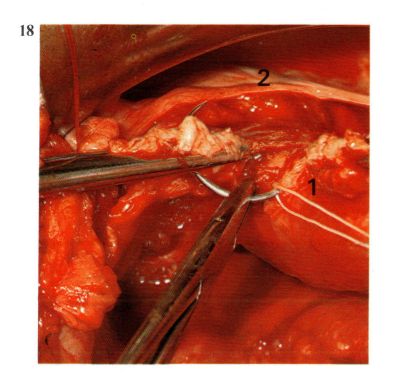

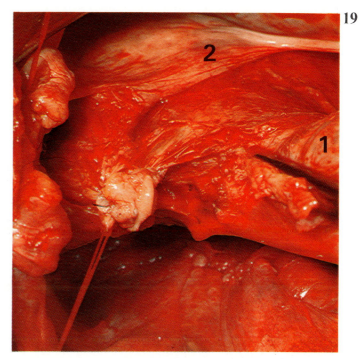

16 to 19 Securing uterine pedicles

The right uterine vessels have been clamped and are being detached from the uterus in such a way as to give a good pedicle in Figure 16. The pedicle with its secure ligature is seen in Figure 17. The left uterine pedicle is being transfixed in Figure 18 and ligated in Figure 19. The uterus is at (1) and the bladder at (2) in each photograph.

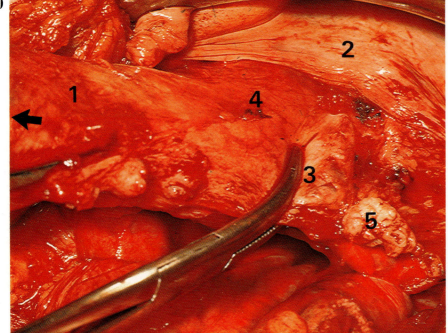

20 Securing right vaginal angle
The uterus (1) is held medially in the direction of the arrow while the right vaginal angle is clamped (3) to include a cuff of upper vagina. The level of the external cervical os is indicated by the stitch (4); the ligated uterine pedicle (5) and the bladder (2) are indicated.

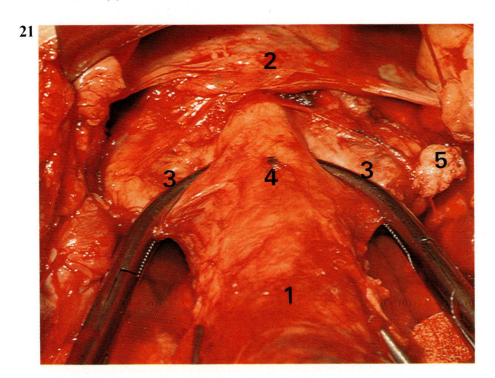

21 Securing both vaginal angles
This photograph shows an anterior view of the uterus with both vaginal angles clamped and the uterus ready for detachment. The numbers are the same as in Figure 20.

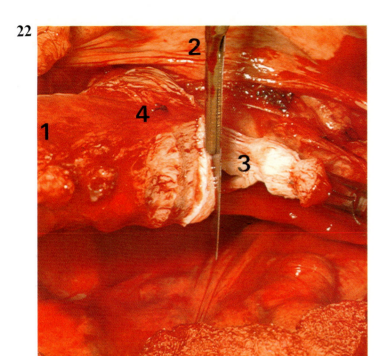

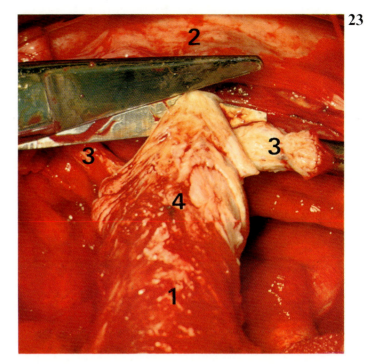

23

22 to 24 Removal of uterus

The uterus is removed by first opening the right vaginal angle proximal to the clamp as shown in Figure 22 and repeating the procedure on the opposite side. The uterus is then attached only to the vagina anteriorly and posteriorly and the anterior attachment is seen divided in Figure 23 and the posterior in Figure 24. The tissue forceps hold the anterior edge of the open vagina in Figure 24. The numbers are the same as in previous photographs.

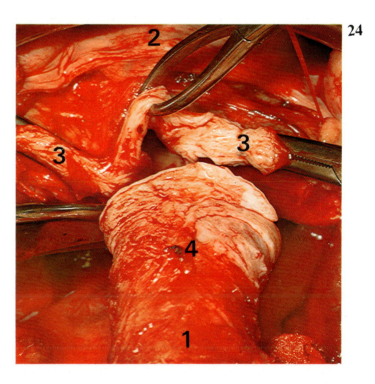

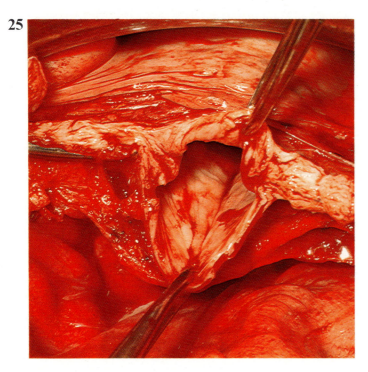

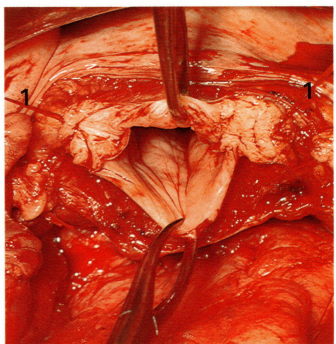

24

25 to 27 Closure of vaginal vault

The vagina is held open by the tissue forceps and the angles are seen secured by the strong curved forceps in Figure 25. In Figure 26 the angles have been ligated and the forceps replaced by the uncut sutures (1) and (1). In Figure 27 closure of the vault has been completed and it will be seen that the utero-sacral ligaments (2) and (2) have been attached to the posterior aspect of the vault by the mattress sutures which are about to be cut (3) and (3).

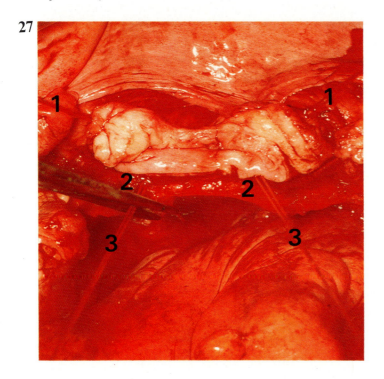

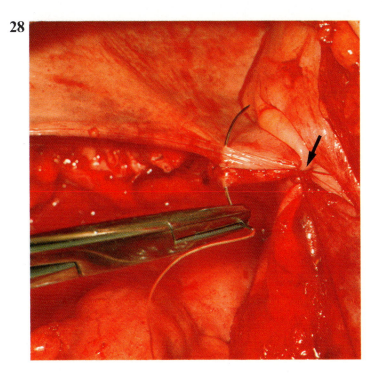

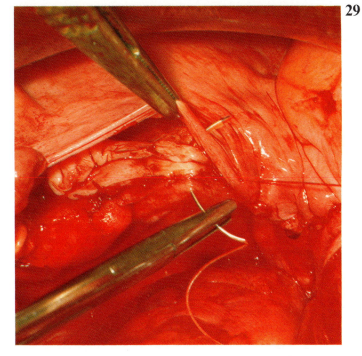

29

28 to 30 Reperitonisation

The peritoneal edges are approximated by a continuous suture in the usual manner. In Figure 28 a half purse string suture has buried the right ovarian and right round ligament pedicles under the anchor knot (arrowed), and the stitch proceeds across the pelvis. The method of picking up the vaginal edges to eliminate dead space is shown in Figure 29 and the pelvic peritoneum is shown completely closed in Figure 30 with the suture line arrowed.

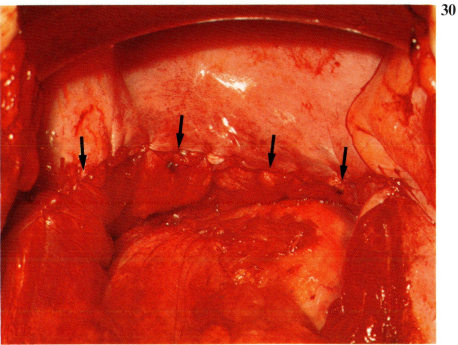

30

2. Conservative operation: Oophorectomy

The case now described is referred to on page 243 of the Introduction. It involves a very complex area of pathology where it is possible to make mistakes and the authors' comment is therefore cautious. It would be correct to say that retention of the uterus is contra-indicated in granulosa-cell tumours and also in the endometrioid group. On the other hand, conservation of the other ovary might be admissible in special circumstances where a young woman was particularly keen to have children, where the growth was encapsulated and considered of borderline malignancy and where the various options had been fully discussed and agreed before operation. The question of conservative management for unilateral Stage 1a carcinoma of the ovary has been reviewed by Munnell (1974 and 1978). An admissible growth for such management would be a pseudomucinous one of borderline malignancy, as in this instance.

The case also gives the opportunity of discussing the question of tapping ovarian cysts, a matter on which the reader will expect some guidance. In removing potentially or probably malignant cysts it is obviously beneficial if that can be done without spilling malignant cells. Most gynaecologists have been taught that they must on no account tap or aspirate cysts and that an adequate incision must be made to allow intact removal of the cyst, no matter how large it may be or whether the incision stretch from xiphisternum to the pubis. This was referred to in Volume 2 in relation to cysts that were clinically assessed as probably, but not necessarily, benign. While agreeing that the teaching is generally correct, it was pointed out that sometimes the price could be too high and that a sense of proportion should be observed. Rupture of the cyst during delivery through the stretched incision or the tearing of the vessels in the pedicle by its unsupported weight were obvious dangers. More serious was the lack of access to intra-pelvic attachments of the cyst and to its pedicle with resultant danger to large blood vessels, ureters and viscera from blindly conducted surgery. The possibility of expressing tumour cells into the circulation during manipulation and the absurd situation when the cyst ruptured during separation were touched on and the case was made for definitive tapping of very large and adherent cysts.

The probability rather than the possibility of malignancy does not affect the need to adopt a common-sense approach. The necessary and inevitable manipulation of a large cyst during its removal will do more harm by expressing malignant cells into the circulation in a blood-borne tumour than a clean controlled aspiration with no leakage of fluid. Where the cyst ruptures during separation it is clear that in the circumstances the worst of both worlds has been achieved. Radiotherapists will attest to their weariness with requests for radiotherapy where removal was thought to be complete but the cyst ruptured during removal. The authors are not advocating a return to tapping of cysts as practised by the pioneer gynaecologists. They are suggesting only that the options be considered pragmatically and without bias. A method of tapping a large cyst without causing spill is illustrated.

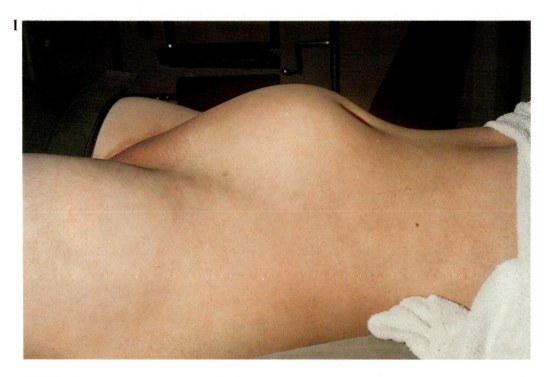

1 Abdominal appearance preoperatively
The abdomen is obviously that of a young woman and the abdominal swelling is localised and of approximately 24 weeks pregnancy size. The swelling was recognised to be cystic and was mobile.

Stage 1: Opening the abdomen

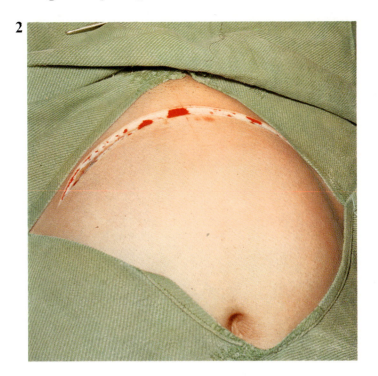

2

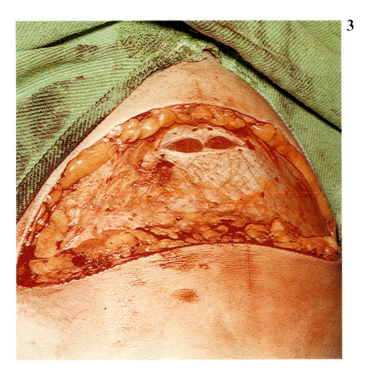

3

2 to 4 Lower transverse abdominal incision

In Figure 2 the incision is made very much at the usual level but with the lateral aspects curving upwards slightly so that they would clear the anterior superior iliac spines if the incision had to be extended. The drapes are secured by stitches placed exactly on each anterior superior iliac spine.

The rectus sheath has been opened to show the fibres of both recti in Figure 3. In Figure 4 retraction of the rectus sheath in the direction of the arrows shows the length of incision available in the midline even without further lateral extension.

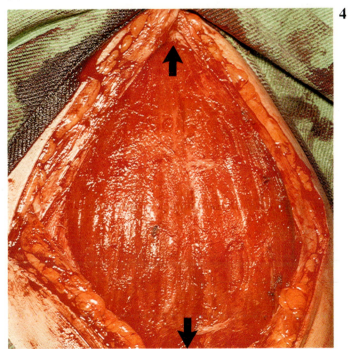

4

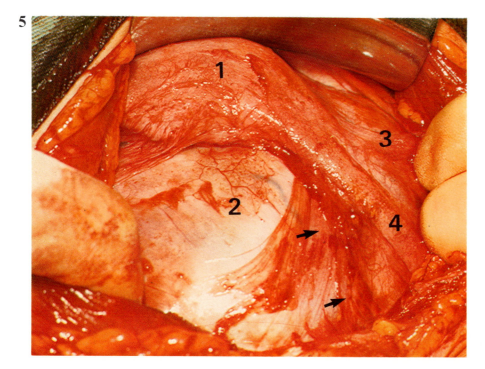

5 Appearance on opening the abdomen
The uterus (1) is pushed forwards and slightly to the left by the cyst (2) and the right round ligament (3) and the right tube (4) are stretched over its upper surface. There are adhesions on both sides posteriorly (arrowed) and particularly involving the right appendages so that access is obviously very limited.

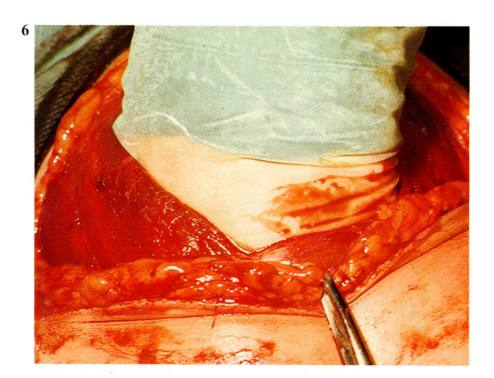

6 Exploration of abdomen
This important step establishes the size, consistency and fixity of the cyst. Examination of the upper abdomen generally needs to await removal of the large cyst which impedes access. In this instance there were multiple adhesions between the cyst and the pelvic floor and side walls so that access would be most dangerous without prior aspiration of the cyst. It was arising from the right ovary.

7
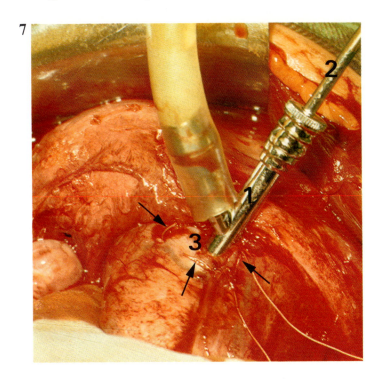

8
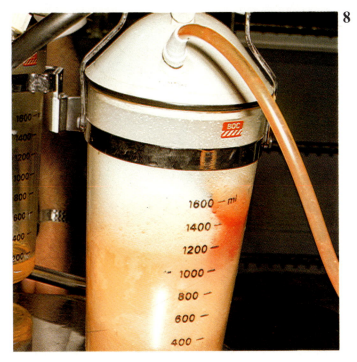

9
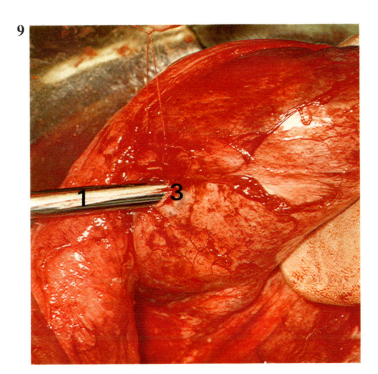

10
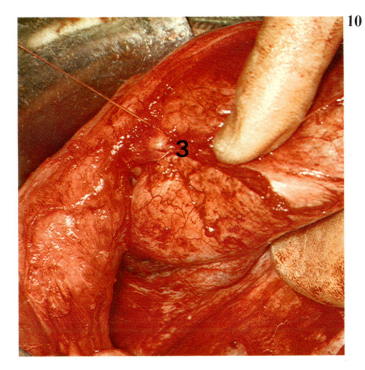

7 to 10 Aspiration of cyst

The policy in relation to aspiration or tapping of the cyst has been discussed. Figure 7 shows the trochar (1) *in situ* with the captive cannula (2) withdrawn and aspiration proceeding. A purse string suture (arrowed) surrounds the point of puncture (3). The suction container shown in Figure 8 already contains 1100 ml of aspirate from this cyst. In Figure 9 the trochar is being withdrawn while the surgeon milks the remainder of the cyst content towards it and the assistant holds the purse string suture ready to be tied off. The stitch is shown tied in Figure 10.

Stage 3: Mobilisation of decompressed ovarian cyst

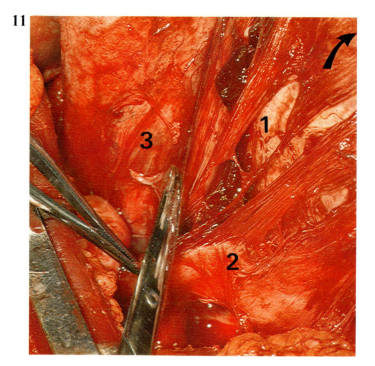

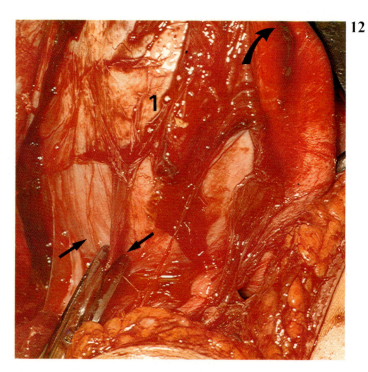

11 and 12 Elevation of cyst from pelvic floor

Where the appendages are enlarged and adherent, thus making pelvic access difficult, the best initial approach is directed between the mass and the intestines towards the pouch of Douglas. In Figure 11 the ovarian swelling is held upwards and forwards by the fingers in the direction of the arrow and throws into relief the adhesions between the cyst (1) and the small and large intestine (2) and (3). The latter is being freed by the scissors and in Figure 12 adhesions to the pelvic floor are being divided (fine arrows).

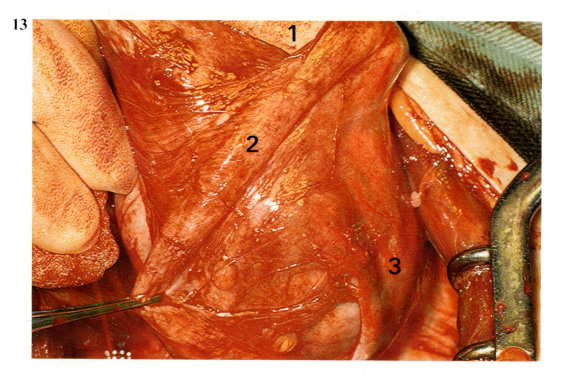

13 Elevation of cyst (continued)

The decompressed cyst has been hooked up into the wound by the finger (1). The tissue forceps hold the fallopian tube (2) taut as it runs over the cyst; the right ovarian pedicle is at (3).

Stage 4: Definition of ureters

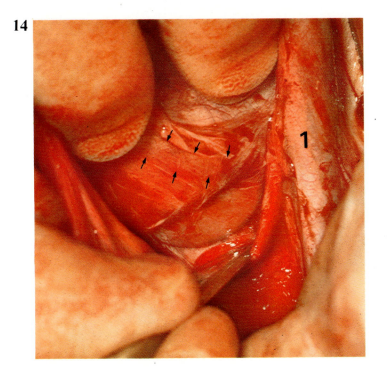

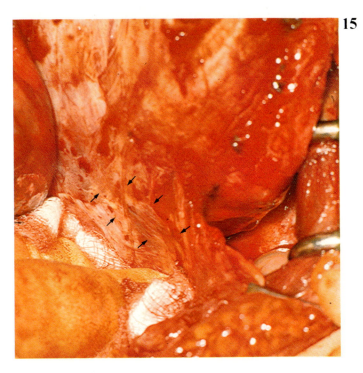

14 and 15 Defining right ureter

As elevation of the cyst and right appendages proceeds, the ureter comes into view in Figure 15 (arrowed) with the ovarian pedicle (1) held taut on the right of the picture. In Figure 16 the ureter has been separated down off the cyst and is again outlined.

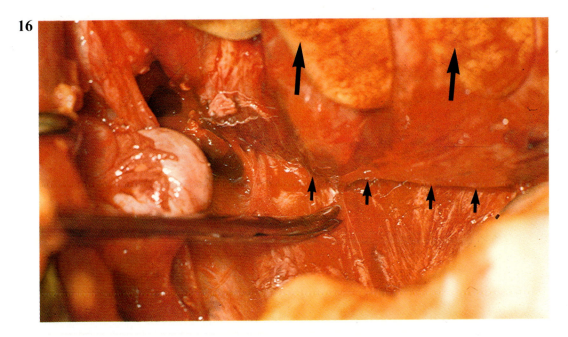

16 Further separation of cyst from pelvic floor

Elevation of the right appendages with the fingers continues in the direction of the arrows, and the scissors find a plane of separation (arrowed) between the cyst and the pelvic floor.

17

18

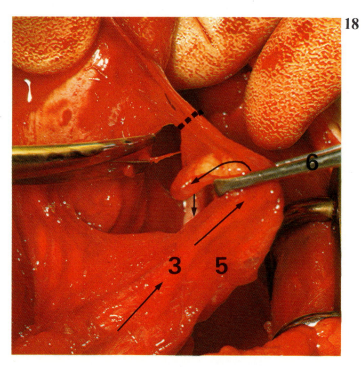

17 and 18 Dissection of right ureter

It is essential to safeguard the ureter in a case like this and in Figure 17 the peritoneal fold (1) of the ovarian pedicle (2) is dissected laterally with the scissors and again brings the ureter (3) into view. In Figure 18 the ureter (3) is about to be completely detached from the cyst with the scissors at the dotted line. It is important to note that the ureter retains its mesentery unimpaired at (5). The photographic angle is a little confusing but the ureter is held laterally as a loop by the tissue forceps (6). The direction of the ureter is indicated by the arrows. The ureter was elongated where adherent to the cyst and so tends to coil on itself when freed.

19

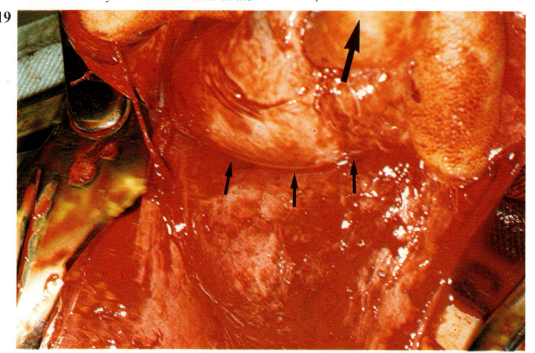

19 Right ovary delivered into wound

The ovarian cyst is now seen being delivered by the fingers into the wound in the direction of the arrows. A clearly defined plane of separation from the pelvic floor is arrowed.

Stage 5: Removal of ovarian cyst

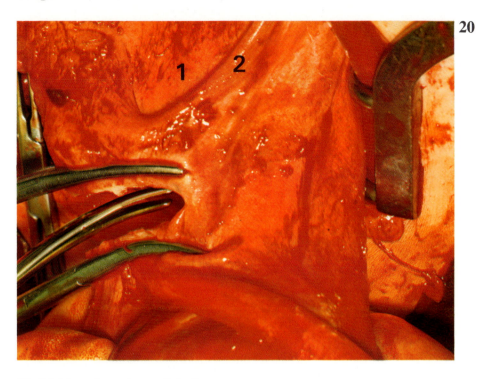

20

20 Division of ovarian pedicle (i)
The rather broad pedicle of the flaccid cyst (1) with the attached tube (2) has now been defined and the scissors cut between the first two pairs of clamps.

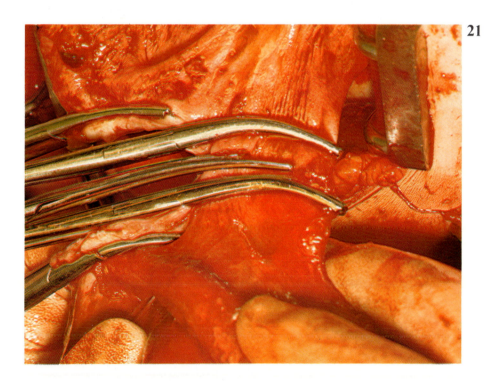

21

21 Division of ovarian pedicle (ii)
A further two pairs of forceps are applied; the scissors cut between to detach the cyst completely.

263

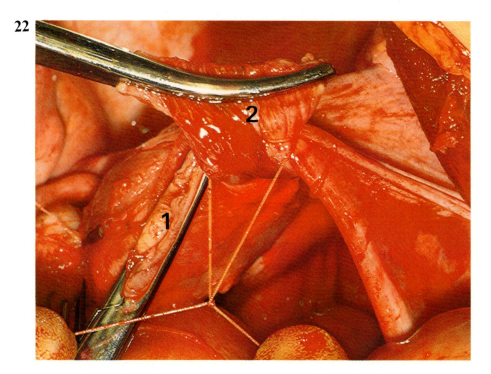

22 Ligation of ovarian pedicle
The two clamped portions of the ovarian pedicle (1) and (2)
are transfixed and tied as shown for (2).

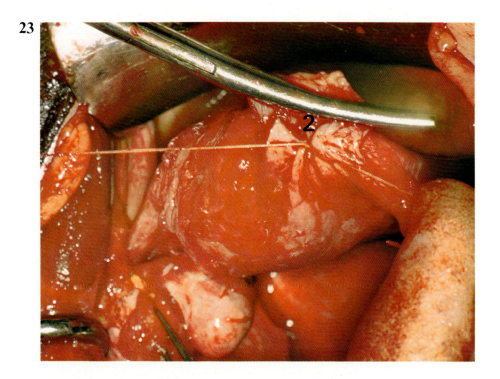

23 Ligation of broad ligament pedicle
In addition to its ovarian pedicle the cyst is attached, of
course, to the uterus by the broad ligament including the
fallopian tube. This attachment was divided between clamps
and the uterine or broad ligament end of the pedicle is seen
being ligated.

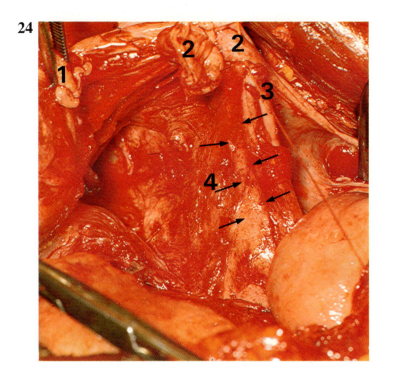

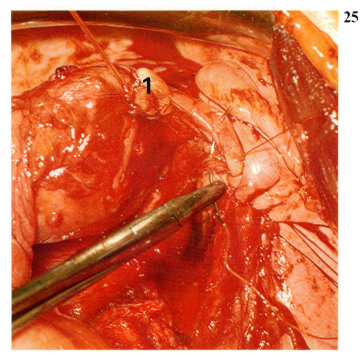

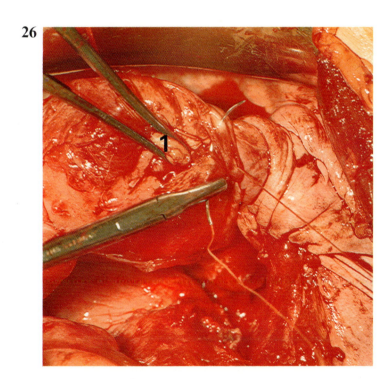

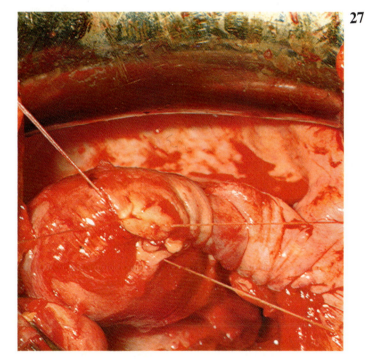

24 to 27 Closure of pelvic peritoneum

In Figure 24 the broad ligament pedicle (1) is held in forceps and the twin ovarian pedicles (2) and (2) are ready to be covered by the peritoneal half purse string stitch (3) anchored just laterally. The ureter is outlined by fine arrows on the raw area of the pelvic floor (4). In Figure 25 the con-

tinuous peritoneal stitch is carried medially; in Figure 26 the needle is about to invert and cover the broad ligament pedicle (1) with peritoneum; in Figure 27 the stitch is being tied off to leave a complete covering of peritoneum at the previous site of the cystic tumour.

II Surgical removal is not possible
1.(i) Radical operation: extensive surgical removal of ovarian primary growth with greater omentum

Complete surgical removal was not possible in this instance and the case therefore belongs to the group referred to on page 243. The growth was difficult to stage but multiple adhesions and metastases on the pelvic peritoneum without obvious spread to the general peritoneal cavity seemed to indicate Stage 2b. The uterus was not involved except for some serious coat adhesion and prior curettage had revealed no endometrial lesion. In all the circumstances the primary ovarian growth was removed as completely as possible and the uterus was not disturbed. The omentum did not appear to contain secondaries but was removed.

The case illustrates an important practical point. There was widespread involvement of the pelvic parietal peritoneum and structures of the pelvic floor on the affected side but there was no evidence of spread to the uterus. Complete removal of the growth was in any case not possible and harm rather than benefit would result from opening up tissue planes of the mid-pelvis and vaginal vault in doing hysterectomy. For these reasons it was omitted; omentectomy carried no such risks and was completed.

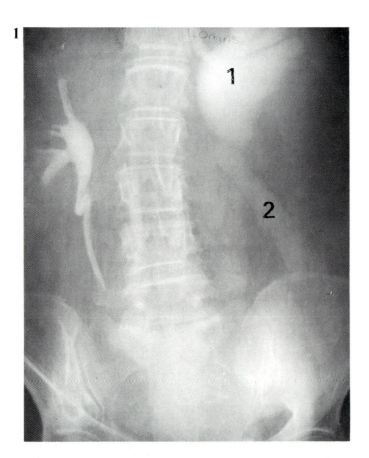

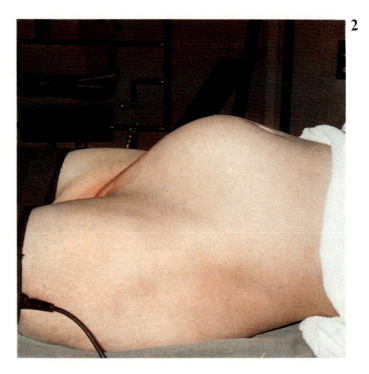

1 Preoperative intravenous urogram
A radiograph of an intravenous urogram taken 40 minutes after injection of contrast medium shows the presence of a large left-sided hydronephrosis (1) secondary to ureteric obstruction caused by the ovarian growth. The obvious hydroureter is seen at (2).

2 Appearance of abdomen preoperatively
The tumour is of 24 weeks pregnancy size and lies mainly towards the left side of the abdomen. On palpatation it was firm, not obviously cystic and just mobile. Note the enlarged skin blood vessels where a collateral circulation is being established. This appearance is always suspicious of malignancy.

Stage 1: Opening the abdomen

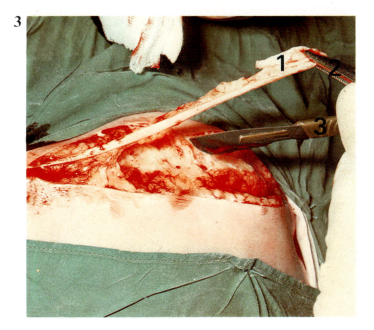

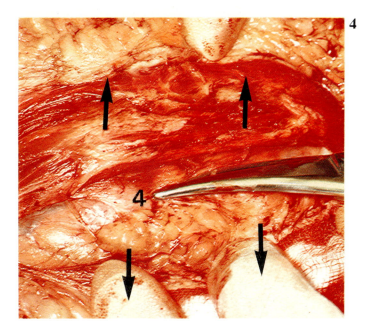

3 to 5 Excision of previous weak midline scar and opening peritoneal cavity

A previous operation had left a wide and weak midline scar with actual herniation just below the umbilicus. The upper end of an excised band of thin skin (1) is held by dissecting forceps (2) and removed with the scalpel (3) in Figure 3, (see Volume 2 page 40 for details of this technique). In Figure 4 the sheath and the fibres of the recti muscles on each side are retracted with the fingers as arrowed, while the scissors define the peritoneum (4). The peritoneum is opened with the scalpel between forceps at (5) in Figure 5.

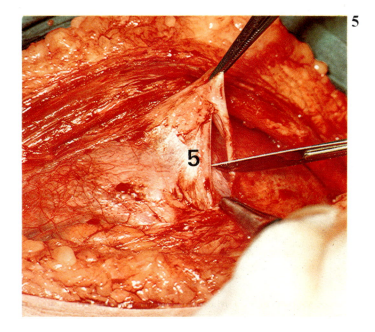

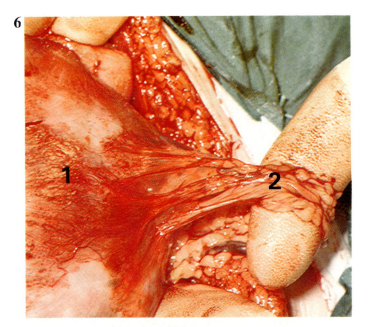

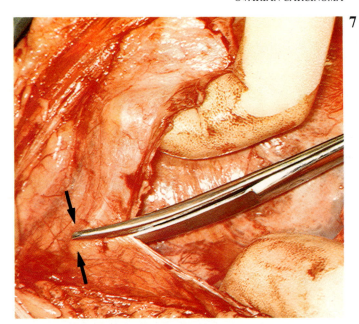

6 and 7 Obtaining access to peritoneal cavity (i)

The ovarian tumour (1) presents in the wound in Figure 6 but is attached to the omentum by a firm adhesion (2) which precludes entry and has to be divided between forceps. This has been done in Figure 7 and allows the scissors to extend the peritoneal incision as far as the upper border of the bladder (arrowed).

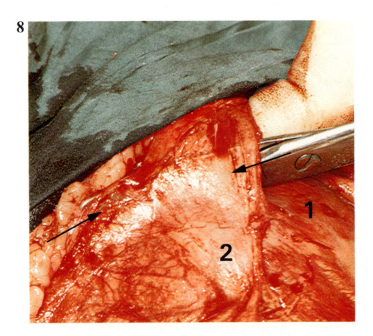

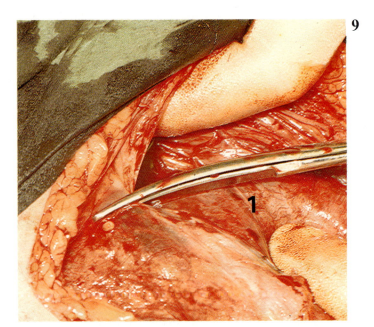

8 and 9 Obtaining access to peritoneal cavity (ii)

Further adhesion between the anterior aspect of the tumour (1) and the parietal peritoneum on the right side of the wound (2) is defined by the scissors in Figure 8 (arrowed). This band of adhesions is being divided in Figure 9 and access to the abdomen is finally obtained.

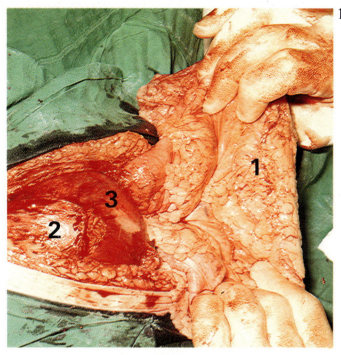

10 Exploration of abdomen
It was established that the growth was completely filling the pelvis and lower abdomen and that it was largely solid in consistency. It was found to be firmly fixed in the pelvis and was adherent to large and small intestine.

11 Examination of omentum
Despite the pelvic findings the omentum did not obviously contain macroscopic metastases. It is held up (1) and the ovarian tumour (2) is seen to be covered by an adherent coil of small intestine (3).

Stage 2: Mobilisation of ovarian tumour

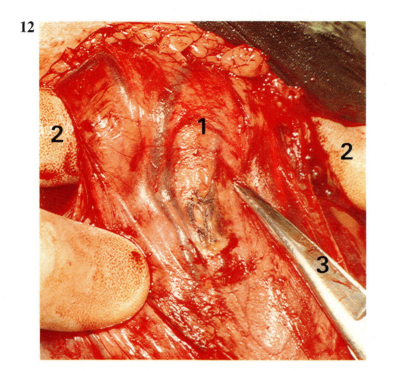

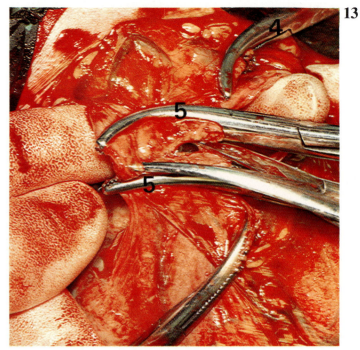

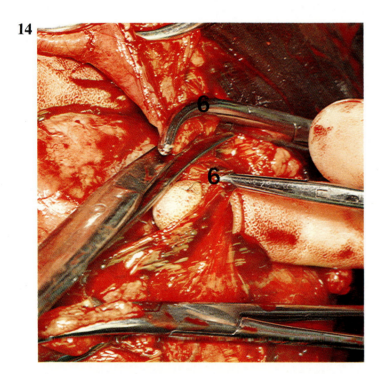

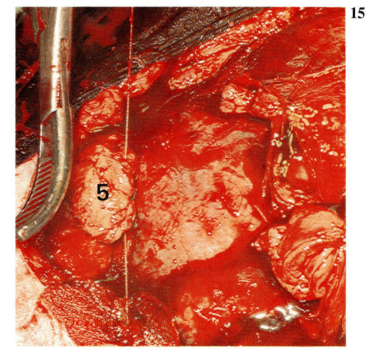

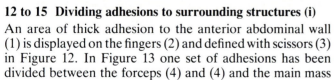

12 to 15 Dividing adhesions to surrounding structures (i)

An area of thick adhesion to the anterior abdominal wall (1) is displayed on the fingers (2) and defined with scissors (3) in Figure 12. In Figure 13 one set of adhesions has been divided between the forceps (4) and (4) and the main mass is being divided between forceps (5) and (5). Further division proceeds (6) and (6) in Figure 14; in Figure 15 all have been tied off except the largest of the divided ends which is in process of being ligated (5).

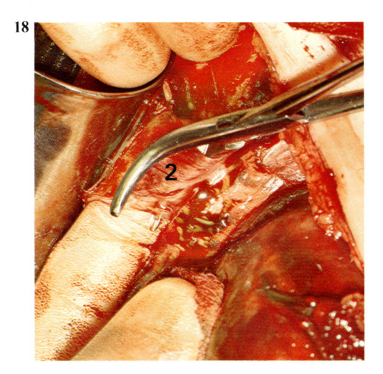

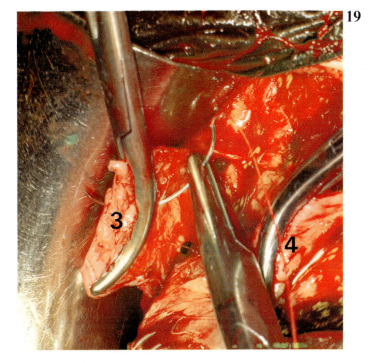

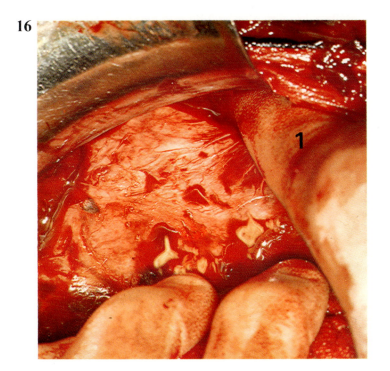

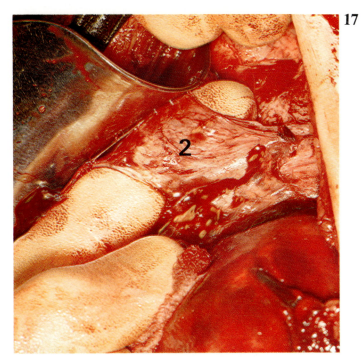

16 to 19 Dividing adhesions to surrounding structures (ii)

The growth had developed adhesions anteriorly over the bladder and in the right inguinal region. These are being defined with the finger (1) in Figure 16, displayed (2) in Figure 17, and clamped in Figure 18. In Figure 19 one cut end (3) is being transfixed prior to ligation; the other (4) will be similarly treated.

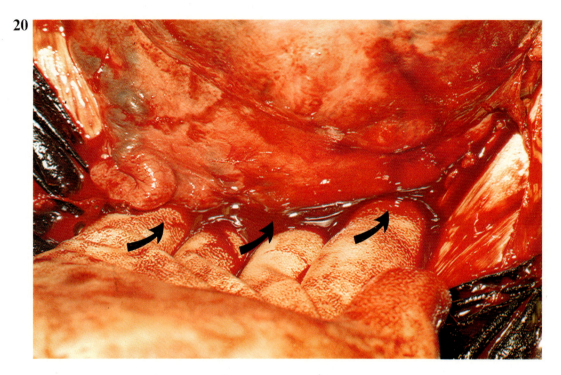

20 Elevation of tumour from pelvic floor

Adhesions to the pelvic floor were less dense and could be broken down with the fingers. The hand is seen sliding under the lower pole of the growth towards the pouch of Douglas, like a large spoon (see page 247), to bring it up into the wound. The hand is inserted in the direction of the arrows.

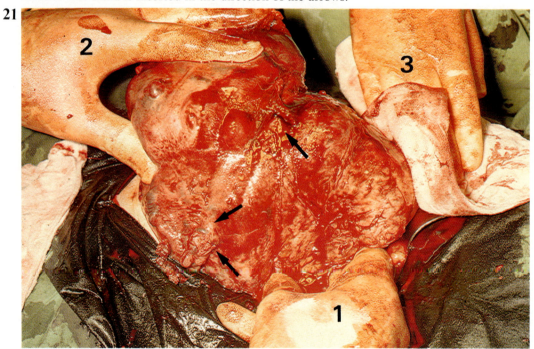

21 Delivery of tumour into wound

The tumour has now been delivered into the wound by the surgeon's right hand (1) and is steadied by his left (2) while his assistant (3) helps to express the mass from the pelvis. The rough areas where it adhered are arrowed.

Stage 3: Salpingo-oophorectomy

22

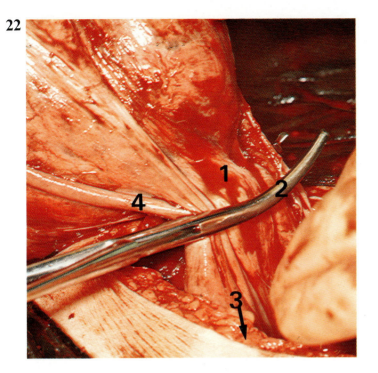

23

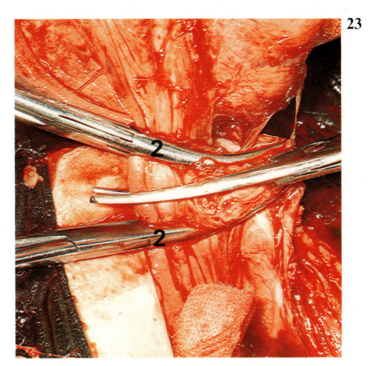

22 to 24 Right salpingo-oophorectomy

The right broad ligament (1) is defined between the jaws of large forceps (2) in Figure 22. The uterus is at (3) and the fallopian tube (4). In Figure 23 the broad ligament is being cut with scissors between forceps (2) and (2) and in Figure 24 the medial part of the broad ligament pedicle is being ligated. The lumen of the fallopian tube (4) and the enlarged vessels in the broad ligament are clearly seen (arrowed). The uterus is at (3) and the rectum (5). A large moist swab (6) acts as a haemostatic aid for the rather vascular bed from which the tumour was raised.

24

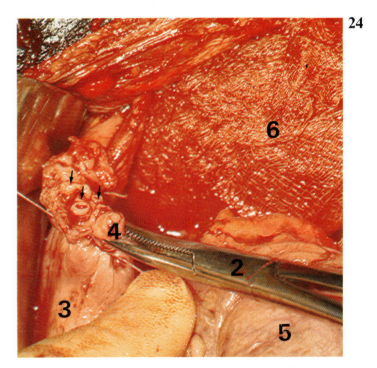

Stage 4: Reperitonisation

25

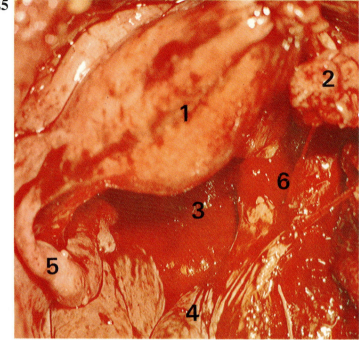

26

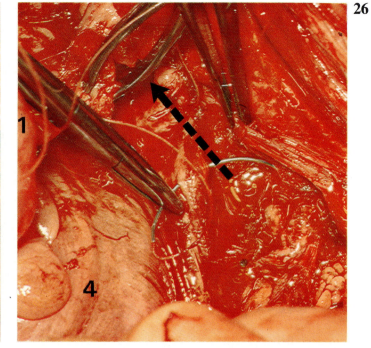

25 to 27 Covering tumour bed with peritoneum

Figure 25 shows the pelvis remarkably clear with the uterus (1) lifted anteriorly and to the left to show the ligated broad ligament pedicle (2), the pouch of Douglas (3), the rectum (4), and the left tube (5). The general bare area where the tumour was adherent is at (6). A continuous peritoneal stitch commences the closure of the raw area by bringing the edges together laterally in Figure 26, and in Figure 27 has progressed medially to complete the closure and is shown being tied off. The broken arrow lines indicate the direction of peritoneal closure in Figures 26 and 27; the photographs are at slightly different angles.

27

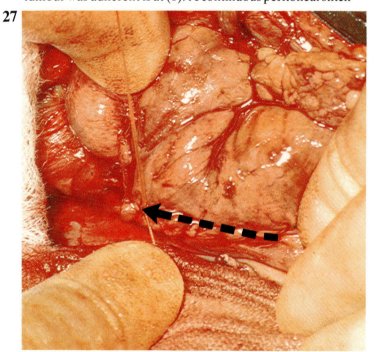

Stage 5: Excision of greater omentum

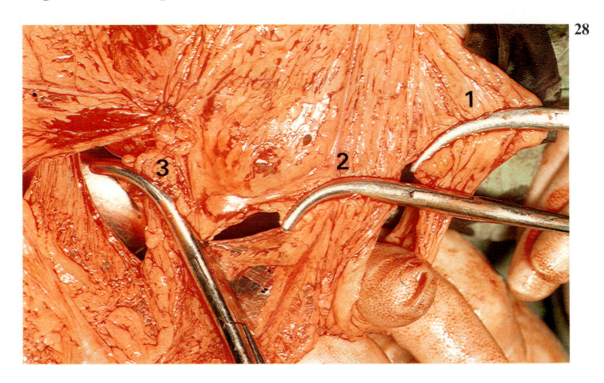

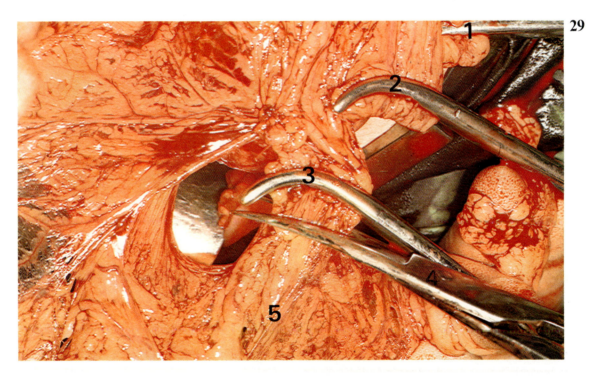

28 and 29 Steps in removal of omentum (i)
The omentum is excised along a line corresponding to the anti-mesenteric border of the transverse colon. Each Spencer-Wells forceps is first pushed antero-posteriorly through the omentum to define a suitably sized pedicle or bite of tissue which it then clamps off; this has been done in three places (1), (2) and (3) in Figure 28. In Figure 29 the scissors (4) have divided and detached the omentum (5) beyond the forceps (1) and (2) and are in process of dividing (3).

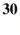

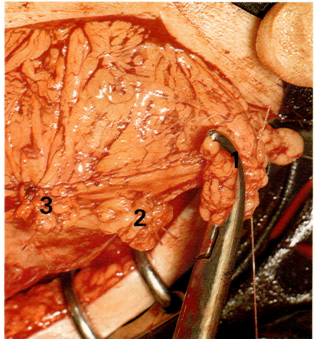

30 Steps in removal of omentum (ii)

The pedicles (2) and (3) have been ligated; the exact technique is shown in relation to (1). This pedicle has already been transfixed and ligation is being completed, first under the toe and then under the heel of the forceps. It is important that the ligatures should be secure as omental vessels have very little tissue support and are liable to bleed if not firmly tied.

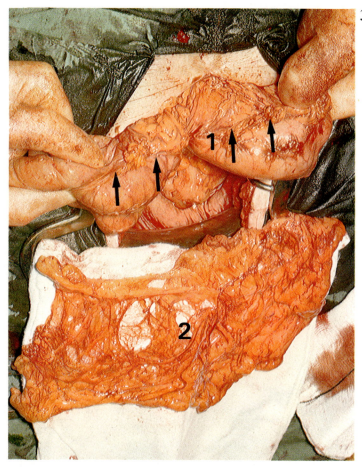

31 Steps in removal of omentum (iii)

The transverse colon (1) is held in an anterior and cephalad direction by the surgeon to show the excision line (arrowed) and the detached omentum (2) lies on a large swab just over the blade of the Balfour retractor.

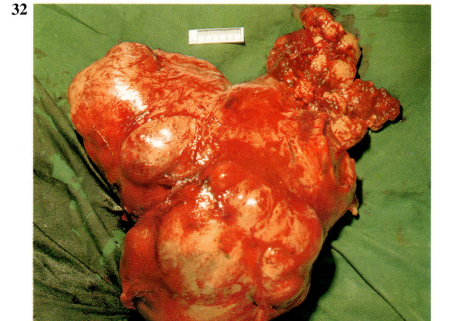

32 Specimen

1.(ii) Radical operation: extensive surgical removal of abdomino-pelvic growth and intestinal metastases (pseudo-myxoma)

The case described here also belongs to the group referred to on page 243. Its inclusion serves to emphasise the large number of ovarian growths which cannot be completely removed surgically. Pseudo-myxomatous growths which also fall into this category are not uncommon and every gynaecologist is faced with the management of these very difficult cases from time to time. The condition can occur when the epithelium is benign, but that was not the case in this instance and the bowel was also involved. The best prospect with this disease is generally to remove the involved pelvic structures while clearing the pelvis of the mucinous mass and to give postoperative chemotherapy, usually in the form of alkylating agents.

1 External appearance preoperatively

The whole lower abdomen shows general distention with a raised firm area on the right side (1). There is a certain amount of skin discoloration (2) suggesting deeper blood extravasation and the enlarged blood vessels on the thighs and loins (arrowed) show that a collateral circulation has been established.

2 Negative of ultrasonic scan

The longitudinal cut of a B-Scan (Ultrasound) from a Diasonograph 4102 shows the general outline and extent of the tumour which is arrowed. Multiple septa (1) can be seen separating the mass which is composed of cystic (2) and solid areas (3). This appearance is highly suggestive of a malignant ovarian lesion. The bladder is seen at (4) and the pubic symphysis marked by a perpendicular arrow.

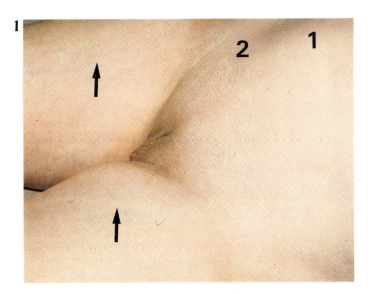

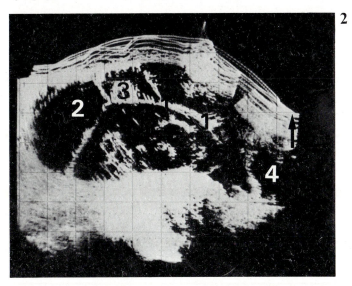

Stage 1: Opening the abdomen

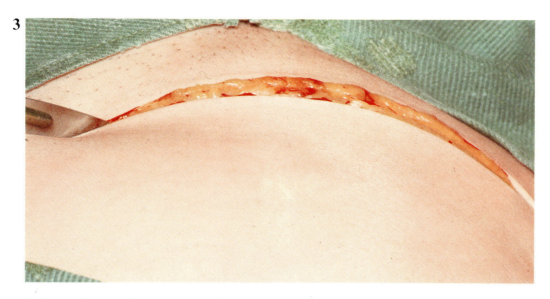

3 Lower abdominal transverse incision
The incision is made slightly higher than usual and the outer ends are curved upwards so that they can be extended laterally above the anterior superior iliac spines if the wound needs to be enlarged.

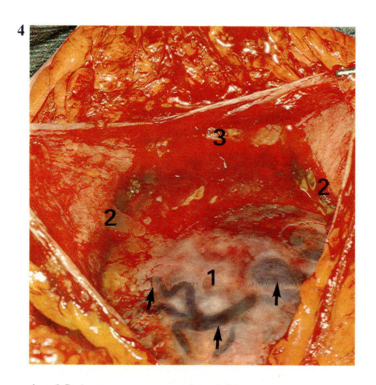 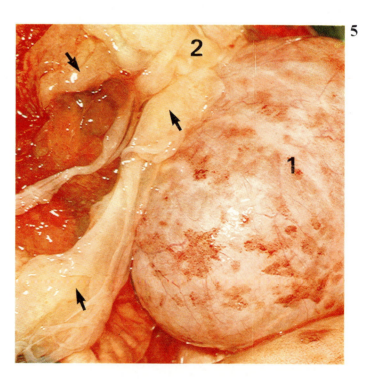

4 and 5 Appearance on opening abdomen
The peritoneal cavity has been opened in Figure 4 and the pseudo-myxomatous condition is immediately apparent. The upper pole of the right-sided swelling (1) has large blood vessels coursing over it (arrowed) and the mucinous mass is adherent to the peritoneum both laterally (2) and over the bladder (3). In Figure 5 the right ovarian cyst (1) has been delivered into the wound and it is apparent that the whole pelvis is filled with sheets of pseudo-mucin (arrowed). There is an accumulation around the pedicle of the cyst (2).

Stage 2: Right salpingo-oophorectomy

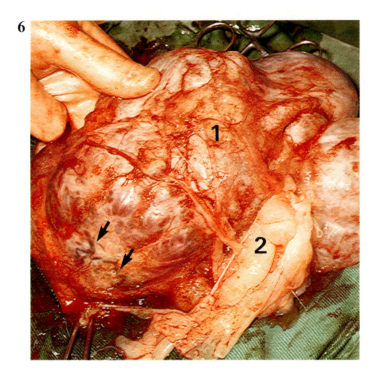

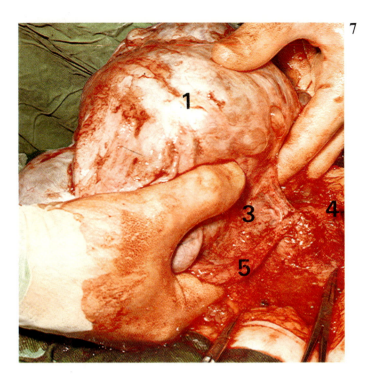

6 to 8 Steps in removal of tumour

The photographs are taken from the patient's right side in the direction of the symphysis pubis. In Figure 6 the whole right-sided mass (1) has now been delivered into the wound and is steadied by the left hand. The sheets of pseudo-mucin (2) are still obvious and the blood vessels noted previously (arrowed). In Figure 7 the right ovarian pedicle has been defined (3) as the tumour is elevated from the pelvis, and the uterus (4) and right fallopian tube (5) lie anteriorly. In Figure 8 the pedicle is being divided with scissors between the first pair of clamping forceps prior to removal of the tumour.

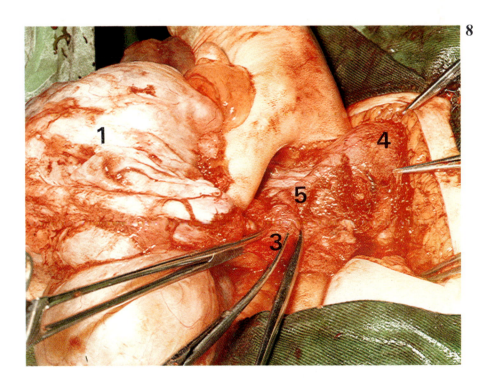

9

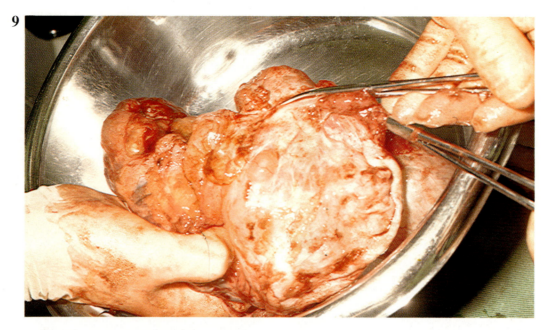

9 Right ovarian cyst removed
The right tube and ovary with the pseudo-mucinous cyst are examined in the specimen bowl. There is a complete mucinous covering. Exophytic growth from the tumour in several places indicates that it is almost certainly malignant.

10

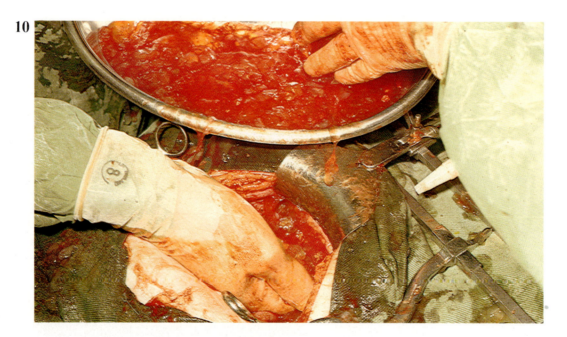

10 Removing pseudo-mucin from pelvic cavity
This photograph shows the mucin being scooped from the pelvis into a specimen bowl by the surgeon's hand. There was approximately one litre and it was almost entirely in the pelvis.

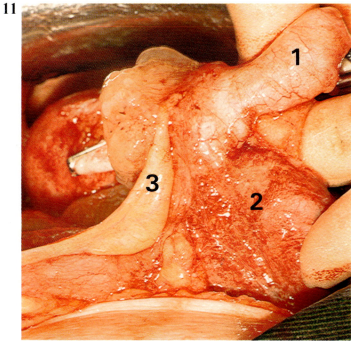

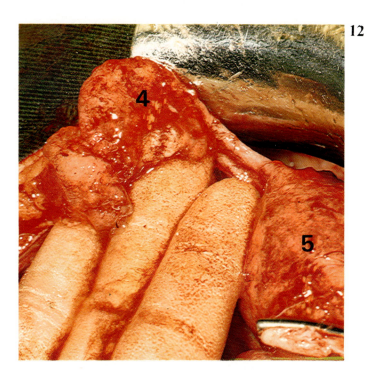

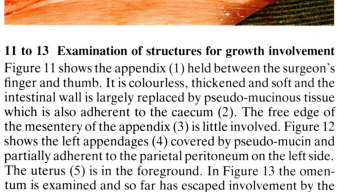

11 to 13 Examination of structures for growth involvement
Figure 11 shows the appendix (1) held between the surgeon's finger and thumb. It is colourless, thickened and soft and the intestinal wall is largely replaced by pseudo-mucinous tissue which is also adherent to the caecum (2). The free edge of the mesentery of the appendix (3) is little involved. Figure 12 shows the left appendages (4) covered by pseudo-mucin and partially adherent to the parietal peritoneum on the left side. The uterus (5) is in the foreground. In Figure 13 the omentum is examined and so far has escaped involvement by the pseudo-myxomatous process.

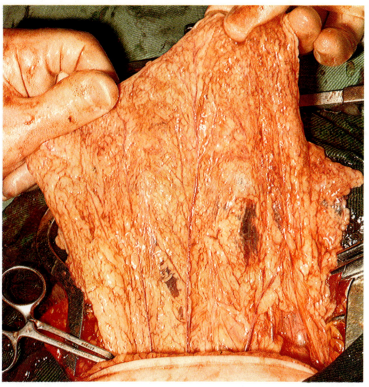

281

Stage 4: Hysterectomy

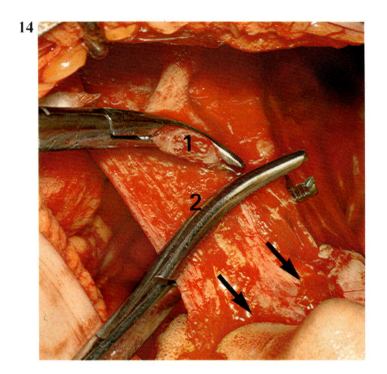

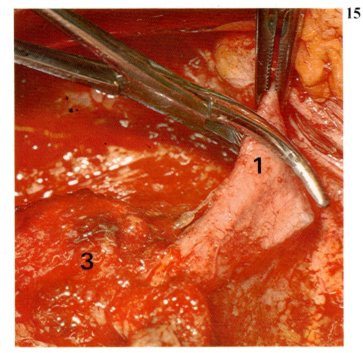

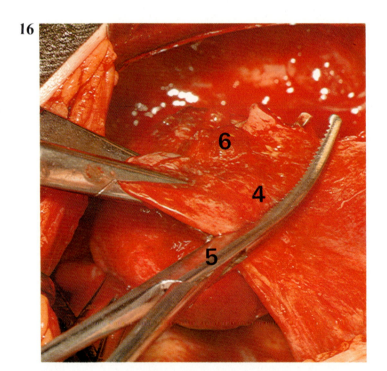

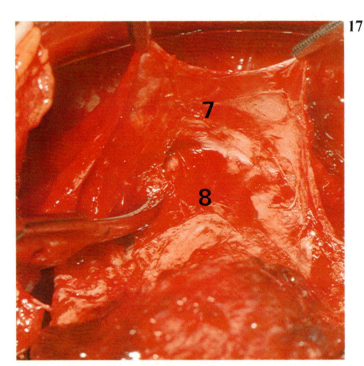

14 to 17 Securing upper uterine attachments

In Figure 14 the uterus is held medially in the direction of the arrows. The left round ligament (1) has been detached and the left ovarian pedicle (2) is being clamped prior to division. The right round ligament (1) is being clamped ready for separation in Figure 15 and the uterus (3) is seen medially. In Figure 16 the ovarian pedicle of the removed growth on the right side (4) is shown being shortened by application of fresh forceps (5) which will allow an affected area (6) to be excised. The position of the ureter is checked before applying this clamp. Figure 17 shows the utero-vesical pouch opened and the bladder (7) being dissected off the anterior aspect of the cervix (8) with the scissors.

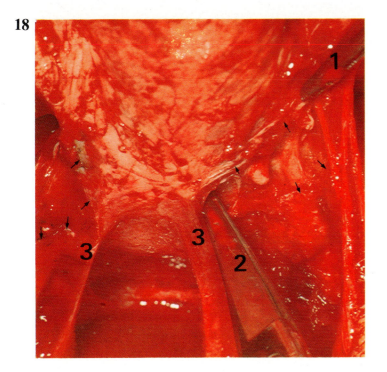

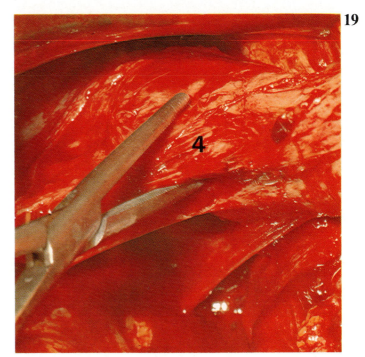

18 to 20 Securing uterine pedicle

In Figure 18 the posterior leaf of the right broad ligament is held by dissecting forceps (1) while the scissors (2) open it up as far as the utero-sacral ligament (3). The same has already been done on the left side and the cut edges of the posterior leaves of the broad ligament are arrowed. In Figure 19 the left uterine vessels (4) are being clamped by a straight Oschner forceps and in Figure 20 the right uterine pedicle (4) held in a similar clamp is being detached from the uterus with the scissors. The forceps (5) is positioned on the uterine end of the pedicle so as to prevent backflow of blood.

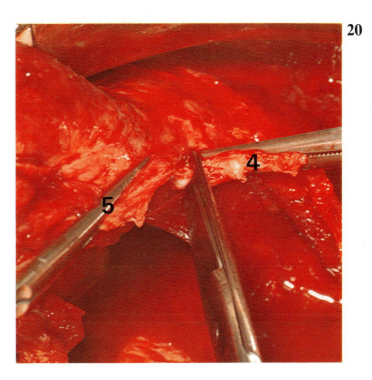

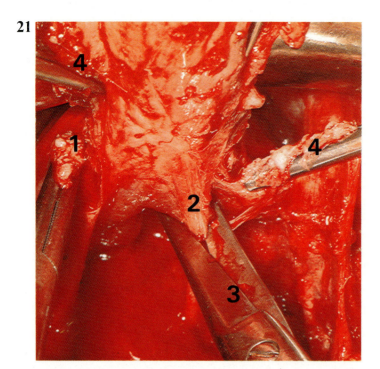

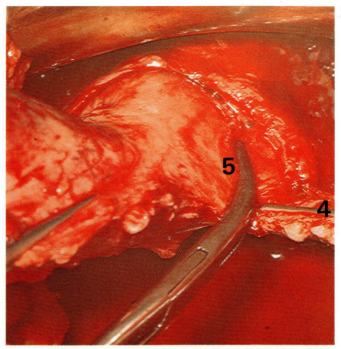

21 to 23 Securing lower uterine attachments

In Figure 21 the left utero-sacral ligament (1) has been detached from the uterus and the right one (2) is being divided by scissors (3). The uterine pedicles are still held in forceps (4) and (4). Figure 22 shows the application of curved forceps to the right vaginal angle (5); Figure 23 to the left vaginal angle (5).

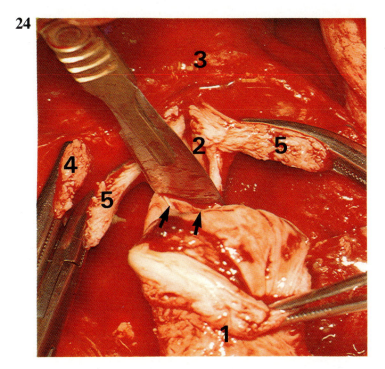

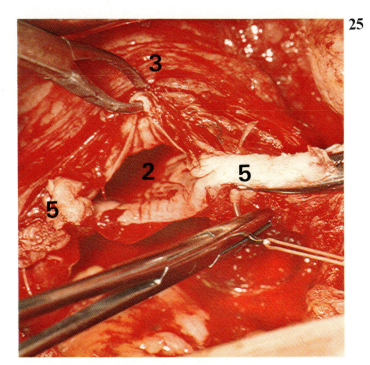

24 to 26 Removal of uterus and closure of vault of vagina

In Figure 24 the scalpel has incised each vaginal angle (5) and (5) and detached the uterus (1) at the vault, except at one place on the posterior wall (arrowed). The open vagina is at (2) and the bladder (3). The uterus has been removed in Figure 25. The left vaginal pedicle (5) is ligated and the right (5) is being transfixed with the needle. In Figure 26 the two lateral uncut mattress sutures (6) and (6) incorporate the utero-sacral pedicles and close the vault, while a central mattress suture is being placed at (7).

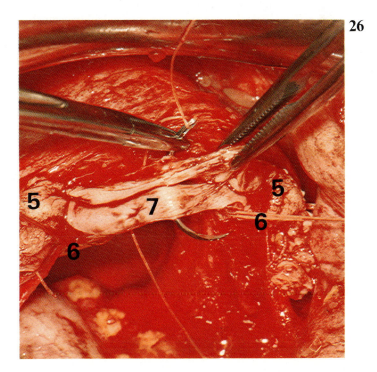

27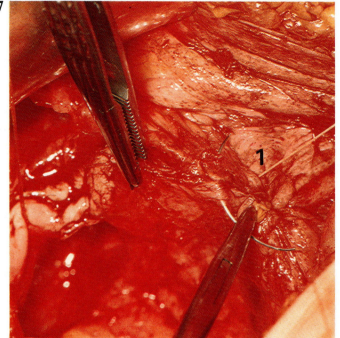

28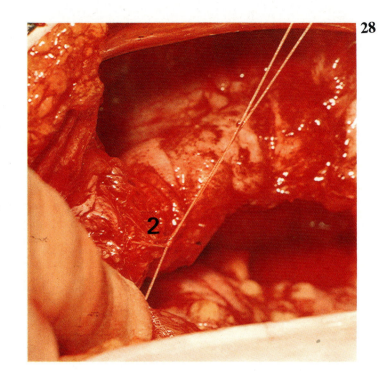

27 and 28 Reperitonisation

In Figure 27 the continuous peritoneal stitch has buried the right ovarian and round ligament pedicles under the anchor stitch (1) which was placed in the usual half purse string fashion; after this manoeuvre the stitch proceeds across the pelvis. In Figure 28 the peritoneum is seen to be closed and the stitch is tied off to cover the left pedicles in the same way as on the right (2).

Stage 5: Removal of mucocele of appendix

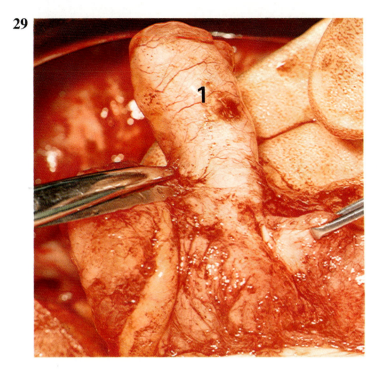

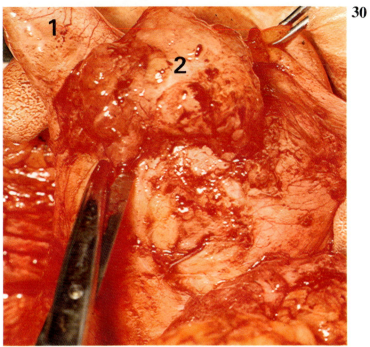

30

29 to 31 Steps in appendicectomy and partial resection of caecum (i)

In Figure 29 the pseudo-myxomatous mucocele of the appendix (1) is supported by the fingers and dissected out with scissors. In Figure 30 there is obviously a mass of pseudo-mucin adjacent to it on the surface of the caecum (2) and this is also being defined with the scissors. In Figure 31 a leash of blood vessels in the relatively unaffected free edge of the appendix mesentery is clamped as shown (3).

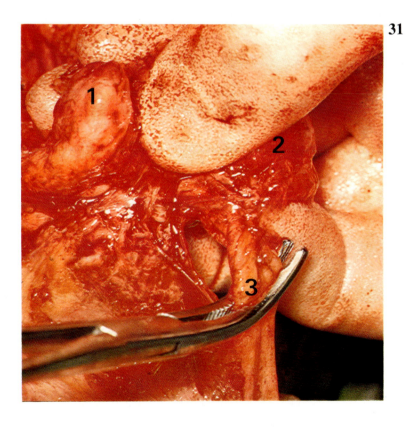

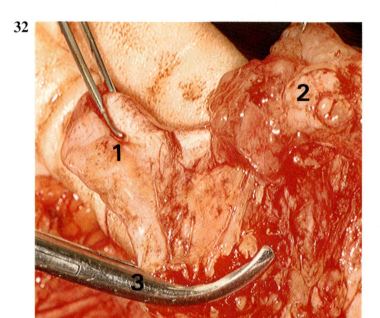

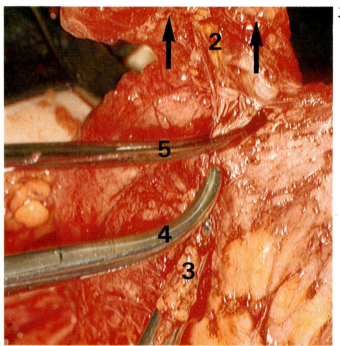

31

32 to 34 Steps in appendicectomy and partial resection of caecum (ii)

The appendix is at (1) and the caecal pseudo-myxoma (2) in Figure 32. The Phillips' forceps (3) clamps the broad base of the appendix but subsequent appendicectomy is not shown. In Figure 33 the forceps on the appendicular stump (3) are joined by others (4) which control a bleeding vessel and the scissors (5) seek a plane of separation between the caecum and the pseudo-mucinous mass (2), held up in the direction of the arrows. In Figure 34 the scissors have inadvertently entered the caecum and the opening into the bowel is outlined by arrows.

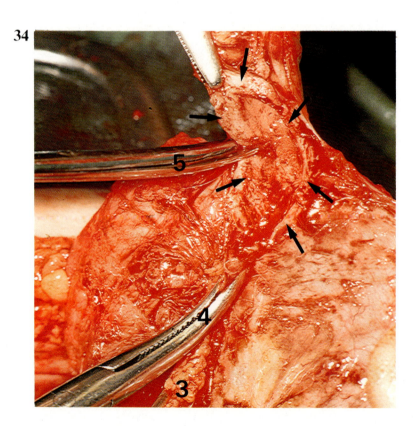

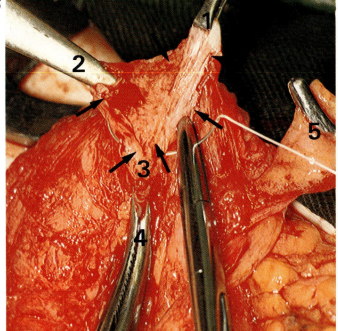

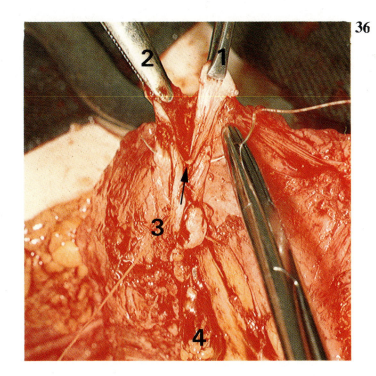

36

35 to 37 Steps in appendicectomy and partial resection of caecum (iii)

In Figure 35, and since the caecum has been opened, the pseudo-myxoma is cleanly excised from the caecum leaving an opening which is outlined by arrows. It is held open by tissue forceps (1), dissecting forceps (2), and the haemostatic forceps (4) already referred to. A first layer closure of the wall of the caecum is commencing at (3); the needle carries a PGA No. 00 suture. The still untied leash of vessels in the appendicular mesenteric edge is at (5). In Figure 36 the haemostatic forceps has been removed and the uncut end of the commencement of the caecal stitch is at (3). The suture which includes all layers of the caecum proceeds in the direction of the arrow. The appendicular stump is at (4); the forceps holding this suture are just excluded from this photograph. In Figure 37 a second inverting suture has closed the opening in the caecum and is being tied off where arrowed. The appendix stump still held in forceps can just be seen at (4).

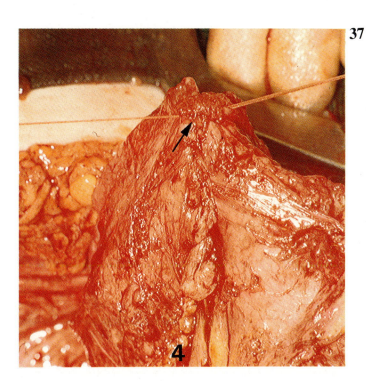

37

38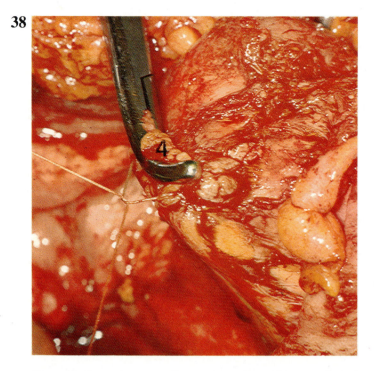

39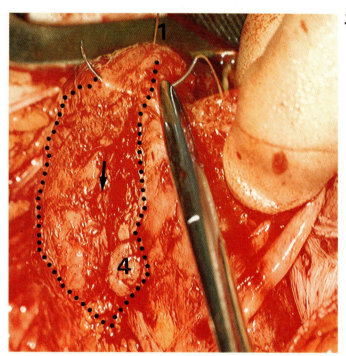

38 to 40 Steps in appendicectomy and partial resection of caecum (iv)

In Figure 38 the broad appendix stump is tied off with PGA No. 0 material. In Figure 39 a Lembert type serous stitch of PGA No. 00 is used to cover the raw area of the caecum which is outlined by a broken line. The anchor knot

is seen at (1). The ligated appendix stump is still numbered (4) and will be inverted by the same stitch which proceeds in the direction of the arrow. Figure 40 shows the serous stitch being tied off (2) at the end of its course (double broken line). The buried appendix stump is approximately in the area (4).

40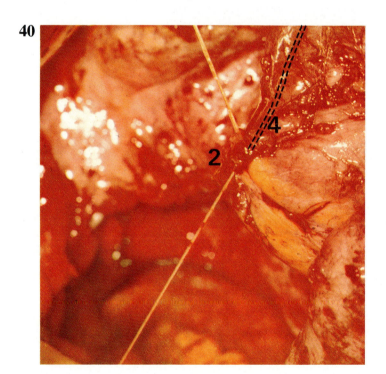

41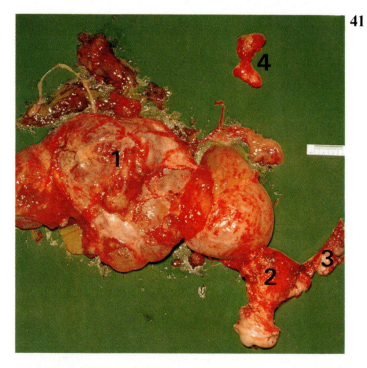

41 Specimen

The large right-sided pseudo-myxomatous mass (1) is typical with its mucin covered surface and rough areas of attachment to other structures. The uterus (2), the left ovary (3), the appendix and part of the caecum (4) are all, to some extent, involved in the process.

Suggested reading

Barber, H. R. K., Graber, E. A. & Kwon, T. H. (1974). Ovarian cancer. *Cancer* (1974), Vol. 24, 339.

Hudson, C. N. (1978). The place of surgery in the treatment of ovarian cancer. *Clinics in Obstetrics and Gynaecology,* 5, 3, 695–708. W. B. Saunders, Philadelphia.

Keegel, W. C., Pixley, E. E. & Bauchsbaum, H. J. (1974). Experience with peritoneal cytology in the management of gynecologic malignancies. *American Journal of Obstetrics and Gynecology,* 120, 174.

Mattingley, R. F. (1977). Staging and treatment of ovarian carcinoma. *Te Linde's Operative Gynecology,* 831–853. Fifth edition. J. B. Lippincott.

Munnell, E. W. (1974). Cancer of the ovary. *Proceedings of the Royal Society of Medicine,* 67, 797.

Munnell, E. W. (1978). *Corscaden's Gynecologic Cancer.* 375–396, edited by S. G. Gusberg & H. C. Frick. Fifth edition. Williams & Wilkins, Baltimore.

6: Surgical management of Recurrent pelvic Malignancy (following failed radiotherapy)

When cases of cervical and endometrial cancer recur following definitive radiotherapy, they present particular problems because there is little more that can be done in the way of further radiotherapy. Recurrence takes various forms but is usually accompanied by marked deterioration in general condition so that further management has to be entirely palliative. When metastases are extra-pelvic, and even if the patient's general condition is good, surgery is out of the question. In these circumstances only chemotherapy or hormone treatment is available.

There are, however, occasions when the recurrence is localised and the general condition of the patient is reasonably good so that there is a possible place for surgery. In one such group there are localised lower vaginal metastases close to the introitus; this is particularly associated with endometrial carcinoma. They usually respond very well to radiotherapy applied locally or by needles and are in an area where the additional necessary dosage is not being superimposed on high previous dosages.

The other and more usual local recurrence is centrally in the pelvis and involves the region of the cervix and the upper vagina. The ectocervix, the cervical canal or even the lower cavity of the uterus may be involved. The patient is distressed and ill with a discharging and bleeding lesion. Full radiotherapy has been given and the patient's hopes of cure are minimal. The radiotherapist, having given maximum treatment, looks to the surgeon for help. Some of these cases are cervical carcinomata but the majority are endometrial and arise because surgery was not considered advisable in the first place, either because of the patient's general medical unfitness or gross obesity.

The main problems in management are the devitalised state of the tissues following radiotherapy and uncertainty regarding the extent of the growth recurrence. Some authorities say that pelvic exenteration is the only possible treatment but we believe that readers should note the less radical approach adopted at the M.D. Anderson Hospital, Houston (Rutledge, Boronow and Wharton, 1976); their experience corresponds with our own. The position of the practising surgeon who is faced with such a case and who has no experience of exenteration and no special facilities at his disposal has already been discussed. We do not believe that he would wish to embark on such a procedure even if it were the sole option.

The other possibility, which has been referred to above, is to do a radical hysterectomy with vaginal vault excision but without attempting pelvic lymphadenectomy. Particular care is taken to avoid trauma or devascularisation of the tissues, the urinary tract is treated with caution and disturbed as little as possible, and every postoperative facility is used to encourage pelvic blood flow and early mobilisation. Such

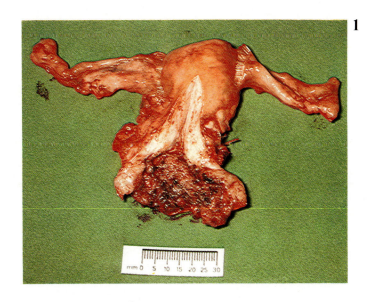

1

1 Operation specimen to indicate the problem

This photograph of the specimen actually removed at the operation to be described illustrates the essential problem. There is recurrence of a moderately differentiated squamous cervical growth with extension to the lower body of the uterus and to the upper third of the vagina. Full radiotherapy had already been given; there was no evidence of distant metastases in the lymphograms.

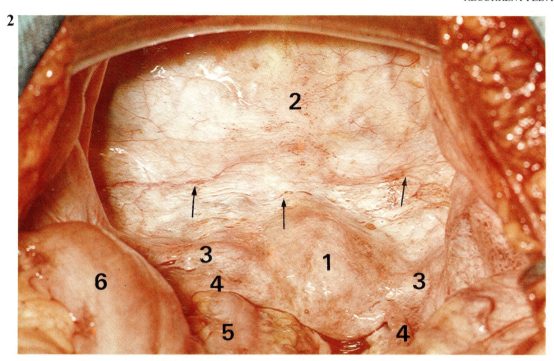

2 Appearance on opening the abdomen

The abdomen has been opened by a transverse lower abdominal incision and a Balfour's self-retaining retractor is in position. The intra-peritoneal appearances show typical post-radiation atrophic changes. The peritoneum is pale and slightly yellow with loss of surface sheen. Small telangiectatic blood vessels course over the surface and the uterus is retroposed and obviously fixed in the pelvis. The uterus is at (1) the bladder (2), round ligaments (3), fallopian tubes (4), small intestine (5) and large intestine (6). The surface blood vessels are indicated by small arrows.

an operation is described in this chapter and the important points are stressed as they are encountered.

By virtue of close association with a regional radiotherapy hospital over many years, the senior author has served as the end referral point for a number of such patients. The type of operation described here has been performed on at least twelve patients with results that are most gratifying. The circumstances have not allowed of really accurate follow-up but all patients were relieved of their symptoms. There were no operative deaths and several patients have survived for over five years. It can be said with conviction that in no instance has such treatment ever been regretted; neither has a urinary fistula developed in any of the cases.

Rutledge, Boronow and Wharton (1976) have published figures which relate to this limited group of patients. They believe that the type of radical hysterectomy under discussion should be used for a lesion restricted to the immediate

vicinity of the cervix and upper vagina but they indicate that a high incidence of fistulae must be expected. They have used the method for the treatment of persistent or recurrent cancer following x-ray therapy in 65 patients. Of the 47 patients treated 5 years ago, 26 (55.3 per cent) are still free of disease. In the 65 cases, there were 12 vesicovaginal, 3 rectovaginal and 1 ureterovaginal fistulae but this high incidence was largely contributed to by eight cases where segmental resection of ureter or resection of a portion of bladder was done, and they do not now advocate such extensions of the operation.

Their success rate has encouraged them to use radical hysterectomy for suitable patients despite the need to do further operations to correct fistulae. In regard to pelvic exenteration, they consider it both formidable and risky and only justified if there is a good chance of long term cancer control.

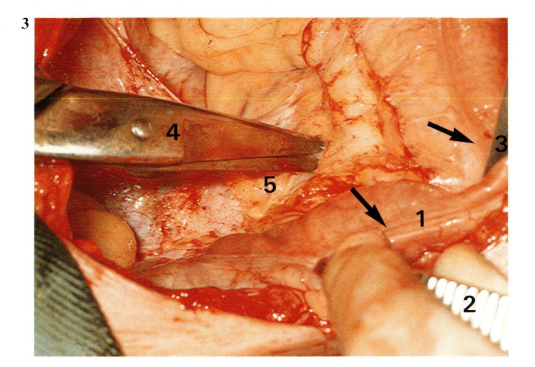

3 Release of pelvic colon from left infundibulo-pelvic ligament

It is very important to have adequate access in such a case and the large bowel (1) is held in a cephalad direction by dissecting forceps (2) and retractor (3), as arrowed, while the scissors (4) free adhesions from the region of the infundibulo-pelvic ligament (5).

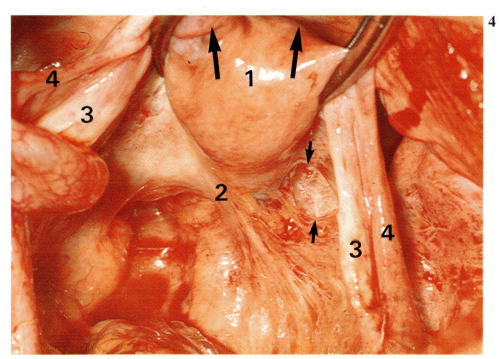

4 Elevation of uterus from pelvic floor

Oschner forceps on the broad ligament are used to elevate the uterus (1) from the pelvic floor in the direction of the arrows and this disrupts a curtain of adhesions in the region of the utero-sacral ligament on the right side (torn edges are indicated by fine arrows). Such adhesions are common following radiotherapy. There is thickening around and below the left utero-sacral ligament (2) corresponding to the extension to the left lateral fornix seen in the specimen. As one would expect, both ovaries (3) and (3) and fallopian tubes (4) and (4) are small and atrophic.

Stage 1: Division of upper uterine attachments

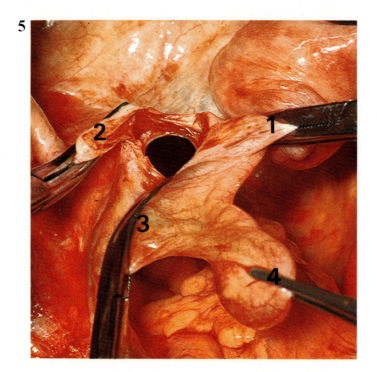

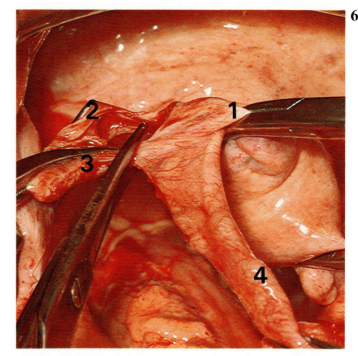

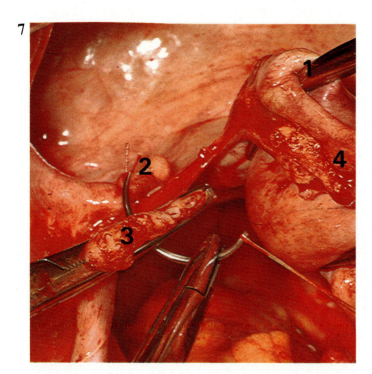

5 to 7 Division of upper uterine attachments (i)

In Figure 5 the left broad ligament is held by forceps (1), the left round ligament (2) has been clamped and detached leaving a gap in the broad ligament and the left ovarian pedicle has been clamped at (3). The left appendages are held by tissue forceps (4). In Figure 6 the ovarian pedicle is being divided with scissors (3). In Figure 7 the left round ligament has been ligated (2) while the ovarian pedicle (3) has been transfixed. The appendages are at (4).

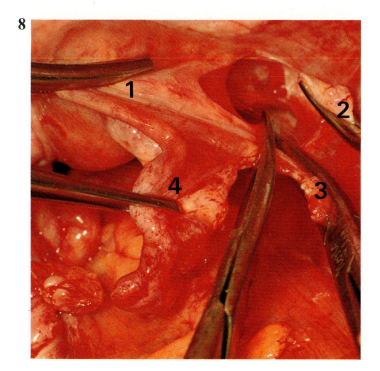

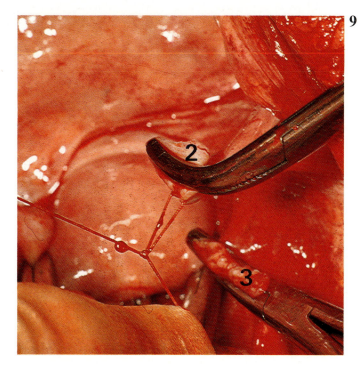

8 to 10 Division of upper uterine attachments (ii)

The procedure is repeated on the right side. In Figure 8 Oschner forceps hold the broad ligament (1) and the right round ligament is detached (2) while the clamped ovarian pedicle (3) is being cut by the scissors and the appendages are held medially (4). In this, as on the other side, it will be noted that the radiotherapy is followed by closure of the fimbrial end of the tube and a degree of hydrosalpinx is present. In Figure 9 the right round ligament pedicle (2) is ligated and in Figure 10 the right ovarian pedicle (3) is similarly dealt with.

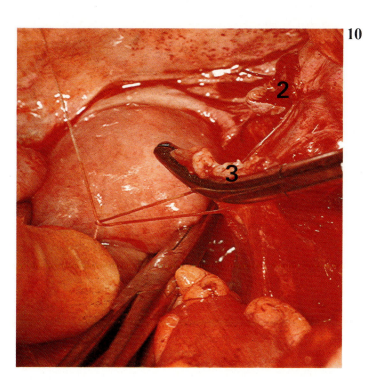

Stage 2: Separation of uterus from bladder anteriorly

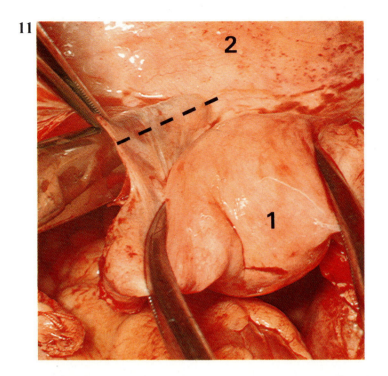

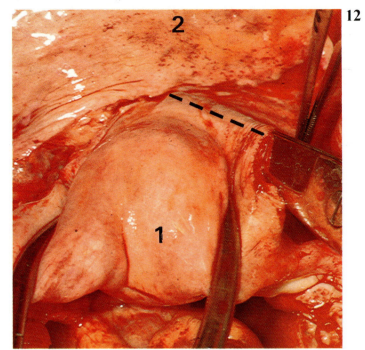

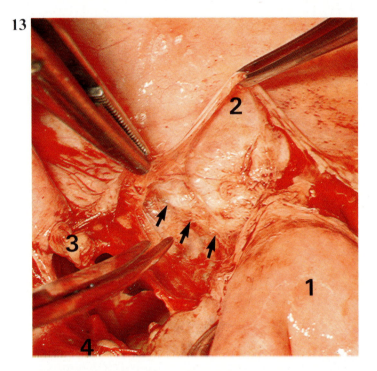

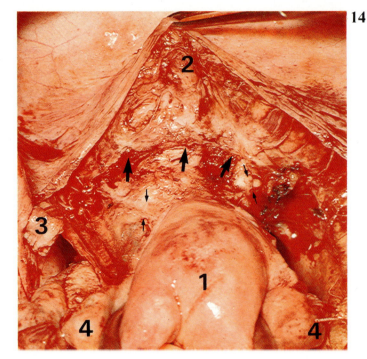

11 to 14 Dissection of uterus from bladder

This is obviously an important and potentially dangerous step, as there is the likelihood of dense adhesions following radiotherapy and the possibility of extension of the growth to the bladder, although that should have been excluded by previous cystoscopy. The surgeon must proceed cautiously and meticulously using sharp dissection under vision. In Figure 11 the left side of the utero-vesical fold is raised on scissors before division along the dotted line. That division has been made in Figure 12 and the process is being repeated with the line again indicated. Sharp dissection under vision

proceeds in Figure 13 and is largely completed in Figure 14. The structures are indicated thus:

  1 Uterus
  2 Bladder
  3 Ligated round ligaments
  4 Ligated ovarian pedicles

The plane of separation at the tip of the scissors in Figure 13 (arrowed) has been carried more distally in Figure 14 (arrowed). The uterine arteries can be seen in both (indicated by fine arrows).

Stage 3: Definition and dissection of ureters

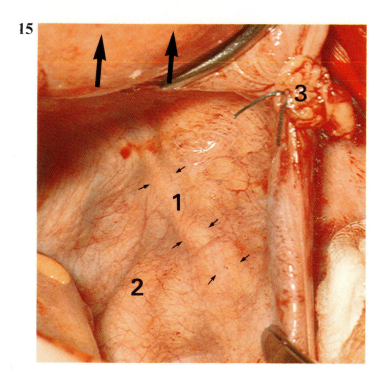

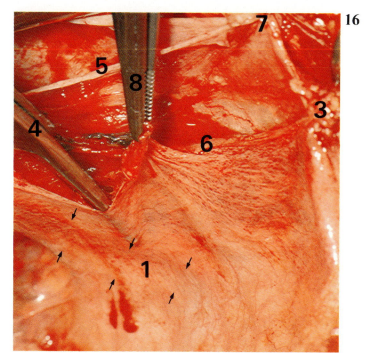

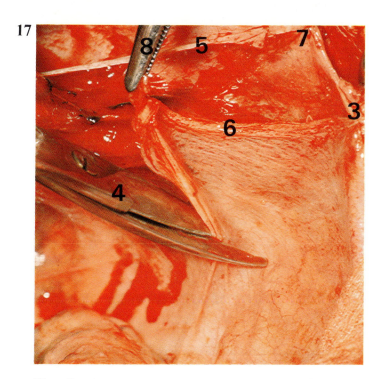

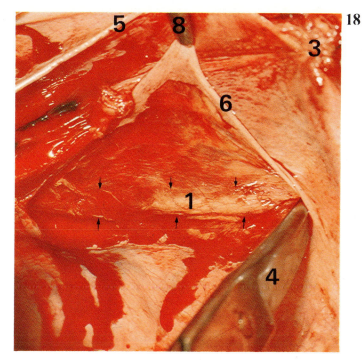

15 to 18 Dissection of right ureter from broad ligament

In Figure 15 the ureter (1) is seen crossing the common iliac artery (2) medial to the ligated ovarian pedicle (3) as the uterus is held upwards, as arrowed. In Figure 16 the anterior (5) and the posterior (6) leaves of the broad ligament are clearly seen; the ovarian pedicle is at (3) and the round ligament pedicle at (7). The posterior leaf is held in dissecting forceps (8) just lateral to the ureter and the scissors (4) elevate the peritoneum parallel and just lateral to it. They incise the peritoneum in that line in Figure 17 and lay bare the ureter on the pelvic side wall in Figure 18. The fine arrows outline the ureter under the peritoneum in Figures 15 and 16 and exposed in Figure 18.

19 to 22 Dissection of left ureter from broad ligament
The same procedure is carried out on the left side, and in this case the ureter is shown being underrun with a tape in Figure 22. The ureter (1) is outlined in each photograph.

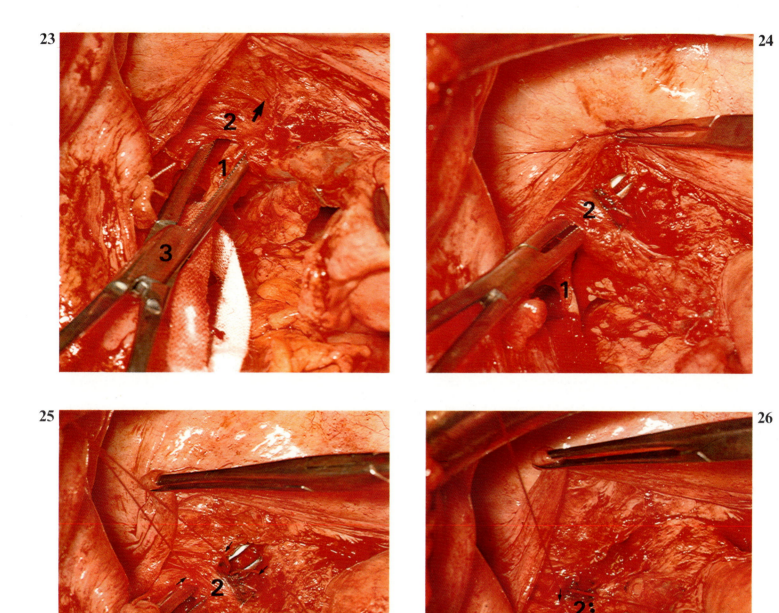

23 to 26 Exposing left ureter in ureteric tunnel (i)

In Figure 23 the ureter (1) lying on the tape is followed into the parametrial tunnel (2) by long curved Spencer-Wells forceps (3) in the direction of the arrow. The tunnel is defined by the forceps in Figure 24 and double ligatures are in place in Figure 25 (arrowed). The proximal ligature is tied in Figure 26 (arrowed) but the distal ligature will be replaced by forceps at the dotted line: this is done so that the lower uterus can be controlled by the forceps while the ureter is displaced laterally.

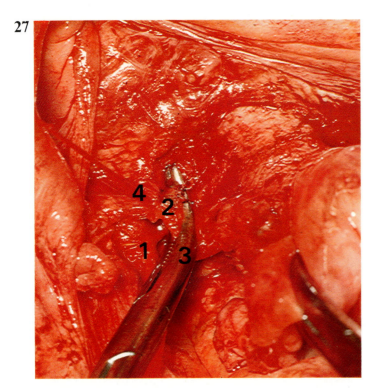

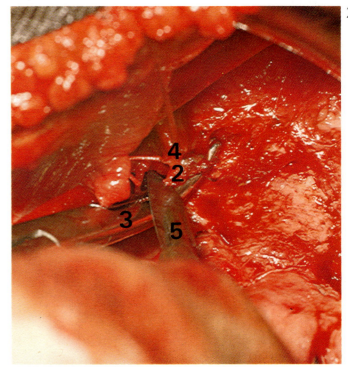

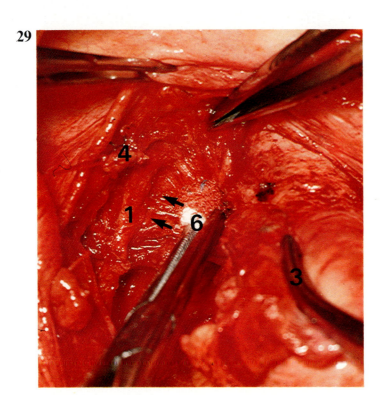

27 to 29 Exposing left ureter in ureteric tunnel (ii)

In Figure 27 the tunnel (2) is ready for division between the Phillips' forceps (3) and the ligature (4); the ureter is at (1). In Figure 28 the scalpel (5) divides the roof of the ureteric tunnel and uterine vessels close to the forceps so as to leave a cuff of 0.5 cm distal to the ligature. Figure 29 shows the ureter (1) clearly exposed with the Phillips' forceps at (3) and the proximal ligature at (4). A forceps holding a pledget of gauze (6) is used to displace the ureter laterally from the uterus in the direction of the arrows.

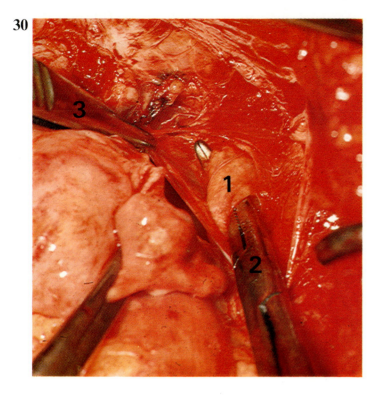

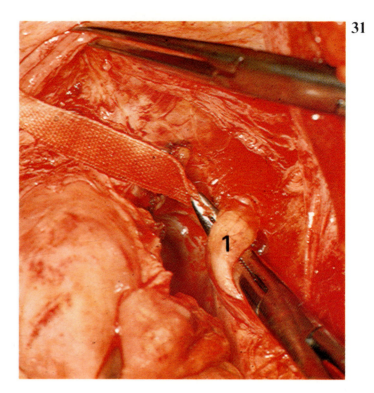

31

30 to 32 Exposing right ureter in ureteric tunnel (i)
In Figure 30 the Phillips' forceps (2) underlies and displays
the ureter (1) while the posterior layer of the broad ligament
is held medially by the dissecting forceps (3). A tape is
drawn under the ureter for identification purposes in
Figure 31. In Figure 32, forceps (4) are used to displace the
bladder angle in the direction of the arrows while scissors (5)
expose the roof of the ureteric tunnel (2). The ureter (1)
which is outlined by fine arrows is seen entering the ureteric
tunnel.

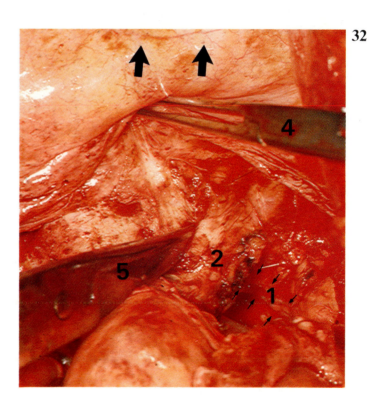

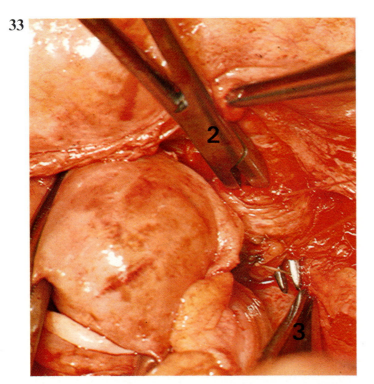

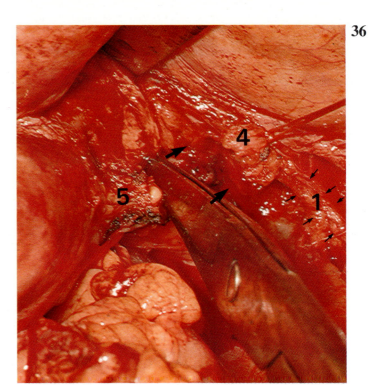

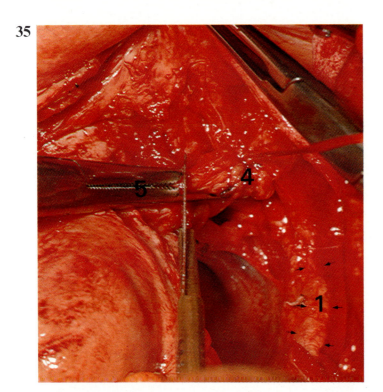

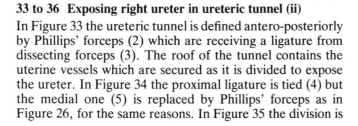

32

33 to 36 Exposing right ureter in ureteric tunnel (ii)

In Figure 33 the ureteric tunnel is defined antero-posteriorly by Phillips' forceps (2) which are receiving a ligature from dissecting forceps (3). The roof of the tunnel contains the uterine vessels which are secured as it is divided to expose the ureter. In Figure 34 the proximal ligature is tied (4) but the medial one (5) is replaced by Phillips' forceps as in Figure 26, for the same reasons. In Figure 35 the division is made with a scalpel close to the Phillips' forceps and leaving a cuff beyond the ligature (4). In Figure 36 both proximal and distal ends of the uterine vessels have been ligated (4) and (5) and the scissors are used to displace the ureter laterally in the direction of the arrows. In Figures 35 and 36 the mid-pelvic portion of the ureter (1), with its marking tape, is clearly seen.

Stage 4: Division of lower uterine attachments

37 Separation of bladder completed

The bladder (2) has been separated down off the uterus, the cervix and the vagina as far as the arrows. The ureters (3) and (3) lie just medial to the ligated uterine pedicles (4) and (4). The uterus is at (1).

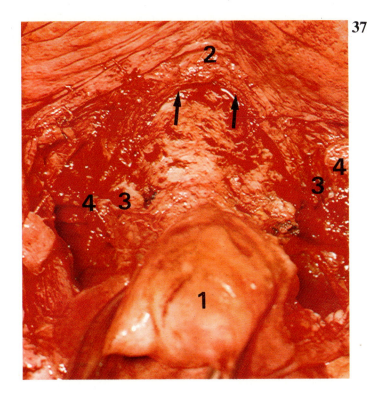

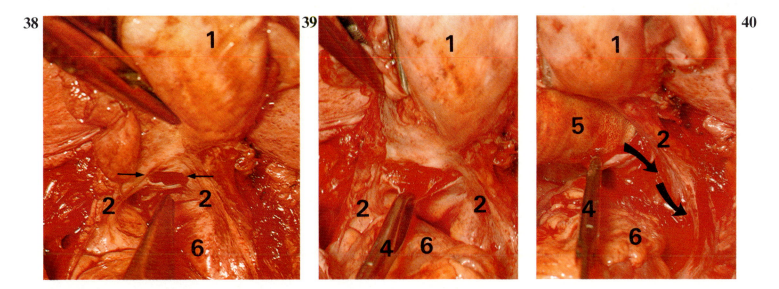

38 to 40 Opening recto-vaginal space

The uterus (1) is held upwards and the peritoneum on the posterior aspect of the cervix just below the utero-sacral ligaments (2) and (2) is incised where arrowed in Figure 38. Tissue forceps (4) hold the lower leaf of the opened peritoneum in Figure 39 and the surgeon's forefinger (5) is introduced distally behind the cervix and into the recto-vaginal space in Figure 40. It follows a downwards and forwards direction, as arrowed, and separating the two structures as far as the pelvic floor. This is as described in the Wertheim operation (page 168) and a firm vaginal pack already in place makes separation easy. The rectum is (6) in each photograph.

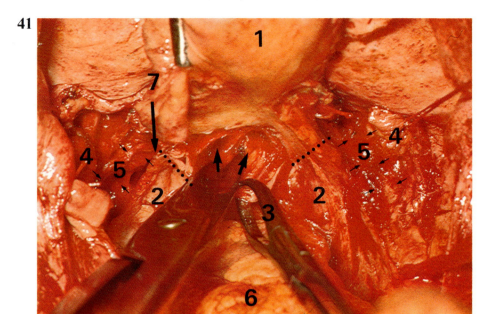

41 Release of uterus posteriorly

The utero-sacral ligaments (2) and (2) are defined and they represent the posterior edge of the fan-shaped ligamentous attachments of the uterus to the pelvic side wall. The opening into the recto-vaginal space is held open by tissue forceps (3) and is being enlarged with scissors where arrowed. The peritoneum overlying the utero-sacral ligaments is divided along the dotted lines and the utero-sacral-cardinal ligaments are clamped by a series of forceps on each side. The extension of the growth in the general area (7) on the left side demands a wider separation on that side. The uterus (1), the rectum (6) and the ureters (5) and (5) are all seen (outlined with arrows) medial to the uterine pedicles (4) and (4).

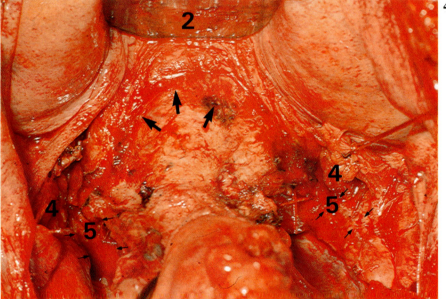

42 Release of uterus anteriorly

It is very important to obtain maximum mobilisation of the uterus without trauma or haemorrhage in a case where the tissues have had maximum radiation, and with the aid of a deep retractor (2) the anterior aspect is again inspected. The bladder is adequately separated anteriorly (the line of separation is arrowed), and the uterine pedicles (4) and (4) are well lateral to expose the ureters (5) and (5), indicated with small arrows.

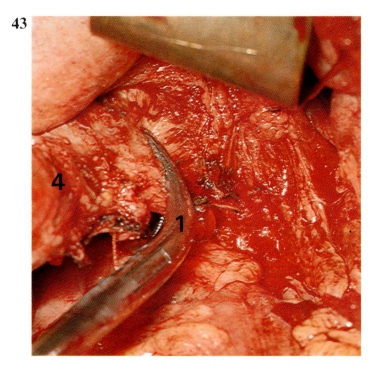

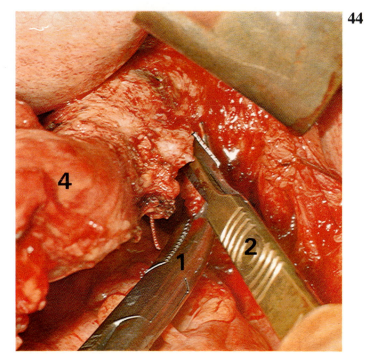

43 and 45 Securing right utero-sacral-cardinal ligament

The utero-sacral and part of the cardinal ligament is grasped with the curved forceps (1) in Figure 43 and the scalpel (2) detaches it from the uterus in Figure 44. This detached pedicle (1) is held laterally in Figure 45, while a second curved forceps (3) grasps the cardinal ligament as far as the lateral wall of the vagina (indicated by a dotted line). The uterus is at (4) in all three photographs.

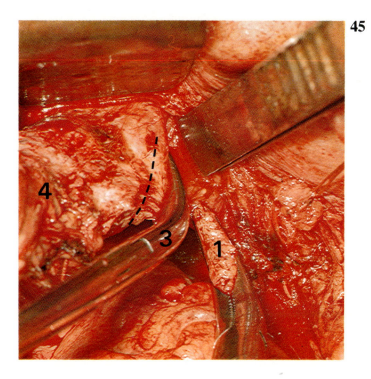

46

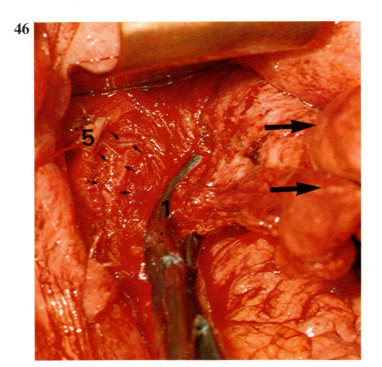

47

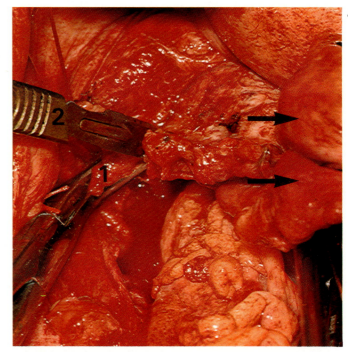

48

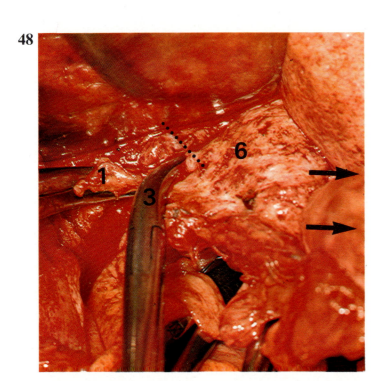

46 to 48 Securing left utero-sacral-cardinal ligament

The same procedure is carried out on the left side but is rendered more difficult by the extension of the growth into the left lateral fornix and the uterus has to be removed more widely. The uterus is held medially by the forceps in the direction of the arrows and the curved forceps (1) grasps the utero-sacral attachment in Figure 46. The uterine pedicle is at (5) and the ureter is outlined medial to it. The scalpel (2) detaches the pedicle in the forceps in Figure 47, and in Figure 48 a second curved forceps (3) secures the cardinal ligament as far as the lateral vaginal edge, indicated by the dotted line. The lateral extension of the growth is in the general area (6). The uterus lies in the direction of the large arrows in these photographs.

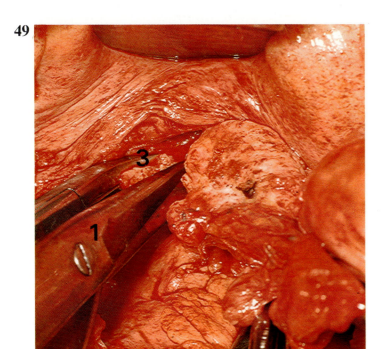

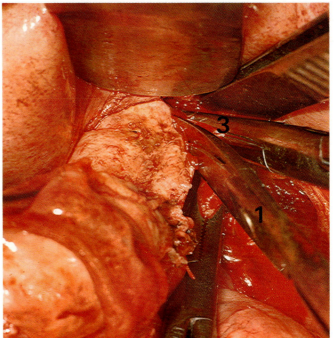

49 and 50 Detaching cardinal ligaments

Two pairs of forceps are still in place on each side. Those holding the utero-sacral ligaments have been separated from the uterus. Those on the cardinal ligaments will now be detached to leave the uterus attached only to the vagina. It is a very important part of the operation to remove the upper half of the vagina with its contained growth, as described in Stage 5 of the operation. In Figure 49 the scissors (1) detach the clamped left cardinal ligament (3) from the uterus and in Figure 50 the scissors (1) separate the right clamped cardinal ligament (3) in similar fashion.

Stage 5: Removal of uterus and upper half of vagina

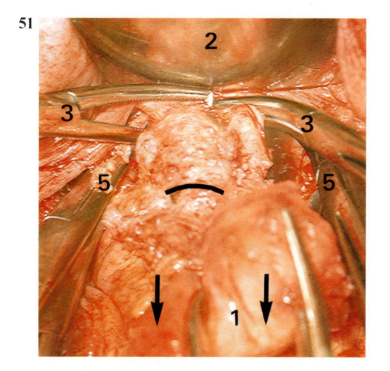

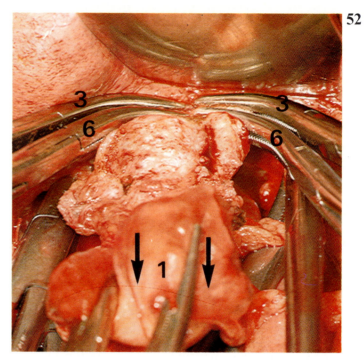

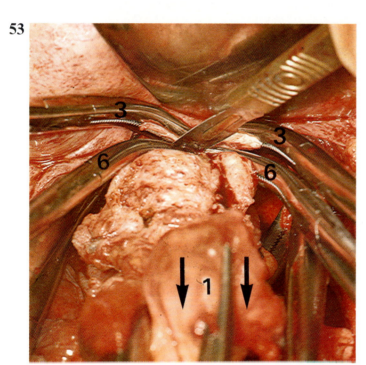

51 to 53 Double clamping and cutting across vagina

In each photograph the uterus (1) is held anteriorly and in a cephalad direction, as arrowed, to put the vaginal wall on the stretch longitudinally. In Figure 51 the retractor (2) protects the bladder while curved Oschner forceps (3) and (3) are applied across the vagina at its mid-point. The level of the external cervical os is indicated by a curved line. The detached cardinal ligaments are at (5) and (5). In Figure 52 two further long curved forceps (6) and (6) are applied, proximal to those in place at (3) and (3) so that the vagina can be transected between them with minimal risk of spilling malignant cells. In Figure 53 the vagina is being cut across with the scalpel to detach the uterus and the upper half of the vagina. The numerals are as before.

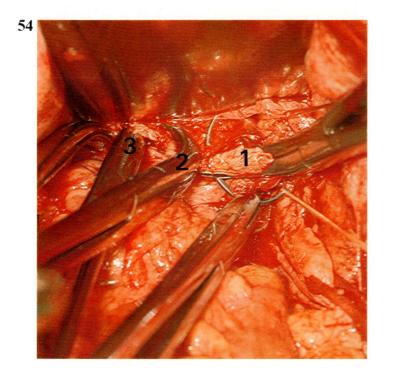

54

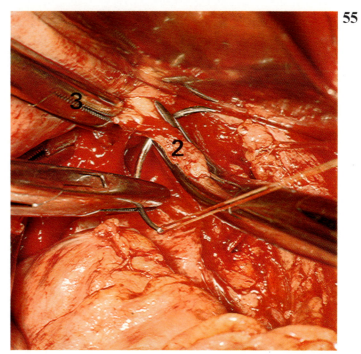

55

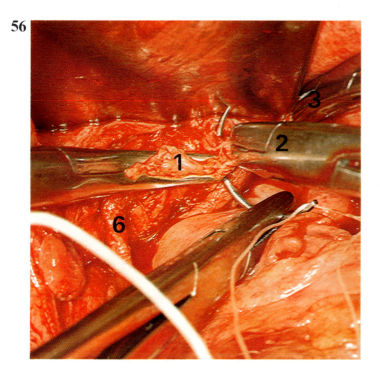

56

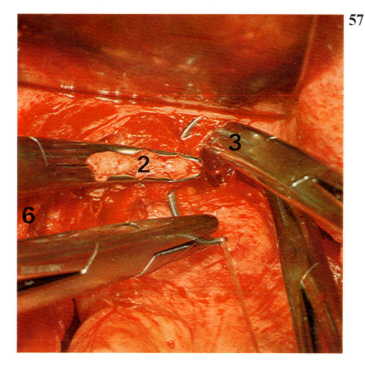

57

54 to 57 Securing utero-sacral-cardinal ligaments
The right utero-sacral pedicle (1) is transfixed in Figure 54 and will be tied off under the heel of the forceps. The forceps on the cardinal ligament is at (2) and on the vaginal angle at (3). In Figure 55 the right cardinal ligament (2) is transfixed

just on the vaginal edge prior to ligation; the clamped vaginal angle lies just medially (3). The procedure is repeated on the left in Figures 56 and 57; the same numbers apply. The line of excision had to be well lateral on the left side but the ureter (6) is under direct vision in Figures 56 and 57.

58

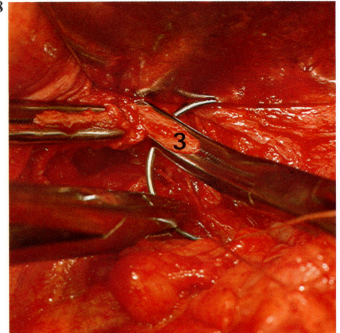

59

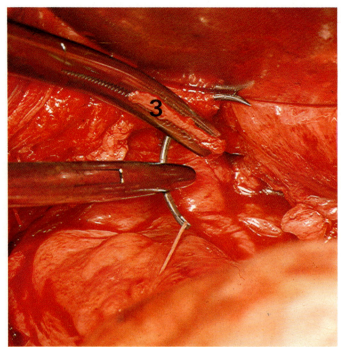

60

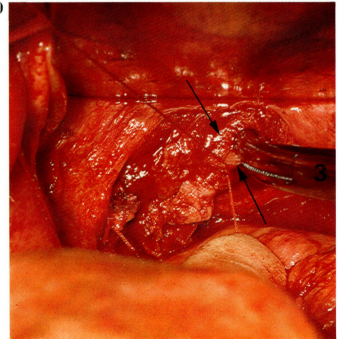

58 to 60 Closure of vaginal vault

It is arguable that the vagina be left open in such a case; there are, however, certain disadvantages in doing so. It would be necessary to place a continuous haemostatic stitch around the vault and that necessarily causes constriction while still leaving a central area which granulates over a period of several weeks or even months. On speculum examination it is always difficult to know whether or not there has been further recurrence. The vagina is shown being closed by transfixion sutures through the vaginal angle pedicles (3) and (3) first on the right side in Figure 58, and on the left side in Figure 59. Note that the stitch does not take the whole half-diameter of the vagina so as not to narrow it transversely. In Figure 60 the stitch is tied off under the heel of the forceps on the left side in such a way as to ensure a cuff of tissue where arrowed and so that it cannot slip off. One, or possibly two, central mattress sutures complete the closure medially and leave a relaxed and neat suture line.

61 and 62 Closure of pelvic peritoneum

The appearance before and after closure of the pelvic peritoneum is shown in the photographs. In Figure 61 the vaginal vault is hidden between the bladder (1) and the rectum (2) but the uncut lateral vaginal sutures are at (3) and (3). The ureters are at (4) and (4) and arrowed, and the operative field is seen to be quite dry. Two extra-peritoneal Redivac drains are inserted and brought out on each side lateral to the wound. Figure 62 shows the peritoneum closed in the manner described for Wertheim and extended hysterectomy operations (page 190, Figures 127–129 and page 219, Figures 60–64). The broken line indicates the transverse peritoneal closure; the dotted lines the sagittal closures. It will be seen that the bladder has partially filled up by the end of the longish operation. This is an embarrassment and can be avoided by having an indwelling Foley catheter in place during the operation.

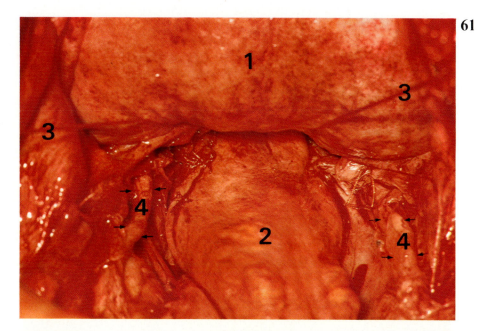

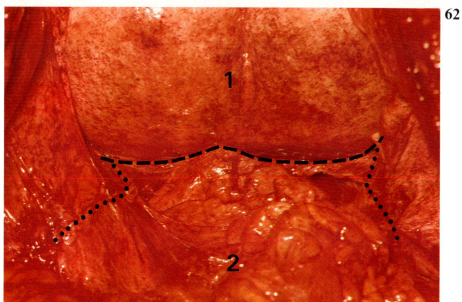

63 Specimen

The uterus is small and generally atrophic and the hydrosalpinges have already been noted. The vaginal excision is adequate and contains the growth extension on the left side. The exophytic growth is filling and distending the whole vaginal vault so that the amount of vaginal skin removed is more than would appear.

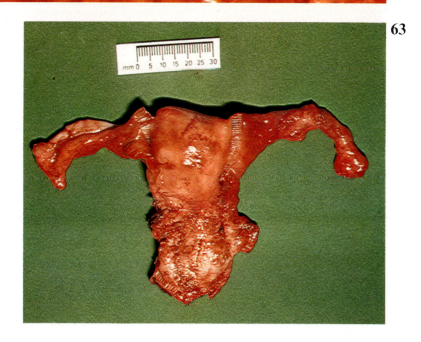

Surgical removal of lower vaginal recurrence

Lower vaginal recurrences in the region of the introitus and lower third of the canal most commonly follow endometrial or intra-cervical growths. They usually respond very well to local radiotherapy by 'needling' and it is convenient that full radiation is unlikely to have been expended in that area.

Since full radiation had been given and had failed to control the primary growth in this case, excision seemed the correct course. The recurrence was in the lower third of the vagina anteriorly and of 2 cm diameter. The steps in the operation are illustrated and described.

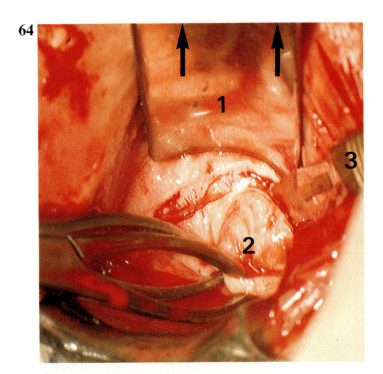

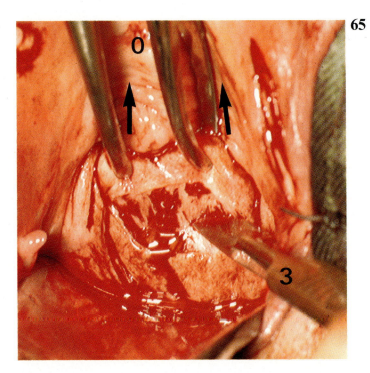

64 and 65 Outlining vaginal skin incision

In Figure 64 the urethral orifice is protected by the retractor (1) acting in the direction of the arrows, while two Little-wood's forceps hold the apex of the growth (2) and the scalpel (3) makes a semi-circular incision transversely across the lower vagina a full centimetre clear of the tumour and through the full skin thickness. In Figure 65 the Littlewood's forceps hold the growth upwards as arrowed and a matching similar incision is made on the other side of the growth (i.e. higher up the vagina). The external urethral orifice is marked (0).

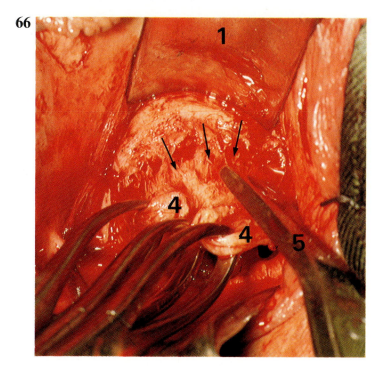

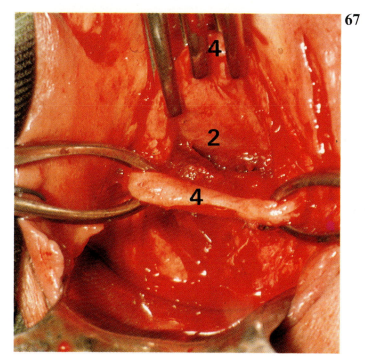

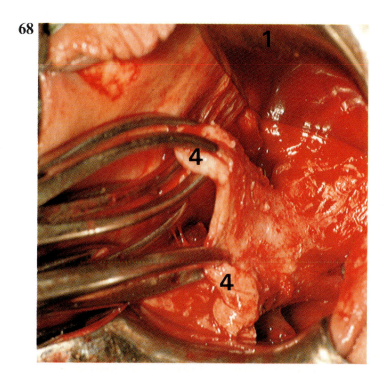

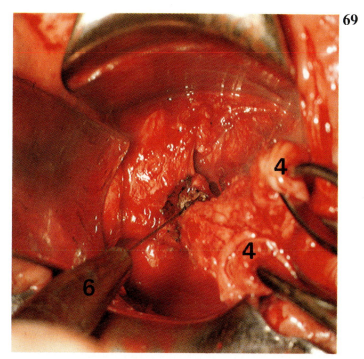

66 to 69 Dissecting growth from vaginal wall

In Figure 66 the edge of the growth-bearing vaginal skin (4) is held in Littlewood's forceps while the angled scissors (5) dissect it clear of the underlying tissues where arrowed. In Figure 67 this has been done both above and below the growth (2) which is now within a pouch of skin. The procedure is shown from the lateral aspect in Figure 68 and the growth is finally detached with the diathermy cutting needle (6) in Figure 69.

70

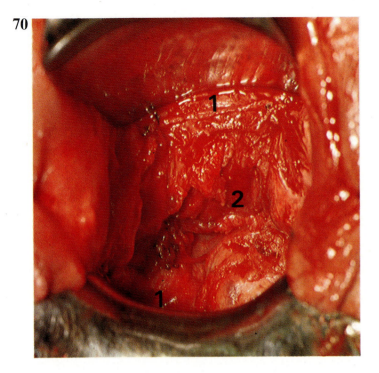

71

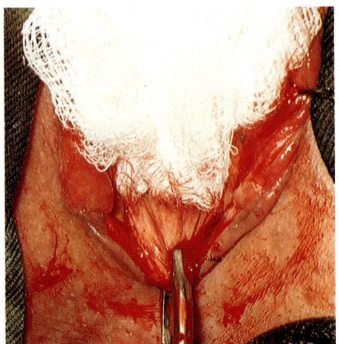

70 Appearance following removal of growth

The anterior vaginal wall is exposed by retractors anteriorly and posteriorly and shows the vaginal skin edges (1) and (1) and the irregular cavity from which the growth was removed (2). Neither the urethra nor the bladder was involved in the growth.

71 Wound unsutured and vaginal gauze pack inserted

It is unwise to insert stitches so close to a recurrent growth and, in any case, the skin edges fall inwards and largely occlude the cavity. This action is aided by the insertion of a light gauze vaginal pack, the end of which is smeared with petroleum jelly to prevent adhesion to the tissues.

72

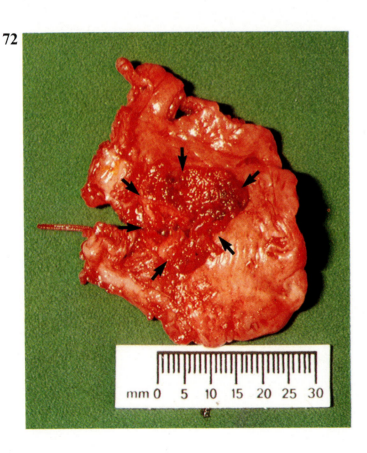

72 Specimen

The surface area of the secondary growth is outlined by arrows and shows a good margin of healthy excised tissue around it. Full thickness vaginal skin and fascia were removed so that excision is also well clear of the base of the nodule.

Suggested reading

Rutledge, F. N. (1976). Management: treatment failures in carcinoma of the cervix. *Gynecologic Oncology*, 86–92, edited by F. N. Rutledge, R. C. Boronow & J. T. Wharton. John Wiley Biomedical Publications, New York, London.

7: Radiation therapy for gynaecological cancer

by **Dr F. E. Neal**
Consultant Radiotherapist,
Weston Park Hospital, Sheffield

Historical background

Ionising radiation has been employed in the management of uterine cancer for over 70 years and was one of the first treatment methods to be developed after the discovery of radium in 1897. The advent of megavoltage external beam therapy in the 1950s made it possible to provide effective radiation to the pelvis and abdomen, thus giving a rational form of radiation therapy for pelvic tumours. In many centres radiation therapy has become the treatment of choice in cervical cancer and it is used extensively in the management of endometrial, ovarian and vaginal malignancy. It has a minor rôle in the treatment of vulvar carcinoma.

The initial techniques were empirical but the realisation that the uterus and vagina were natural radium holders and the discovery that the cervix, upper vagina and paracervical tissues could tolerate large radiation doses without damage to normal tissues led to the adoption of various treatment methods, some of which have been in use for over half a century.

Biological action of radiation

The effect of radiation on living tissue is non-specific, producing equal damage to normal and abnormal cells. As a result of the physical process of ionisation at therapy levels, chemical and biological cell changes are produced which inhibit reproduction. Normal tissue defences are responsible for the removal of dead and dying cells.

The differential therapeutic effect of radiation treatment is achieved through the ability of normal tissue to recover from radiation damage more rapidly than tumour tissue. This may be aided by fractionation regimes or by using a 'local' radiation technique which reduces the exposure of normal tissue to a minimum. The objective of radiation therapy is to produce a high uniform deposition of energy within the tumour volume while irradiating as small an amount of normal tissue as possible.

Unit of radiation

The Rad is the unit in current use and defines the amount of radiation absorbed per unit mass of tissue, i.e. 100 ergs per gram. The biological effect varies according to the time over which the radiation is delivered and treatment regimes must always state the length of time, e.g. 6,000 rads in a space of five weeks. The energy of the radiation and the fractionation regime should always be stated, e.g. megavoltage irradiation daily or three times per week. (It has been suggested that SI Units would be preferable – if introduced the standard unit would be the Gray.)

Methods of radiation therapy

In the management of gynaecological tumours it is essential to have effective local treatment and megavoltage irradiation and the available radiation treatments are as follows:

'Local' techniques
Solid isotopes
   i interstitial
   ii intracavitary
Liquid isotopes
   i intracavitary
External beam therapy
X or gamma rays
   i superficial therapy 100 to 140 k.v.
   ii orthovoltage therapy 200 to 600 k.v.
   iii megavoltage therapy over 2 m.v.
Particulate irradiation
   i electron beam
   ii neutron therapy

Local methods

These techniques traditionally utilised naturally occurring isotopes such as radium, but in modern practice the artificially prepared isotope of cobalt (Co^{60}) and the fission product radioactive caesium (Cs^{137}) are more readily available and are preferred. These isotopes all have an effective gamma emission and can be prepared either in the form of needles for interstitial implantation or as tubes for intracavitary use. The latter may be placed in the uterus or mounted in special applicators or moulds for insertion into the vagina.

The advantage of local placement is the high concentration of energy achieved in a small volume of tissue with minimal irradiation of surrounding normal tissues. The form in which these sources are used and the method of application depends on the lesion being treated and will be described in relation to the individual malignancies. There is a problem in relation to radiation safety and this has led to the development of after-loading or remote-loading techniques, such as the cathetron, to safeguard staff and other patients and to cut down radiation generally.

External beam therapy

The only effective form of external irradiation for gynaecological purposes is a megavoltage beam. X-rays may be produced by some form of electrical apparatus, e.g. Linear accelerator (Figure 1) or by gamma rays obtained from a large radioactive source, e.g. Telecobalt unit (Figure 2).

The penetration of a radiation beam is proportional to its energy and at megavoltage levels it is technically possible to achieve effective and accurately defined cancericidal doses at depth with minimum upset to the patient. The body surface receives a relatively low dose and unpleasant skin reactions are avoided.

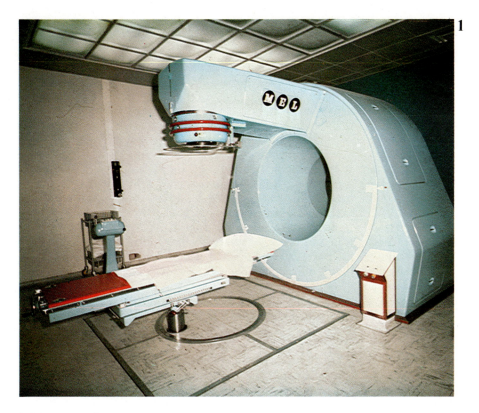

1 Linear accelerator
M.E.L. S.L. 75, 8 Me V Linear accelerator.

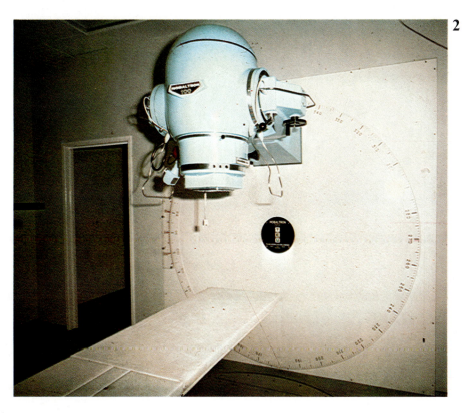

2 Telecobalt unit
Mobaltron 100 Telecobalt unit, Source = 5000 curies.

Radiation dosage

Local treatment by internal sources delivers a high radiation dose to the primary tumour which is generally in the centre of the pelvis. The dose falls off rapidly from a source placed in the uterus or vaginal vault in accordance with the inverse square law. Nodal tissue in the pelvis therefore receives a relative low dose. This is illustrated by reference to the diagram of internal sources in position where the area of high radiation is enclosed within the thick broken line (Figure 3). The diagrammatic graph (Figure 4) shows the dose distributions from the internal and the external sources separately and the combined total dosage when they are added together. The broken line shows the central area of high irradiation from the solid sources with the dosage falling steeply as it moves away from the midline. This unequal distribution of irradiation to the pelvis from a solid source is balanced by using special techniques of external irradiation, which provide a high energy deposition at the pelvic side wall and a lower dose in the centre of the pelvis. This is effected by using a pair of opposed fields (anterior and posterior) across the pelvis but with a central shielding strip (lead) which effectively adjusts the irradiation reaching the cervical and para-cervical tissues, the bladder and the rectum. These have already been irradiated to a high level by the Cs^{137}. The central wedge is specially shaped and assorted thicknesses may be used to enable the desired doses to be delivered at the appropriate point. The type of dosage curve from external irradiation is shown by the dotted line on the diagram and it is seen to contribute mainly to the side walls of the pelvis. The combination of the two dosages gives the total dosage which is shown by the solid line on the graph. This indicates the total dosage given to each part of the pelvis.

In order to ensure that adequate radiation is delivered to relevant parts of the pelvis, a number of physical points are used to compute the doses. The most useful of these is designated Point A and is defined as a point 2 cm lateral and 2 cm above the external cervical os. It is convenient to know how many rads have been delivered at point A. The total dosage is the most important information and in a case of cervical carcinoma, for example, it is described as 6000 rads delivered locally by Cs^{137} and 1500 rads by MXR (megavoltage therapy), making a total of 7500 rads. The lateral location of points A and B is indicated on the base line in Figure 4, and it will be seen that the combined curve shows a dosage of 7500 rads delivered to point A.

There is also an important matter of tolerance in relation to the bladder base and rectum. Even with adequate screening it is sometimes difficult to reduce the dose to the rectum and bladder base to acceptable levels. The tolerance levels are 5000 rads in the rectum and 6000 rads at the bladder base in the four to five-weeks treatment period.

3 Idealised geometry of uterine and vaginal sources
The broken line shows the high dose volume.

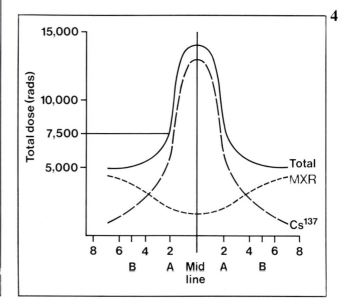

4 Diagrammatic graph to show dose distribution from internal sources, external megavoltage irradiation and the combination of both.

Radiation reactions

Because of the non-specific biological effect of irradiation, side effects from normal tissue reaction accompany treatment whatever the site. The severity of the reaction varies from individual to individual; during pelvic irradiation the problems are those of local discomfort and the effect on the lower bowel. Ideally those receiving treatment for pelvic malignancy should be inpatients in a specialised hospital or unit.

There may be considerable local soreness of the vulva and vagina and this is likely to be accompanied by symptoms of cystitis and proctitis. The production of fibrin from mucous membranes results in a yellowish vaginal discharge which persists until the reaction settles. Persistent diarrhoea is a frequent and troublesome symptom and may be associated with anorexia, nausea and vomiting. It is essential to maintain fluid intake at a high level throughout treatment, by using intravenous infusion if necessary, and maintaining nutrition by the provision of nourishing meals which the patient can tolerate. Diarrhoea and vomiting can generally be controlled by the use of drugs although treatment sometimes has to be discontinued until the fluid loss has ceased. Reactions usually subside over four to six weeks following completion of treatment.

Radiation safety

Hazards accompany all radiation exposure but when treatment is given by solid isotopes, radiation protection is a particular problem. Small amounts of ionising radiation inevitably 'escape' from the patient and produce 'scattered' irradiation in the atmosphere. The main danger is its contribution to general radiation background with the possibility of genetic changes in future generations.

Reduction of these radiation levels to a minimum depends to a large extent on the expertise of the operators. Solid isotopes should be handled only by expert clinicians and technicians who are aware of the dangers involved, and they should be stored in a special room in charge of a responsible custodian.

The dosage received by individuals working in radiotherapy departments can be kept at low levels by suitable shielding (as illustrated in Figure 7), by the use of long-handled instruments and by ensuring that every action is performed in the shortest possible time.

Cleaning, preparation, packing and sterilisation of sources is carried out by remote control and they are placed in a special safe built into the wall between the caesium preparation room (Figure 5) and the operating theatre.

When required for clinical use they are removed from the lead-lined safe and assembled behind screens prior to insertion into the appropriate part of the patient (Figure 6). On the ward the patient is nursed behind lead screens (Figure 8) and, following removal, the source is immediately placed in a lead-lined trolley and conveyed to a special lead-lined hoist for return to the safety of the preparation room.

5

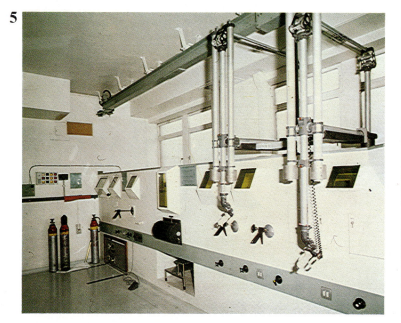

5 Preparation room for Caesium[137] sources
Lead walls protect the preparation bench and sources are handled by remote control.

6

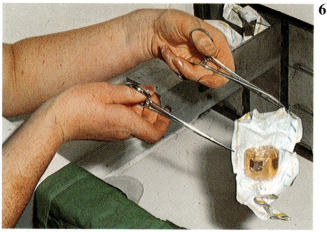

6 Theatre storage safe
Prepacked sterile sources are passed through the wall from the preparation room and assembled in the lead well.

7

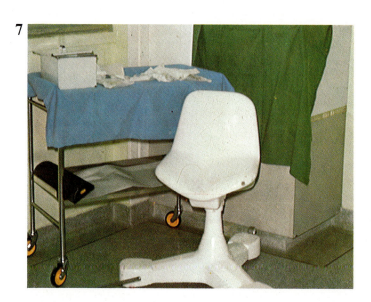

7 Operating stool
The surgeon sits behind the protective shield.

8

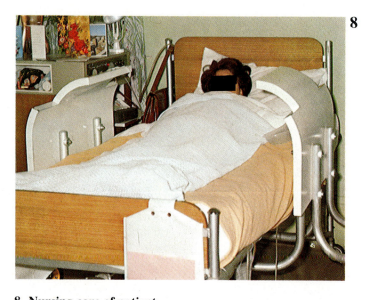

8 Nursing care of patient
The patient is nursed between lateral lead screens to reduce exposure of nursing staff.

Lymphography

The radiological examination of the pelvic and para-aortic lymph nodes by injection of contrast medium is considered by many as an essential part of the investigation of most pelvic tumours. Although a relatively simple technique, it requires practice and delicate handling to dissect out a lymphatic vessel and cannulate it with a suitably prepared catheter. In expert hands, the procedure is without complication although an allergy to the dye (patent blue) is sometimes exhibited.

Lymphography has three main applications. It may be used as an investigative technique to look for partial or non-filling of lymph nodes as evidence of metastases. It can be used as an aid to more effective lymphadenectomy by taking radiographs immediately the gland excision has been completed. The patient is still on the operating table so that it is possible to go back and look for glands which are still visible radiologically. A third use of the method is in the follow-up of treated cases of cancer. The oil-based contrast medium is retained in the lymph nodes for many months and serial lymphograms at successive follow-up visits provide evidence of whether or not the disease is controlled.

In all three applications there are pitfalls and difficulties of interpretation, so that some experienced clinicians are not convinced that it has great value. In this centre we have found it particularly helpful in the follow-up of cancer cases and if it is available it certainly ought to be used as a clinical investigative method.

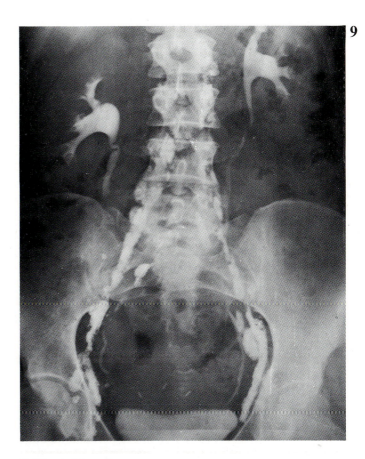

9

9 Normal lymphogram

An A.P. radiograph, lymphogram and I.V.U. of a 48 year-old patient with a stage 1 carcinoma of the cervix. On both sides, the lymph node groups are clearly shown and are normal in size with no filling defects or other evidence of tumour deposits. The I.V. urogram is also normal.

10

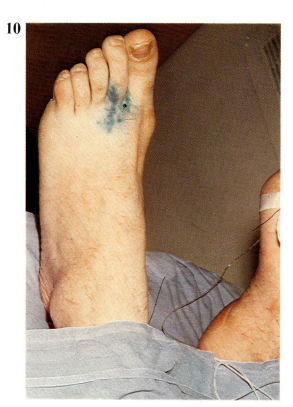

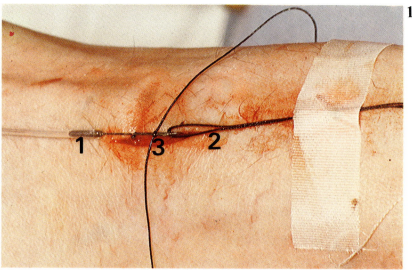

12

10 The main lymph channels on the dorsum of the foot are outlined by introducing vital blue dye superficially between the first two toes.

Surgical technique of lymphography

It is not proposed to describe this specialist minor operation in detail. Figures 10, 11, 12 and 13 show the principal steps in the procedure.

12 A cannula (1) has been introduced into the lumen of the lymph vessel which is supported on the untied suture (2) and tied into the vessel by suture (3).

11

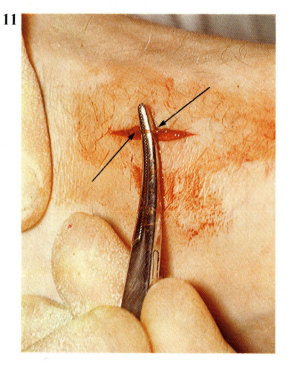

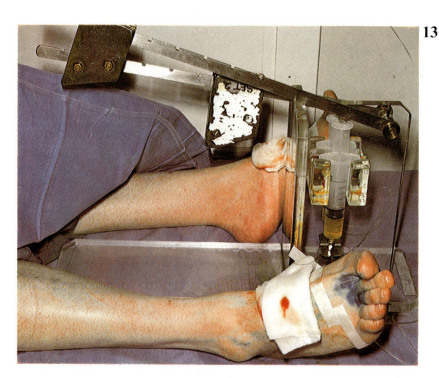

13

11 Under local anaesthesia a major lymph vessel has been isolated and raised on forceps as arrowed.

13 A pump is injecting the radio-opaque oily contrast medium into the lymph stream.

Lymphograms showing filling defects due to gland metastases

14
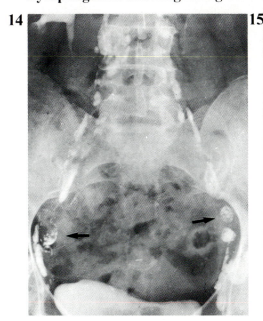

15
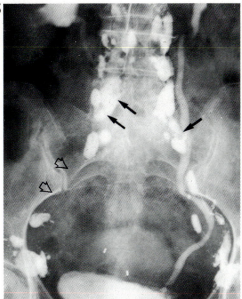

16
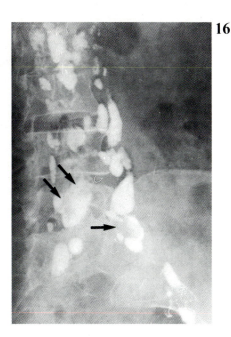

14 Carcinoma of cervix

A 50 year-old patient with a stage 1 carcinoma of the cervix (poorly differentiated epidermoid carcinoma). Lymphogram shows filling defects due to metastatic deposits in external iliac lymph nodes on both sides (arrowed). The common iliac and para-aortic lymph nodes are normal; I.V.U. is normal.

15 and 16 Carcinoma of cervix

A.P. and oblique radiographs of a 61 year-old patient with a stage 2 carcinoma of the cervix (pleomorphic poorly differentiated squamous carcinoma). Clinically the growth was confined to the cervix, apart from minimal involvement of the left parametrium. Filling defects due to metastatic deposits are seen in lymph nodes at the upper ends of both common iliac groups (solid arrows). The lymph nodes in the right external iliac chain are not opacified (open arrows). This is likely to be due to complete tumour replacement of these nodes. The I.V. urogram shows minimal dilatation of the left ureter indicating early obstruction at its lower end.

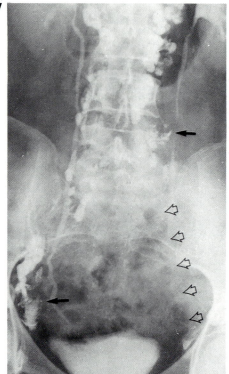

17 Carcinoma of vulva

A 45 year-old patient with a carcinoma of the left side of the vulva and clinically palpable lymph nodes in the left inguinal region (histologically a very poorly differentiated squamous carcinoma). The lymphogram shows filling defects due to metastases in the right external iliac group and in the lower end of the left para-aortic group (solid arrows). The left external and common iliac groups are not opacified (open arrows). This appearance may indicate complete tumour replacement of these lymph nodes. The I.V. urogram is normal.

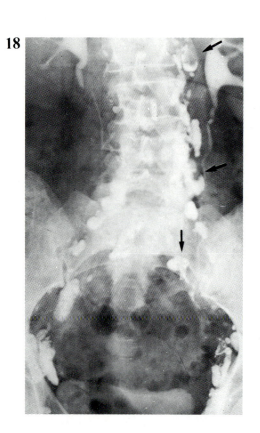

18 Carcinoma of body of uterus

A patient aged 69 years with an endometrial adenocarcinoma (well differentiated). The lymphogram shows filling defects due to metastatic deposits in the upper part of the left common iliac node group and in the left upper para-aortic region (arrowed). The I.V. urogram is normal.

Radiotherapy in the treatment of individual gynaecological cancers

Cervical cancer

Radiation treatment for cervical malignancy relies on an integrated treatment regime of internal solid isotope therapy and external beam irradiation. The initial treatment generally consists of an intracavitary insertion of a radioactive source into the uterus and vagina. There are many methods of providing this local radiation and the Sheffield technique described here has been in use for 25 years.

1. Local technique: internal sources

Two internal sources are used. One consists of an isotope tube or isotope tubes in tandem in a nylon envelope which lies longitudinally in the cavity of the uterus and cervical canal. The other is a high vaginal one and is housed in a plastic container designed to fit into the posterior vaginal fornix. It is referred to as the Sheffield applicator. Figure 19 shows both types.

The Sheffield isotope holder or applicator is kidney-shaped so that it lies in the posterior fornix with the concave side towards the cervix. It holds two radiation sources and contains two specially-shaped tungsten screens which reduce the amount of radiation received by the rectal mucosa.

These applicators can be used singly, or doubly if required, and they fit on to a central rod which has different sizes of distance pieces to match the length of the vagina. There is a non-rotating handle to complete a rigid assembly, which facilitates accurate placement of the source container (Figure 20).

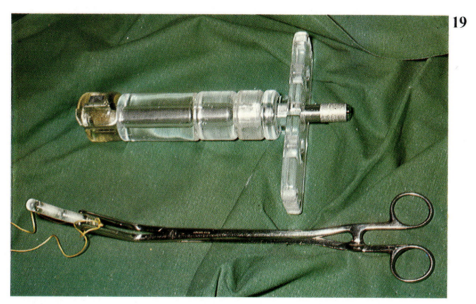
19

20 1 Source carrier
2 Central rod
3 Distance piece
4 Non-rotating handle
5 Fixing screw
6 Radiation source
7 Tungsten rectal screen

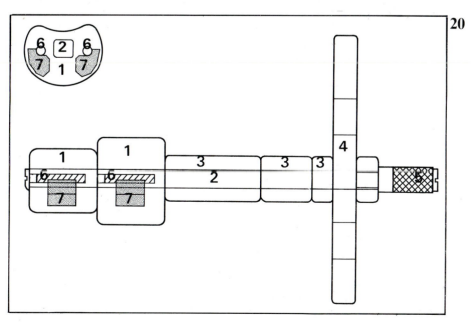
20

21

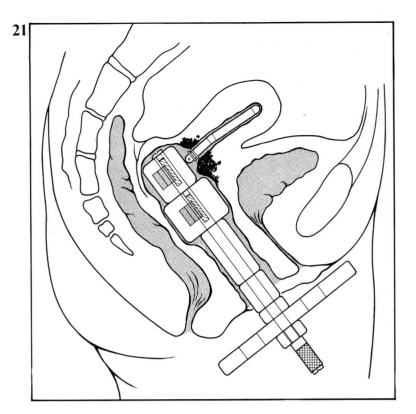

This position is maintained by attaching the handle to elastic straps which, in turn, are attached to a belt around the patient's waist. The rectal mucosa is adequately protected by the screens and the diameter of the applicator approximates to that of the vagina, so that packing with gauze is not required (Figure 21). The applicators are in position for the number of hours required for the estimated total dosage. As we have already seen, this part of the treatment delivers a high radiation dose to the primary tumour but very little to the sides of the pelvis.

2. External beam therapy

External beam therapy is used in such a way as to balance the total dosage to the pelvis in the manner already described; before commencing treatment the radiotherapist will have worked out the dosage to be given. The dosage is planned for each individual case but the following general examples can be given. In stages 1 and 2 growths separate applications of Cs^{137} are given at an interval of one week and followed by three weeks of megavoltage radiation treatment. In stage 3 growths one application is given and followed by four weeks of megavoltage radiation. In stage 4 growths treatment is usually entirely by megavoltage radiation. The actual doses in stages 1 and 2 amount to 6000 rads at point A with

1500 rads of megavoltage radiation, making a total of 7500 rads. Stage 3 growths receive 4000 rads at point A followed by 2500–3500 rads by megavoltage radiation, making a total of 6500 to 7500 rads. In stages 1, 2 and 3 the radiation dose to point B – the pelvic wall – is 5000 rads. Stage 4 growths would possibly have a total of 5000 rads by megavoltage radiation only. The overall treatment time in all stages is four weeks with daily fractionation of megavoltage radiation.

When irradiation is used prior to surgery, internal sources only are used. These are applied in exactly the same way although the dosage is less, being approximately two-thirds of full treatment. This is always given in a single application.

3. Larger field external beam therapy

Routine lymphangiography sometimes reveals that patients who are thought to have an early carcinoma have demonstrable metastases in the para-aortic lymph nodes. These cases are treated with external beam irradiation by adding a vertical arm to the pelvic field (anterior and posterior) and extending it to the level of the diaphragm. With modern megavoltage apparatus it is possible to irradiate this large area as one field. A total dosage of 4500 rads in four weeks is delivered.

4. Results of radiotherapy

Treatment of cervical cancer in the Sheffield Area is predominantly by radiotherapy; and the five-year survival rates achieved in the very large number of patients treated indicates what can be expected from such management. Table 1 gives the five-year survival rate by clinical stages in a group of 534 patients treated in the years 1968 to 1972 at Weston Park Hospital, Sheffield, England.

Table 1
Results of Radiation Treatment in Carcinoma of Cervix
(Sheffield Area)
(1968–1972)

Clinical Stage	Number Treated	Number Free of Disease After 5 Years %	
1	121	92	(76)
2	236	123	(52)
3	125	41	(33)
4	52	2	(4)
Total	534	258	(50)

Endometrial cancer

The treatment of choice for early adenocarcinoma of the uterine body is hysterectomy with the addition of some form of radiation therapy. This may be given either pre- or postoperatively and the principal aim is to reduce the incidence of vault recurrence. In the more advanced stages it may be necessary to use both pre- and postoperative radiation.

The preoperative technique is identical with that used in the treatment of cervical cancer with solid isotopes: one insertion only is used and is in place for a period of approximately 48 hours.

Hysterectomy is performed during the same week, or after an interval of six weeks, and the discovery of involved nodes at operation is an indication for lymphography and external irradiation as for cervical cancer.

If surgery is precluded by advanced disease or because of the poor general condition of the patient, treatment is entirely by irradiation. In the Sheffield centre this treatment would be identical with that for carcinoma of cervix but another method is to pack the cavity of the uterus with solid sources after the method of Heyman. This can be combined, if necessary, with external irradiation.

The results that can be achieved by surgery and adjuvant radiotherapy are referred to in Chapter 4.

Technique for insertion of internal isotope sources for treatment of uterine carcinoma (applicable to cervical and endometrial lesions)

The following illustrations and legends show the important points in the application of the internal isotope sources.

22
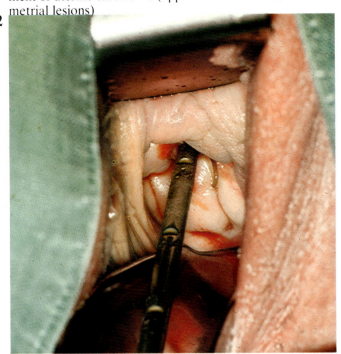

23
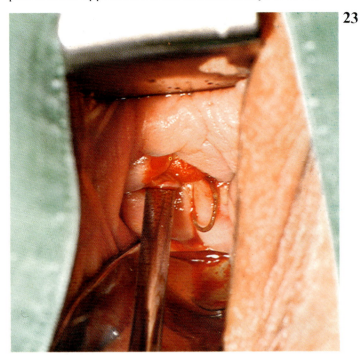

22 to 25 Insertion of caesium – uterine source
Preparation for and insertion of intrauterine source.

24
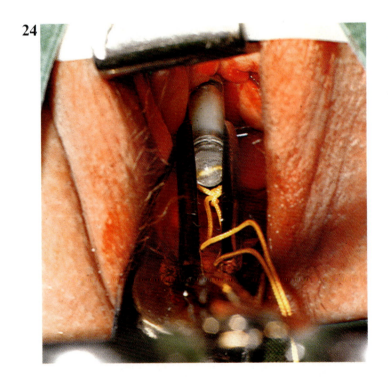

25
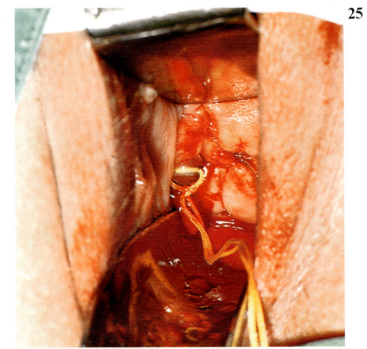

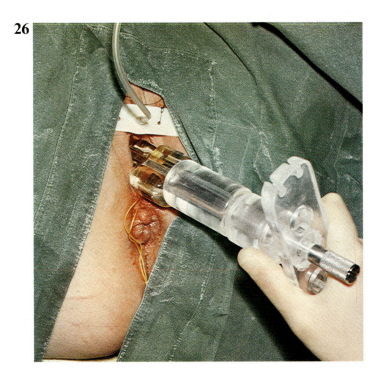

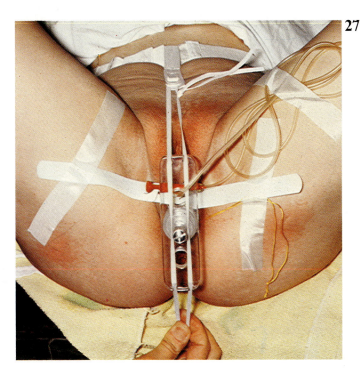

26 to 29 Insertion of caesium – vaginal source
26 Insertion of vaginal applicator.

27 Securing vaginal applicator.

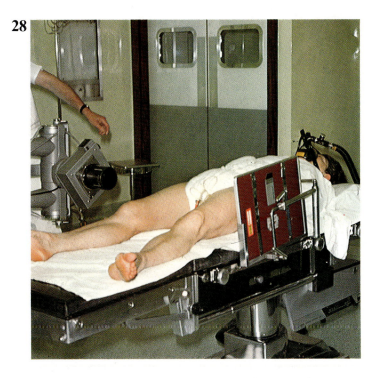

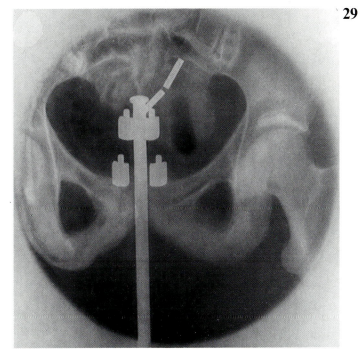

28 and 29 Radiological confirmation of source placement.

Vaginal cancer

This growth is very suitable for treatment by radiotherapy and the technique depends on the site of the lesion. Fortunately it is often localised and can be treated exclusively by a local irradiation method. If general spread is thought likely, then lymphography should be done and any involved nodes treated by supplementary external beam therapy to the pelvic and, if necessary, to the para-aortic nodes.

Upper vaginal tumours are treated in identical fashion with that described for cervical malignancy.

Midvaginal tumours require a special applicator (Figures 30 and 31) containing a 'line' source without rectal shielding which is used either alone or combined with an intrauterine tube. Two insertions, with an interval of one week between each insertion, are appropriate and give a 'mucosal' dose of approximately 10,000 rads (i.e. 2 insertions of 50 hours).

Lower vaginal tumours can be treated with a central source but if localised to the introitus it may be preferable to use an implant of interstitial needles. These sources have to be accurately positioned to deliver a uniform dose. The method of placing the needles is shown below and a dosage of 6000 rads delivered over one week is considered to be adequate.

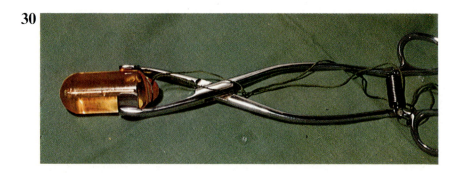

30 Central vaginal applicator ready for insertion

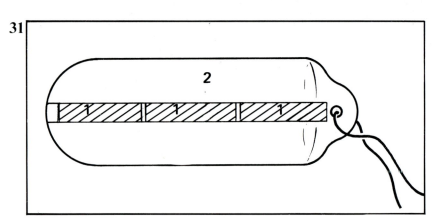

31 Longitudinal section of central vaginal source without rectal protection

1 Cs^{137} sources

2 Perspex spacer

32

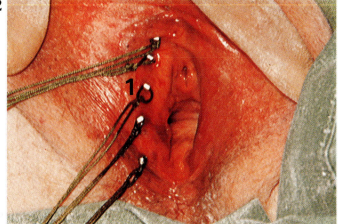

33

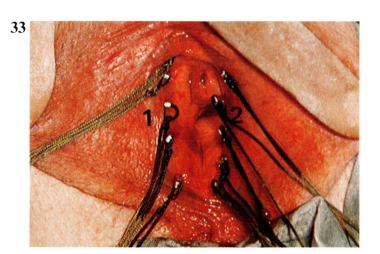

34

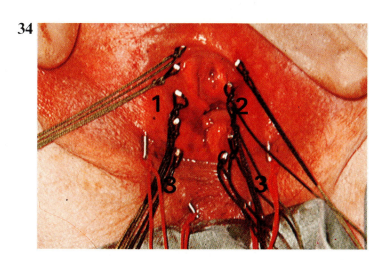

32 to 34 Demonstration of the method of implantation of Cs^{137} interstitial needles

32 Differentially loaded Cs^{137} needles are inserted in a single plane on the right side of the introitus. These needles should be parallel to the vaginal wall and to each other. There is a distance of 1 cm between needles.

33 An identical plane is inserted on the left side parallel to the existing needles.

35 Radiograph to demonstrate the distribution of sources in a combined treatment using interstitial needles and a central source

35

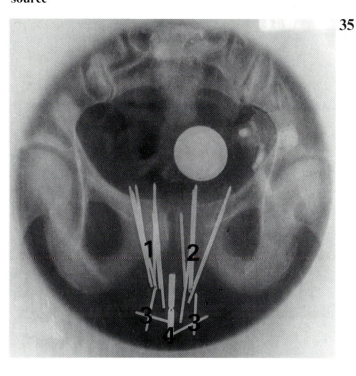

34 Each plane is completed, by inserting two uniformly loaded Cs^{137} needles (numbered 3) which are at right angles to the existing needles but in the same plane. These 'crossing' needles are required to ensure uniformity of dose throughout the treatment volume.

Each Cs^{137} source (needle) contains 2 mgm equivalent of radium. The total amount of isotope used is therefore 28 mgm equivalent of radium i.e. 14 needles.

1 Plane of parallel needles on right of introitus
2 Plane of parallel needles on left of introitus
3 'Crossing' needles
4 Central source
The circular shadow is a standard 2.5 cm metal disc to enable a magnification factor to be derived. From this information it is possible to calculate an accurate dose rate from the combined sources.

Vulvar cancer

The accepted treatment of primary carcinoma of the vulva is by surgery but irradiation has a part to play in the palliative management of advanced disease or recurrence after radical surgery. A combination of surgery and irradiation may be used occasionally as a primary treatment, but the vulva tolerates radiation badly and necrosis is easily produced.

Solid isotopes may be used as a central source in the vagina, as an interstitial implant or even in both capacities. External beam therapy can be used as a single direct field applied to the vulva and perineum, or a pair of parallel opposed fields designed to include the vulvar tumour and inguinal lymph nodes.

The reaction to treatment is usually severe and painful and control of the disease tends to be temporary. Doses of 4500 to 5000 rads over three to four weeks given by megavoltage irradiation are tolerated reasonably well and do not produce necrosis.

Ovarian cancer

Radical removal of the tumour by surgery is the treatment of choice but the number of patients who are able to have such treatment is small. In a number of patients, the malignancy has progressed to an inoperable stage before medical advice is sought and then palliation may be achieved by external beam therapy. This consists of a localised treatment using two opposed fields across the pelvis (anterior and posterior) or treatment to the whole abdomen. The dose varies from 4500 to 5000 rads in four weeks for local pelvic irradiation, to 3000 rads in five weeks for the large abdominal field.

There are many patients who have been treated surgically but removal of the growth has been incomplete or there has been spill of tumour tissue at operation. Each of these presents an individual problem in management and requires the attention of a specialist radiotherapist. The most difficult decision can be whether or not to give any treatment in the first instance, and previous experience of large numbers of cases is sometimes the only worthwhile criterion.

Appendix

Clinical staging of carcinoma of the cervix, corpus, and ovary

1. Carcinoma of cervix

A Clinical staging

PRE-INVASIVE CARCINOMA

Stage 0 Carcinoma *in situ* (CERVICAL INTRAEPITHELIAL NEOPLASIA, CIN III).

Cases of Stage 0 should not be included in any therapeutic statistics for invasive carcinoma.

INVASIVE CARCINOMA

Stage 1 Carcinoma strictly confined to the cervix (extension to the corpus should be disregarded).

Stage 1a Microinvasive carcinoma (early stromal invasion).

Stage 1b All other cases of Stage 1. Occult cancer should be marked 'occ'.

Stage 2 The carcinoma extends beyond the cervix, but has not extended on to the pelvic wall. The carcinoma involves the vagina, but not the lower third.

Stage 2a No obvious parametrial involvement.

Stage 2b Obvious parametrial involvement.

Stage 3 The carcinoma has extended on to the pelvic wall. On rectal examination there is no cancer-free space between the tumour and the pelvic wall. The tumour involves the lower third of the vagina. All cases with a hydro-nephrosis or non-functioning kidney.

Stage 3a No extension on to the pelvic wall.

Stage 3b Extension on to the pelvic wall and/or hydro-nephrosis or non-functioning kidney.

Stage 4 The carcinoma has extended beyond the true pelvis or has clinically involved the mucosa of the bladder or rectum. A bullous oedema as such does not permit a case to be allotted to Stage 4.

Stage 4a Spread of the growth to adjacent organs.

Stage 4b Spread to distant organs.

B Notes to the staging

Stage 1a (microinvasive carcinoma) represents those cases of carcinoma *in situ* in which histological evidence of early stromal invasion is unambiguous. The diagnosis is based on microscopical examination of tissue removed by biopsy, conisation, portio amputation, or on the removed uterus. Cases of early stromal invasion should thus be allotted to Stage 1a.

The remainder of Stage 1 cases should be allotted to Stage 1b. As a rule these cases can be diagnosed by routine clinical examination.

Occult cancer is an histologically invasive cancer which cannot be diagnosed by routine clinical examination and is more than early stromal invasion. It is as a rule diagnosed on a cone, the amputated portio, or the removed uterus. Such cases should be included in Stage 1b and should be marked Stage 1b 'occ'.

As a rule it is difficult clinically to estimate whether a cancer of the cervix has extended to the corpus or not. Extension to the corpus should therefore be disregarded.

A patient with a growth fixed to the pelvic wall by a short and indurated, but not nodular parametrium should be allotted to Stage 2b. It is impossible at clinical examination to decide whether a smooth and indurated parametrium is truly cancerous or only inflammatory. Therefore, a case should be placed in Stage 3 only if the parametrium is nodular out on the pelvic wall or the growth itself extends out on the pelvic wall.

The presence of hydronephrosis or non-functioning kidney due to stenosis of the ureter by cancer permits a case to be allotted to Stage 3 even if according to the other findings the case should be allotted to Stage 1 or Stage 2.

The presence of a bullous oedema as such should not permit a case to be allotted to Stage 4. Ridges and furrows into the bladder wall should be interpreted as signs of sub-mucous involvement of the bladder if they remain fixed to the growth at palposcopy (i.e.

examination from the vagina or the rectum during cystoscopy). A cytological finding of malignant cells in washings from the urinary bladder requires further examination and a biopsy from the wall of the bladder.

The clinical staging of carcinoma of the cervix should be based on the examination methods mentioned in the text. A conisation or amputation of the cervix should be regarded as a clinical examination and an invasive carcinoma of the cervix diagnosed in this way should be reported as invasive carcinoma. If in a case of early invasive carcinoma the gynaecologist considers it appropriate only to perform an amputation or conisation this should be considered as therapy.

Cases of Stage 1a and Stage 1b 'occ' which are revealed by histological examination of the removed uterus should be included in therapeutic statistics on invasive carcinoma of the cervix.

Cases who have been operated upon under the wrong diagnosis and where an advanced invasive carcinoma is found in the removed uterus cannot be clinically staged. Such cases should not be included in therapeutic statistics, but it is desirable that they be reported separately.

It is important to follow the above principles in order to secure comparability of therapeutic statistics. The Editorial Committee is well aware of the fact that the clinical observations do not always agree with the anatomical findings and that many patients of, for instance, Stage 1 and Stage 2 might at operation be found to have metastases to the lymph nodes or spread of the tumour beyond the true pelvis. It may also in rare cases be found that a Stage 3 carcinoma of the cervix at laparotomy proves to be operable. In order to secure a reliable uniformity in the clinical staging such incidents should have no influence on the staging.

2. Carcinoma of the corpus

A Clinical staging

Stage 0 Carcinoma *in situ*. Histological findings suspicious of malignancy.

Cases of Stage 0 should not be included in any therapeutic statistics.

Stage 1 The carcinoma is confined to the corpus including the isthmus.

Stage 1a The length of the uterine cavity is 8 cm or less.

Stage 1b The length of the uterine cavity is more than 8 cm.

The Stage 1 cases should be sub-grouped with regard to the histological type of the adenocarcinoma as follows:
G1 – highly differentiated adenomatous carcinoma.
G2 – differentiated adenomatous carcinoma with partly solid areas.
G3 – predominantly solid or entirely undifferentiated carcinoma.

Stage 2 The carcinoma has involved the corpus and the cervix, but has not extended outside the uterus.

Stage 3 The carcinoma has extended outside the uterus, but not outside the true pelvis.

Stage 4 The carcinoma has extended outside the true pelvis or has obviously involved the mucosa of the bladder or rectum. A bullous oedema as such does not permit a case to be allotted to Stage 4.

Stage 4a Spread of the growth to adjacent organs.

Stage 4b Spread to distant organs.

B Notes to the staging

Studies on large series of endometrial carcinoma limited to the corpus have shown that the prognosis to some extent is related to the size of the uterus. However, enlargement of the uterus may be caused by fibroids, adenomyosis, etc. Therefore, the size of the uterus cannot serve as a basis for sub-grouping Stage 1 cases. The length and the width of the uterine cavity may be related to the prognosis. The great majority of cases of corpus cancer belong to Stage 1. A subdivision of these cases is desirable. Therefore the Cancer Committee recommends a subdivision of the Stage 1 cases, especially with regard to the histopathological examination of curettings.

The extension of the carcinoma to the endocervix is confirmed by fractional curettage, hysterography, or hysteroscopy. Scraping of the cervix should be the first step of the curettage and the specimens from the cervix should be examined separately. Occasionally it may be difficult to decide whether the endocervix is involved by the cancer or not. In such cases the simultaneous presence of normal cervical glands and cancer in the same section will give the final diagnosis.

The presence of metastases in the vagina or in the ovary permits, as such, to allot a case to Stage 3.

3. Carcinoma of the ovary

Ovarian carcinoma is a common malignant tumour. It cannot be regarded as an entity. Therapeutic statistics on ovarian cancer are of limited value if attention is not paid to the histological type of the growth. Experience has shown that there is no clear correlation between clinical and histological malignancy in ovarian tumours. This holds valid for various types of neoplasms, but especially for epithelial tumours, granulosa cell tumours, and virilizing tumours.

The Cancer Unit of the WHO has published a 'Histological typing of ovarian tumours' which certainly will help to understand the pathology and behaviour of ovarian neoplasms. The histopathological classification of epithelial tumours adopted by the WHO corresponds in principle with that proposed by F.I.G.O.

It should be noted that cases of germ cell tumours, hormonal producing neoplasms, and metastatic carcinomas should be excluded from therapeutic statistics on ovarian epithelial tumours.

A Histological classification of the common primary epithelial tumours of the ovary

1 Serous cystomas
  (a) Serous benign cystadenomas.
  (b) Serous cystadenomas with proliferating activity of the epithelial cells and nuclear abnormalities, but with no infiltrative destructive growth (low potential malignancy).
  (c) Serous cystadenocarcinomas.

2 Mucinous cystomas
  (a) Mucinous benign cystadenomas.
  (b) Mucinous cystadenomas with proliferating activity of the epithelial cells and nuclear abnormalities, but with no infiltrative destructive growth (low potential malignancy).
  (c) Mucinous cystadenocarcinomas.

3 Endometrioid tumours (similar to adenocarcinomas in the endometrium)
  (a) Endometrioid benign cysts.
  (b) Endometrioid tumours with proliferating activity of the epithelial cells and nuclear abnormalities, but with no infiltrative destructive growth (low potential malignancy).
  (c) Endometrioid adenocarcinomas.

4 Mesonephric tumours
  (a) Benign mesonephric tumours.
  (b) Mesonephric tumours with proliferating activity of the epithelial cells and nuclear abnormalities, but with no infiltrative destructive growth (low potential malignancy).
  (c) Mesonephric cystadenocarcinomas.

5 Concomitant carcinoma, undifferentiated carcinoma (tumours which cannot be allotted to one of the groups 1, 2, 3, or 4).

6 No histology
In some cases of inoperable widespread malignant tumour it may be impossible for the gynaecologist and for the pathologist to decide the origin of the growth. In order to evaluate the results obtained in the treatment of carcinoma of the ovary it is, however, necessary that all patients are reported, also those who are thought to have a malignant ovarian tumour. If clinical examination cannot exclude the possibility that the lesion is a primary ovarian carcinoma a case should be reported in the group 'special category' (below) and it will belong to either of the histological groups 5 or 6.

Cases where explorative surgery has shown that obvious ovarian malignant tumour is present, but where no biopsy has been taken, should be classified as ovarian carcinoma 'No histology'.

It is desirable to have a clinical stage-grouping of ovarian tumours similar to those already existing for other malignant tumours in the female pelvis. Sometimes it is impossible to come to a final diagnosis by inspection or palpation or by any of the other methods recommended for clinical staging of carcinoma of the uterus and vagina.

B Clinical staging for primary carcinoma of the ovary

Based on findings at clinical examination and surgical exploration. The final histology after surgery is to be considered in the staging, as is cytology as far as effusions are concerned.

Stage 1 Growth limited to the ovaries.

Stage 1a Growth limited to *one* ovary; no ascites.
    (i) No tumour on the external surface; capsule intact.
    (ii) Tumour present on the external surface or/and capsule ruptured.

Stage 1b Growth limited to *both* ovaries; no ascites.
    (i) No tumour on the external surface; capsules intact.
    (ii) Tumour present on the external surface or/and capsule(s) ruptured.

Stage 1c Tumour either Stage 1a or Stage 1b, but with ascites* present or positive peritoneal washings.

Stage 2 Growth involving one or both ovaries with pelvic extension.

Stage 2a Extension and/or metastases to the uterus and/or tubes.

Stage 2b Extension to other pelvic tissues including the peritoneum and the uterus.

Stage 2c Tumour either Stage 2a or Stage 2b, but with ascites* present or positive peritoneal washings.

Stage 3 Growth involving one or both ovaries with intraperitoneal metastases outside the pelvis and/or positive retroperitoneal nodes.
Tumour limited to the true pelvis with histologically proven malignant extension to small bowel or omentum.

Stage 4 Growth involving one or both ovaries with distant metastases.
If pleural effusion is present there must be positive cytology to allot a case to Stage 4.
Parenchymal liver metastases equals Stage 4.

Special category: Cases which are thought to be ovarian carcinoma, but where it has been impossible to tell the origin of the tumour.

*Ascites is peritoneal effusion which in the opinion of the surgeon is pathological or/and clearly exceeds normal amounts.

Therefore the Cancer Committee of F.I.G.O. has recommended that the clinical staging of primary carcinoma of the ovary should be based on clinical examination, i.e. curettage and roentgen examination of the lungs and skeleton, as well as on findings by laparoscopy or laparotomy.

Acknowledgement

Reproduced from the Annual report on the results of treatment in carcinoma of the uterus, vagina and ovary (Vol. 16, 1976), edited by H. L. Kottmeier. Radiumhemmet, Stockholm, with kind permission of the Editor.

Index

Index

Contents of other volumes in the
Gynaecological Surgery series

Volume 1: Vaginal Operations

1 **Dilatation and Curettage**

2 **Diathermy Coagulation of the Cervix**

3 **Cryosurgical Treatment of Cervical Erosion**

4 **Removal of Sub-mucus Fibroid Polyp**
   Vaginal excision

5 **Manchester Repair**
   Anterior and posterior wall repair

6 **Repair of Enterocele**

7 **Repair of Rectocele**

8 **Vaginal Hysterectomy**

9 **Post-Hysterectomy Prolapse**

10 **Surgical Treatment of Stress Incontinence**
   Cruciate bladder sling technique

11 **Vaginoplasty**
   Repair of localised vaginal constriction

12 **Repair of Vesico-Vaginal Fistula**

Volume 2: Abdominal Operations For Benign Conditions

Volume 4: Surgery Of Vulva And Lower Genital Tract

1 **Instruments and Surgical Anatomy**

2 **Urethral Operations**
  Excision of caruncle
  Excision of prolapsed urethra
  Excision of para-urethral cyst

3 **Surgery of Bartholin Duct/Gland**
  Excision of gland
  Marsupialisation of cyst abscess

4 **Surgery of Vaginal Introitus**
  Fenton's operation
  Vaginoplasty with full thickness labial graft

5 **Surgery for Absent or Shortened Vagina**
  Vulvo vaginoplasty (Williams operation)

6 **Surgery for Woolfian Duct Remnants**
  Excision of paravaginal cyst
  Marsupialisation of paravaginal cyst

7 **Treatment of Vulva Condylomata**
  Excision diathermy
  Cryosurgery

8 ***Surgery of Imperforate Hymen***

9 ***Haemorrhoidectomy***

10 ***Closure of Recto-Vaginal Fistula***

Volume 5: Infertility Surgery

Volume 6: Surgery Of Conditions Complicating Pregnancy